Concise
Guide to
Hematology

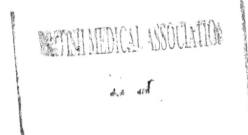

Dr. Schmaier dedicates this book to his life partner Linda and to Alec and Lauren who are contributing to the next generation of physicians.

Dr. Lazarus dedicates this book to his loving wife Joan and sons Jeffrey and Adam and spouses Jana and Sarah for their unwavering support.

Concise Guide to Hematology

EDITED BY

Alvin H. Schmaier MD

Robert W. Kellermeyer Professor of Hematology/Oncology
Case Western Reserve University
University Hospitals Case Medical Center
Cleveland, OH, USA

Hillard M. Lazarus MD, FACP

Professor of Medicine
Case Western Reserve University
University Hospitals Case Medical Center
Cleveland, OH, USA

WILEY-BLACKWELL

A John Wiley & Sons, Ltd., Publication

This edition first published 2012 © 2012 by Blackwell Publishing Ltd.

Blackwell Publishing was acquired by John Wiley & Sons in February 2007. Blackwell's publishing program has been merged with Wiley's global Scientific, Technical and Medical business to form Wiley-Blackwell.

Registered office: John Wiley & Sons, Ltd, The Atrium, Southern Gate, Chichester, West Sussex, PO19 8SQ, UK

Editorial offices: 9600 Garsington Road, Oxford, OX4 2DQ, UK
The Atrium, Southern Gate, Chichester, West Sussex, PO19 8SQ, UK
111 River Street, Hoboken, NJ 07030-5774, USA

For details of our global editorial offices, for customer services and for information about how to apply for permission to reuse the copyright material in this book please see our website at www.wiley.com/wiley-blackwell

The right of the author to be identified as the author of this work has been asserted in accordance with the UK Copyright, Designs and Patents Act 1988.

Library of Congress Cataloging-in-Publication Data

Concise guide to hematology / edited by Alvin H. Schmaier, Hillard M. Lazarus.
    p. ; cm.
  Includes bibliographical references and index.
  ISBN-13: 978-1-4051-9666-6 (hardcover : alk. paper)
  ISBN-10: 1-4051-9666-1 (hardcover : alk. paper)   1. Blood–Diseases.
2. Hematology.   I. Schmaier, Alvin H.   II. Lazarus, Hillard M.
  [DNLM: 1. Hematologic Diseases.   2. Hematopoiesis.   3. Neoplasms, Plasma Cell. WS 39]
  RC633.C66 2011
  616.1'5–dc23

                                                            2011015323

A catalogue record for this book is available from the British Library.

This book is published in the following electronic formats: ePDF 9781444345223; Wiley Online Library 9781444345254; ePub 9781444345230; Mobi 9781444345247

Set in 9.5/12 pt Palatino by Toppan Best-set Premedia Limited

Printed and bound in Singapore by Markono Print Media Pte Ltd

1   2012

Contents

Contributors

Archana M. Agarwal MD
Assistant Professor, Pathology
University of Utah and ARUP Laboratories
Salt Lake City, UT, USA

Sanjay P. Ahuja MD, MS
Assistant Professor, Pediatric Hematology/
Oncology
Director, Hemostasis and Thrombosis Center
Rainbow Babies and Children's Hospital
Case Western Reserve University
Cleveland, OH, USA

Aśok C. Antony MD, FACP
Professor of Medicine
Indiana University School of Medicine
Indianapolis, IN, USA

Makiko Ban-Hoefen MD
Hematology/Oncology Fellow
James P. Wilmot Cancer Center
University of Rochester Medical Center
Rochester, NY, USA

Niels Borregaard MD, PhD
Professor of Hematology and Internal Medicine
University of Copenhagen;
Department of Hematology
Rigshospitalet
Copenhagen, Denmark

Laurence A. Boxer MD
Henry and Mala Dorfman Family Professor of
Pediatric Hematology/Oncology
Department of Pediatrics and Communicable
Diseases
University of Michigan
Ann Arbor, MI, USA

Amy Chadburn MD
Professor of Pathology
Division of Hematopathology
Department of Pathology
Northwestern University, Feinberg School of
Medicine
Chicago, IL, USA

Yi-Hua Chen MD
Assistant Professor of Pathology
Division of Hematopathology
Department of Pathology
Northwestern University, Feinberg School of
Medicine
Chicago, IL, USA

David W. Essex MD
Associate Professor of Medicine
Sol Sherry Thrombosis Research Center and
Division of Hematology
Temple University School of Medicine
Philadelphia, PA, USA

Richard I. Fisher MD
Director, James P. Wilmot Cancer Center
Samuel E. Durand Chair in Medicine
Professor of Medicine
University of Rochester Medical Center
Rochester, NY, USA

Jonathan W. Friedberg MD, MMSc
Professor of Medicine and Oncology
Chief, Hematology Oncology Division
James P. Wilmot Cancer Center
University of Rochester Medical Center
Rochester, NY, USA

Stanton L. Gerson MD
Director, Case Comprehensive Cancer Center
Director, Seidman Cancer Center
Asa and Patricia Shiverik Professor of
Hematology and Oncology
Case Western Reserve University
University Hospitals Case Medical Center
Cleveland, OH, USA

Scott D. Gitlin MD, FACP
Associate Professor of Internal Medicine
Division of Hematology/Oncology
University of Michigan
Ann Arbor VA Health System
Ann Arbor, MI, USA

Lawrence Tim Goodnough MD
Professor of Pathology and Medicine
Director of Transfusion Service
Department of Pathology
Stanford University Medical Center
Stanford, CA, USA

Philip R. Greipp MD
Professor of Medicine
Division of Hematology
Mayo Clinic
Rochester, MN, USA

Christopher D. Hillyer MD
President and Chief Executive Officer
New York Blood Center
Professor of Medicine
Department of Medicine
Weill Cornell Medical College
New York, NY, USA

Hillard M. Lazarus MD, FACP
Professor of Medicine
Case Western Reserve University
University Hospitals Case Medical Center
Cleveland, OH, USA

Howard A. Liebman MD
Professor of Medicine and Pathology
Jane Anne Nohl Division of Hematology
Department of Medicine
University of Southern California-Keck School of
Medicine
Los Angeles, CA, USA

Yuan Lin PhD
Division of Hematology and Oncology
Case Western Reserve University
University Hospitals Case Medical Center
Seidman Cancer Center
Cleveland, OH, USA

Alice Ma MD
Associate Professor of Medicine
Department of Medicine
Division of Hematology/Oncology
University of North Carolina
Chapel Hill, NC, USA

Sumit Madan MD
Research Fellow
Division of Hematology
Mayo Clinic
Rochester, MN, USA

Peter W. Marks MD, PhD
Associate Professor of Medicine
Department of Internal Medicine/Hematology
Yale University School of Medicine
New Haven, CT, USA

Kevin T. McDonagh MD
Markey Foundation Chair
Chief, Division of Hematology, Oncology and
Blood and Marrow Transplantation
University of Kentucky College of Medicine
Lexington, KY, USA

Howard J. Meyerson MD
Director of Hematopathology and Flow
Cytometry
University Hospitals Case Medical Center;
Associate Professor of Pathology
Case Western Reserve University
Cleveland, OH, USA

Gabriela Motyckova MD, PhD
Hematology/Oncology Fellow
Dana-Farber Cancer Institute
Boston, MA, USA

Lilli M. Petruzzelli
Sr. Medical Director, Oncology Translational
Medicine
Novartis Institutes for BioMedical Research, Inc.
Cambridge, MA, USA

Steven W. Pipe MD
Associate Professor of Pediatrics and Pathology
Laurence A. Boxer Research Professor of
Pediatrics and Communicable Diseases
Director, Division of Pediatric Hematology and
Oncology
Pediatric Medical Director, Hemophilia and
Coagulation Disorders Program
Director, Special Coagulation Laboratory
C.S. Mott Children's Hospital
University of Michigan
Ann Arbor, MI, USA

Josef T. Prchal MD
Professor of Medicine, Genetics and Pathology
University of Utah and ARUP Laboratories;
Huntsmar Cancer Hospital
George E. Waheln VA Medical Center
Salt Lake City, UT, USA

A. Koneti Rao MBBS, FACP
Sol Sherry Professor of Medicine
Chief, Hematology Section
Co-Director, Sol Sherry Thrombosis Research
Center
Temple University School of Medicine
Philadelphia, PA, USA

Jacob M. Rowe MD
Professor of Hematology
Director, Department of Hematology and Bone
Marrow Transplantation
Rambam Medical Center and
Bruce Rappaport Faculty of Medicine
Technion—Israel Institute of Technology
Haifa, Israel

Alvin H. Schmaier MD
Robert W. Kellermeyer Professor of Hematology/
Oncology
Case Western Reserve University
University Hospitals Case Medical Center
Cleveland, OH, USA

Anjali A. Sharathkumar MD, MS
Medical Director of Hemophilia and
Thrombophilia Program
Assistant Professor of Pediatrics
Children's Memorial Hospital
Northwestern University, Feinberg School of
Medicine
Chicago, IL, USA

Beth H. Shaz MD
Chief Medical Officer
New York Blood Center
New York, NY, USA;
Clinical Associate Professor
Department of Pathology and Laboratory
Medicine
Emory University School of Medicine
Atlanta, GA, USA

Richard M. Stone MD
Professor of Medicine
Dana-Farber Cancer Institute
Boston, MA, USA

Andrew E. Warkentin BHSc(Hon)
Medical Student
Faculty of Medicine
University of Toronto
Toronto, ON, Canada

Theodore E. Warkentin MD,
BSc(Med), FRCP(C), FACP
Professor, Department of Pathology and
Molecular Medicine, and Department of
Medicine
Michael G. DeGroote School of Medicine
McMaster University
Hamilton, ON, Canada

Tsila Zuckerman MD
Director, Bone Marrow Transplantation Unit
Department of Hematology and Bone Marrow
Transplantation
Rambam Medical Center and
Bruce Rappaport Faculty of Medicine
Technion—Israel Institute of Technology
Haifa, Israel

Preface

This volume originally arose from the need to redesign the hematology course curriculum for second-year medical students at the University of Michigan. The first version was published as *Hematology for Medical Students* in 2003. I was pleased to hear favorable comments by medical students and also some colleagues in the field who used the text for their own medical school courses. In preparing for the second version, we were very pleased that Wiley-Blackwell took an interest in having a book like this prepared for an American audience. In re-designing the text, we realized that its appeal is greater than just medical students. Residents in pediatrics, internal medicine, and pathology found the first version of the text useful and our fellows in hematology and oncology at the University of Michigan and Case Western Reserve University also used it as a handy quick review of basic hematology and hematologic malignancy. Thus, the name was changed to *Concise Guide to Hematology*. In preparing the second version I recruited Dr. Hillard Lazarus as a co-editor. Hillard has a terrific background in classic hematology and is an expert in hematologic malignancies. He also is a critical reader and writer and I have appreciated his efforts in helping me to make this edition possible. Together, we agreed to recruit experts in the various fields of hematology as authors of the chapters. We personally thank the authors for the quality of their contributions to this volume. Lastly, we thank the key personnel at Wiley-Blackwell, Maria Khan, Deirdre Barry, Jennifer Seward, and Cathryn Gates for their focus and contributions to the preparation of this text.

Alvin H. Schmaier
Cleveland, OH, USA
July, 2011

1   Introduction to Hematology

Alvin H. Schmaier

Case Western Reserve University, University Hospitals Case Medical Center, Cleveland, OH, USA

I. Introduction

Hematology is the study of the normal and pathologic aspects of blood and blood elements. Blood is a unique fluid compromised of many cellular elements as well as a liquid portion consisting of proteins, amino acids, carbohydrates, lipids and elements. The hematopoietic system is characterized by turnover and replenishment throughout life. The pluripotent hematopoietic stem cell (HSC) is the progenitor of the cells in blood. The cellular elements that arise from this stem cell that circulates in blood include red blood cells, white blood cells, and platelets. Normal white blood cells in the peripheral circulation include neutrophils, monocytes, eosinophils, basophils and lymphocytes. Since the HSC also gives rise to cells of the lymphoid system, the study of hematology also includes the lymph nodes and lymph tissue. There is no specific organ for hematologic disorders and its diseases arise within the bone marrow, lymph nodes, or the intravascular compartment. The intravascular compartment where these cells circulate includes the endothelial cell lining of blood vessels and the proteins in the blood plasma. The circulating cell–endothelial cell interface and the rheologic aspects of blood coursing through the intravascular compartment also influence "hematology" and its many parts.

This text has been structured to introduce the trainee to the area of hematology. Since the vast majority of medical students and residents do not become hematologists, there are certain essential items that all trainees must learn about this area of medicine. The trainee will learn the physician's approach to anemia and red blood cell disorders and be able to fully evaluate a complete blood count (CBC). Screening tests for bleeding disorders for the diagnosis of an individual who has a defect in the proteins or cellular elements that prevent bleeding will be addressed. The trainee also will be exposed to the clinical, biologic, and genetic risk factors that contribute to thrombosis. Finally,

Concise Guide to Hematology, First Edition. Edited by Alvin H. Schmaier, Hillard M. Lazarus.
© 2012 Blackwell Publishing Ltd. Published 2012 by Blackwell Publishing Ltd.

the student will be introduced to those white cell disorders that are diagnosed and treated by non-hematologists and the uncommon but serious white blood cell disorders where a hematology consultation is needed.

II. Origins of hematopoietic cells

Hematopoiesis begins early in embryonic development. The HSC and the blood vessel lining cells or endothelial cells are thought to be derived from the same precursor cell in the aorto-gonad mesonephros (AGM) system. The common precursor to the HSC and the endothelial cell is the hematoblast. It has been proposed that this cell has the capacity to differentiate into both cell classes. The HSC is present in small numbers and retains its ability to differentiate into all blood cells as well as proliferate. In the earliest stages of embryogenesis, these cells circulate through the embryo to supply oxygen and deliver nutrients. The stem cells that arise from the AGM later in embryogenesis give rise to the blood system that seeds the liver and then the bone marrow. These cells demonstrate the ability to "travel" from the time they leave the yolk sac to populate tissues and still circulate in small numbers even in adults, a property exploited in clinical hematopoietic cell transplantation. These cells regress in the liver, kidney, and spleen, but in times of stress, they can resume blood product production as seen in myeloproliferative disorders and myelofibrosis. Under the influence of specific growth and transcription factors, cells become committed to specific lineages.

A. The myeloid system

Cells of this group arise in the central marrow cavity (called the "medullary" cavity). Myeloid lineage blood cells arising elsewhere in the body are designated as "extramedullary" in origin. The myeloid system consists of the following cells: red blood cells (erythrocytes), white blood cells (neutrophils, monocytes, eosinophils, basophils) and platelets (thrombocytes). Neutrophils, eosinophils and basophils have been collectively called "granulocytes" because the presence and nature of their cytoplasmic granules define their function; however, when physicians use the term "granulocytes", they are often referring just to neutrophils.

1. Erythrocytes (red blood cell, RBC)

An erythrocyte is a specialized anucleated cell that packages hemoglobin, the protein that is a respiratory gas transport vehicle that carries oxygen from the lungs to and carbon dioxide from tissues and back to the lungs to dispel. Erythrocytes undergo erythropoiesis whereby they mature from an early progenitor cell to the non-nucleated, biconcave disk, the erythrocyte, that with the absence of its nucleus and the flexibility of its membrane is able to bend to traverse 2–3 micron capillaries. It is regulated by the growth factor, erythropoietin. The process of erythropoiesis takes 4 days to produce a non-nucleated biconcave disk that enters the circulation with residual RNA in its cytoplasm. A new RBC in the circulation is slightly bigger than older cells.

The reticulocyte count as identified by a special stain represents the percentage of early RBC of the total number of RBC in the circulation. Red blood cell RNA remains in the erythrocyte about 1 day, so a normal "reticulocyte count" is <2%. The red cell life span is 120 days, and normally there are about 5 million RBC/μL in whole blood in adult males and 4.5 million RBC/μL in adult females. Old RBCs lose their energy-producing (ATP) capacity, develop stiff membranes, and are removed from circulation by the macrophages of the mononuclear–phagocytic system of the spleen. Their hemoglobin is normally retained in the reticuloendothelial (RE) system but can be lost when there is brisk shortened red blood cell survival, i.e., hemolysis.

2. Neutrophils

Neutrophils are also referred to as polymorphonuclear neutrophils, PMN or polys, segmented neutrophils, or segs (Atlas Figure 2; see also Chapter 3). The neutrophil contains a nucleus that is usually a 3–4 lobed or "segmented" structure that stains a bluish color with Wright Giemsa stain. An early form of a neutrophil is a "band" that shows an unsegmented nucleus. A neutrophil normally takes 12–13 days to be produced in bone marrow. Its life span in the circulation is about 12 hours and they can live in tissues for several days. The marrow pool of mature neutrophils is 30–40 times that seen in the circulation. In the circulation, half are "marginated" or adherent to the endothelial cells and half flow of the blood stream. Margination of neutrophils allows them to serve as a "reserve" to be released in time of stress such as infection. Only one half of the neutrophils that circulate are reflected in the "white blood cell count" (WBC). In the adult, neutrophils constitute 50–80% of the total WBC analyzed (4000–10,000/μL). Neutrophils exit the circulation via diapedesis into tissue through the capillary junctions in response to chemotactic stimuli. Their functions are to phagocytize and digest bacteria, cellular debris, and dead tissue. Both neutrophils and monocytes are part of the body's innate immunity in contrast to adaptive or learned immunity of lymphocytes (see below; see also Chapter 16).

3. Monocytes

Monocytes are large, mononuclear cells with an indented (kidney-shaped) nucleus that form the circulating component of the mononuclear phagocyte system (Atlas Figure 3). The nucleolus in mature monocytes circulating in the peripheral circulation is usually not identified on blood by light microscopy. Monocytes spend 1–3 days in bone marrow and 8–72 hours in the peripheral blood. They have a similar functional role to neutrophils in host defense against organisms. Once they traverse into tissues, they can differentiate into *macrophages* that can survive in tissues for long periods (up to 80 days). Macrophages are tissue-resident as opposed to circulating monocytes. Macrophages are characterized and named for their tissue origin: alveolar macrophages in lung, Kupffer cells in liver, splenic macrophages, and oligodendrocytes/glial cells in brain. They function to phagocytize pathogens, cellular debris and dead tissue.

4. Eosinophils

Eosinophils are characterized by their prominent orange-reddish (refractile) granules seen on Wright–Giemsa stain (Atlas Figure 6). Eosinophils usually have bilobed nuclei. Eosinophils increase in reaction to foreign protein and thus are seen in parasitic infection (especially larva of roundworms, helminths), allergic conditions, cancer and certain drugs. Granules contain several proteins, most notably major basic protein (MBP). Normally eosinophils constitute 0–2% of WBC differential cell count.

5. Basophils

Basophils are equally colorful with very dark, bluish prominent granules following Wright–Giemsa stain (Atlas Figure 7). Granules contain: histamine, heparin, and hyaluronic acid. Histamine release (basophil degranulation) is part of the allergic reaction. Normally basophils are 0–1% of WBC differential blood count. They are often increased in patients with chronic myelogenous leukemia and other myeloproliferative disorders. Mast cells which are tissue basophils also have prominent granules and play a role in host defenses against parasites.

6. Platelets (thrombocytes)

Platelets bud off from the cytoplasm of the bone marrow megakaryocytes. The "mega" karyocyte in the bone marrow is recognized by its large size. Uniquely, the cell doubles its nuclear and cytoplasmic material but does not divide. Megakaryocyte growth and platelet segmentation is regulated by thrombopoietin. Platelets are anucleated cell fragments that contain remnant mRNA. They have a 7–10 day half-life and their first 1–2 days are spent in the spleen. Platelets can be entrapped by an enlarged spleen as seen in congestive and inflammatory disorders. They play a central role in hemostasis as they contain many hemostatic cofactors and inhibitors in their granules. They also have a role in inflammation since they contain many growth factors. At the megakaryocyte level, plasma proteins can be adsorbed and packaged into platelet granules (see Chapter 13).

B. Mononuclear phagocytic system

The mononuclear phagocyte system consists of circulating monocytes derived from the myeloid progenitor cell in the bone marrow that migrate from the circulation into tissues and differentiate into macrophages. The mononuclear phagocytic system is also called the reticuloendothelial (RE) system. These cells are found in bone marrow, thymus, lymph nodes, spleen, serosal surfaces, adrenal cortex, Peyer's patches, and Waldeyer's ring. They function as a "clean-up system" for circulating debris, microorganisms and aged, defective or antibody-coated RBC.

C. Lymphocyte system

Lymphocytes are mostly in lymph nodes, but are also a large blood and bone marrow component. As already mentioned above, they are part of our adaptive immunity system. The major lymphocyte subsets are B and T cells. NK (natural killer) cells are a specialized lymphoid population. All cells arise in the bone marrow, but T cells mature in the thymus and B cells mature in the lymph nodes, spleen or other lymphoid tissue, e.g., Peyer's patches in the gut and Waldeyer's ring in the throat. Immunosurface markers are used to classify lymphocytes. B cells are identified by CD19 and CD20. T cells are identified by CD3, CD4 or CD8. NK cells comprise 10% of circulating lymphocytes and are identified by the CD3–CD56+ phenotype.

III. The physical states of blood

(i)   Blood is a *suspension* of cells in a solute of water, water-soluble proteins, and electrolytes.
(ii) The *viscosity* of blood = 1.1–1.2 centipoise. The viscosity of blood is highly influenced by red blood cell and protein concentration. Increased viscosity can occur from an elevation in the cellular components as is seen in polycythemia (increased numbers of red blood cells) and protein as seen in disorders such as multiple myeloma (elevated IgG levels) and Waldenström's macroglobulinemia (elevated IgM levels)]. Red cell size (smaller size increases viscosity) and the speed of blood flow in a given vessel also influence viscosity (viscosity in the aorta is much less than in a small arteriole).
(iii) Blood volume averages 70 mL/kg of body weight; thus the 70 kg adult has roughly 5 liters of blood. The blood volume of an individual (man, dog, etc.) is approximately 7% of the total body weight. Children may have a slightly higher % (~10%) blood volume to total body weight.
(iv) Cellular composition of blood averages 38–42% in women, 40–44% in men; the percent volume contributed by red blood cells is called the *"hematocrit"* or packed cell volume.
(v)   *Plasma* is anticoagulated blood (i.e., blood where the calcium chloride has been chelated [i.e., bound] and not available for interaction with proteins) from which the cellular components (red cells, white cells, and platelets) have been removed by centrifugation. It contains the blood coagulation proteins. *Serum* is the liquid in blood that has been collected without an anticoagulant. Many of the proteins have "clotted" and form a precipitate along with the cellular components of the blood. It is usually yellow in color unless the red blood cells lyse (hemolyze) releasing free hemoglobin that gives a red color in visible light. Plasma coagulation studies can only be performed on blood that has been obtained with a proper anticoagulant (usually sodium citrate in clinical medicine) and the plasma separated from the blood cells.

2 Hematopoiesis

Yuan Lin and Stanton L. Gerson

Case Western Reserve University, University Hospitals Case Medical Center, Seidman Cancer Center, Cleveland, OH, USA

I. Introduction

Hematopoiesis is the process of the development of blood cell lineages throughout life. Hematopoiesis in necessary to replenish dying cells with new blood cells. The key role of hematopoietic cells in maintaining hematopoietic homeostasis, host immunity and tissue oxygenation requires that they are highly regulated.

II. Definitions

1. **The hematopoietic system:** the hematopoietic system includes the elements of the blood, marrow, lymph nodes, endothelial cells, thymus and spleen that are involved in the production of all blood lineages. This system further includes cytokine-producing cells and stromal elements of the bone marrow and spleen. In human physiology, the hematopoietic system supplies various cells in the body with oxygen, contributes to the formation of blood clots when needed, and provides protection against infection and pathogens.
2. **Blood cells:** Blood cells include red blood cells (erythrocytes, RBCs), white blood cells (leukocytes) and platelets which provide a variety of functions within the body. RBCs carry oxygen, platelets contribute to hemostasis, thrombosis and the inflammatory response, and white blood cells are involved in immunity.
3. **Hematopoietic homeostasis:** Hematopoiesis is in a delicate state of homeostasis—the process of maintaining balanced production to offset ongoing destruction of blood cells. Some cell lineages such as neutrophils only survive for several hours after release from the bone marrow into the circulation. RBCs can survive longer, lasting 60 to 120 days, and terminally differentiated lymphocytes, plasma cells, may survive for up to 20 to 30

years. Hematopoietic cell production is regulated by cytokines and growth factors and monitored by tissue sensors (tissue oxygenation for red blood cells for example). The specific regulators and sensors for all hematopoietic elements, however, have not been clearly elucidated.

III. Mature hematopoietic cells and their functions

Mature RBCs carry hemoglobin bound oxygen to tissues and release that oxygen under the hypoxic conditions of tissues. Hemoglobin delivery of oxygen is dependent on pH and a number of other metabolic functions that alter the confirmation of the tetramer and the cooperative discharge of oxygen. RBCs also transport and release CO_2 generated from body metabolism in tissues to be expelled from the body via the lungs (see Chapter 3).

Platelets contain a high concentration of proactive inflammatory, hemostatic cofactors, proangiogenic proteins, inhibitors of blood coagulation, inflammation, and fibrinolysis inside their granules. These components are actively secreted on or about the activated platelet surface when an appropriate stimulus arises (see Chapter 13).

White blood cells consist of many cell types including granulocytes (neutrophils, eosinophils and basophils), monocytes, lymphocytes and dendritic cells. Neutrophils are the most common cells.

Neutrophils migrate into tissues in response to inflammation or infection where they may ingest or phagocytose particles and bacteria. These cells contain oxidases and myeloperoxidase within granules that can be activated to produce superoxide to kill ingested bacteria (see Chapter 16).

Eosinophils, basophils and mast cells respond to IgE to produce acute allergic responses. Mast cells are specialized long-lived tissue resident cells similar to basophils that are the initiators of the allergic response. They secrete histamine and vasoactive proteins and recruit eosinophils and basophils in response to antigens bound to IgE. Activated eosinophils express IgE receptors and amplify the allergic response. Eosinophils also contain granules with specialized proteins important for the immune reaction to parasites. Basophils also have IgE receptors and granules containing histamine and mediate allergic inflammation. These cells are present in low numbers in the peripheral blood.

Monocytes enter tissues and become resident macrophages in the lung, liver or other tissues where they also participate in the inflammatory and immune response. These cells produce a wide variety of small chemicals, such as chemokines (small peptide chemicals) and cytokines, for chemoattraction and immune modulation of all immune cells. In disease states, these cells can form clusters that result in granulomas and mediate chronic inflammation. Monocytes can also be antigen-presenting cells for the lymphoid cell population, inducing an immune response.

Dendritic cells are important mediators of innate and adaptive immune responses and are the main antigen presenting cell in the body. They have been suggested to derive from both common myeloid progenitor and common lymphoid progenitor.

B lymphocytes produce antibodies in response to stimulation. The initial response results in secretion of IgM immunoglobulin. The binding specificity towards the antigen is often modest at the initiation of an immune response. Upon antigen exposure, B cells migrate to specific regions within lymph nodes termed germinal centers where the cells proliferate and generate daughter cells with higher affinity for antigen through a mutational process referred to as somatic hypermutation. During this process the cells may switch to produce a different antibody isotype, usually IgG to carry out specific effector functions. B cells mature into long-lived plasma cells and memory B cells to maintain immunologic memory.

T lymphocytes produce cells with cytotoxic, helper or suppressor functions that mediate responses to viral infections or inflammatory conditions. The cytotoxic cells are particularly important to rid the body of virally infected cells. T cells produce cytokines and chemokines that modulate most immune responses including granuloma formation and are required for B-cell antibody production.

IV. Hematopoiesis during development and in adult

1. Hematopoiesis during development

The earliest forms of blood cells are observed in the yolk sac. These cells emanate from a primitive precursor population and produce both cells with oxygen-carrying capacity and a small number of primitive lymphocytes. More definitive hematopoiesis takes place later in development in fetal liver, and during the third trimester, production is transferred to the bone marrow in the developing embryo.

RBC production is unique in development because of the complex evolution in the hemoglobin locus resulting in a structured sequence of distinct hemoglobin produced during fetal life. Because of the oxygen requirements in the fetus and the absence of direct air exchange in the lung, different hemoglobins are produced during gestation. Most significant is fetal hemoglobin or hemoglobin F, a unique tetramer that disappears normally within a few months after birth. It is the main type of hemoglobin in the fetus. It has greater oxygen-affinity than adult hemoglobin A, allowing for the extraction of oxygen from the maternal blood stream. A small percentage of adult hemoglobin or hemoglobin A appears late in gestation and becomes the dominant form within 6 months of birth, reflecting the change in oxygen requirements after birth. Interestingly, fetal hemoglobin ameliorates the disease manifestations of homozygous hemoglobin S, the cause of sickle cell anemia. For this reason, erythropoietin and hydroxycarbamide (hydroxyurea), which promotes the generation of hemoglobin F, are used to treat sickle cell anemia.

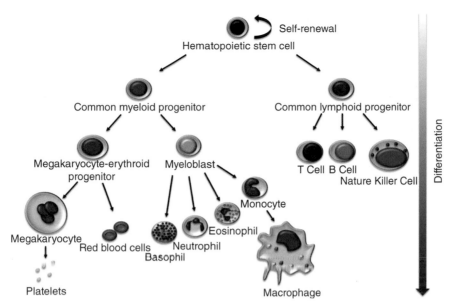

Figure 2.1 Human hematopoiesis. Hematopoietic cell lineages are based on a hierarchical system. Hematopoietic stem cell is one of the most primitive adult stem cells, which can self-renew and differentiate to progenitors that can give rise to all types of blood cells and platelets.

2. Hematopoiesis in adult

In adults, hematopoiesis mainly occurs in bone marrow and thymus. Myelopoiesis (non-lymphoid) and lymphopoiesis diverge during the early stage of differentiation. The hematopoietic stem cell's first lineage commitment is to differentiate to a common myeloid progenitor or a common lymphoid progenitor (Figure 2.1). The common myeloid progenitor produces megakaryocytic, erythroid (RBC), granulocytic and monocytic lineages. The granulocytes, the neutrophils, eosinophils and basophils, are the most phylogenetically related. Monocytes arise from a common granulocyte-monocyte progenitor.

Erythropoiesis is the process of generating RBC. Thrombopoiesis refers to the formation of platelets from their precursor megakaryocytes. Erythrocytes and megakaryocytes both develop from a common precursor cell. RBC production is stimulated by the growth factor, erythropoietin. Megakaryocytes are unusual in that the cell undergoes nuclear division without cytoplasmic division; the generating cell contains a high amount of DNA content, 32n–64n, compared to 2n of normal diploid cell. Each megakaryocyte can generate large numbers of platelets by "budding" off pieces of cytoplasm. The process is stimulated by thrombopoietin (TPO), a cytokine hormone mainly produced by liver and kidney.

Since leukemias often recapitulate the normal developmental process, it is not uncommon to encounter a leukemia with both granulocyte and macrophage differentiation capable of recapitulating the common granulocyte-macrophage progenitor or less often a leukemia demonstrating erythrocyte and megakaryocyte differentiation simulating the common megakaryocyte–erythrocyte progenitor.

The common lymphoid progenitor cell differentiates into B-cell, T-cell and natural killer cells. B-lymphoid development remains localized in the bone marrow, whereas developing T cells emigrate from the bone marrow to the thymus to undergo terminal differentiation. B and T-lymphoid development requires rearrangement of the DNA in the maturing cells; the immunoglobulin locus for B cells and T-cell receptor locus for T cells. DNA recombination in the developing lymphocytes randomly combines _v_ariable, _d_iversity and _j_oining gene segments (VDJ) to generate antibody and T-cell receptor proteins with tremendous diversity ($>1 \times 10^7$) to match potential antigens from a wide variety of infectious or noxious agents. The DNA rearrangement process is intimately related to T and B-cell survival and maturation as lack of effective DNA recombination results in cell death. B-lymphopoiesis occurs under the influence of IL-7. The effects of IL-15 and IL-2 are important later in lymphopoiesis.

V. Hematopoietic stem and progenitor cells and their functions

1. Hematopoietic stem and progenitor cells

An HSC represents approximately one in 10,000 hematopoietic cells in the bone marrow space. During the normal hematopoietic steady state, the HSC is quiescent. When an activation signal reaches the HSC microenvironment, usually due to proliferative stress, the HSC enters into a proliferation state. It may then undergo asymmetric replication, producing another HSC capable of self-renewal and a "daughter" progenitor cell, which begins to differentiate, rapidly divide, and proliferate into mature blood cells (Figure 2.1). The differentiation of HSCs into progenitor cells is accompanied by changes in cell surface molecule expression. As HSCs lose their quiescent state, they acquire growth factor receptors and increase the production of certain messenger RNAs. This process occurs by altering transcription factor-mediated expression of genes for differentiation and lineage commitment.

When HSCs leave the bone marrow niche (a specialized regulatory environment), they usually lose the HSC phenotype and irreversibly begin lineage commitment. However, some can lodge in another niche and resume the quiescent HSC phenotype. A single HSC may produce more than 1 million progeny over the course of this continuous process of proliferation and differentiation.

Hematopoietic progenitor cells, such as common myeloid or lymphoid progenitors, are all differentiated from HSCs. Traditional understanding of hematopoiesis is that the process is unidirectional. Once a progenitor cell has committed to a lineage, there is no turning back, although some researchers argue that hematopoietic progenitor cells are more versatile.

2. Phenotypic and functional analysis of hematopoietic stem and progenitor cells

With the discovery and utilization of surface markers to distinguish hematopoietic cells, a hierarchal map of hematopoiesis was quickly established. The expression of specific surface marker, which is often identified and given a CD (cluster of differentiation) number, defines a stage of hematopoietic stem and progenitor cells. A short list of unique markers to identify and provide lineage specificity to human hematopoietic stem and progenitor cells are is given in Table 2.1.

In vitro assays provide clear identification of hematopoietic precursor populations. Samples of blood or bone marrow can be grown artificially *in vitro* in methylcellulose with appropriate cytokines to produce cell type specific colonies, which represent progeny from a specific progenitor cell (Figure 2.2a). For instance, cells grown in the presence of erythropoietin results in CFU-E (colony forming unit-erythroid) or BFU-E (burst forming unit-erythroid) colonies indicative of erythroid precursors. These colonies contain hemoglobin-producing cells devoid of other lineages. Cells grown in cultures containing G-CSF (granulocyte colony-stimulating factor) or GM-CSF (granulocyte–macrophage colony-stimulating factor) with or without other early phase cytokines such as stem cell factor (SCF), Flt3 or IL-3 result in granulocytic or monocytic colonies, respectively. In some instances these growth factors plus thrombopoietin are used to produce megakaryocytic colonies. Likewise exposure to IL-7 will produce B lymphocytes and growth with IL-2 will stimulate T-lymphocyte colonies.

Another *in vitro* assay is the long-term culture initiating cell assay (LT-CIC), which reflects an earlier progenitor cell. This *in vitro* test, in addition to those described above, only assays hematopoietic progenitors. In order to assess the production of long-term stem cells *in vivo*, bone marrow cell transplantation is needed. One approach is to inject CD34+ human bone marrow cells into

Table 2.1 Surface markers to identify hematopoietic stem and progenitor cells	
Stem and progenitor cells	*Identified surface markers*
HSC	CD 34, CD133,
Common myeloid progenitor	CD33, CD13, CD117
Common lymphoid progenitor	CD135
Megakaryocytic progenitor	CD41/CD61
Erythroid progenitor	Glycophorin A (CD235A)
T-lymphoid progenitor	CD3, CD7, TDT
B-lymphoid progenitor	CD19, CD79a, TDT

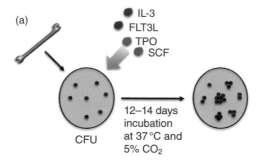

(a)

IL-3
FLT3L
TPO
SCF

CFU

12–14 days
incubation
at 37 °C and
5% CO_2

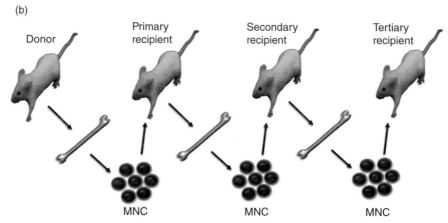

(b)

Donor

Primary
recipient

Secondary
recipient

Tertiary
recipient

MNC

MNC

MNC

Figure 2.2 Hematopoietic stem and progenitor cell assays. (a) *In vitro* hematopoietic progenitor CFU (colony forming unit) assay; (b) Serial transplantation assay for testing long-term hematopoietic stem cells. IL-3, Interleukin-3; FLT3L, FLT-3 ligand; TPO, thrombopoietin; SCF, stem cell factor; MNC, mononuclear cell.

NOD-SCID (non-obese diabetic severe combined immunodeficiency) mice. These immunodeficient mice cannot reject foreign cells and allow human progenitor cells to grow in the murine bone marrow. The "gold standard" for true long-term hematopoietic stem cells is the serial transplantation assay (Figure 2.2b).

VI. Hematopoietic microenvironment

Hematopoietic microenvironments have important roles in regulating HSC activity and the process of hematopoiesis. There are two types of microenvironments in the bone marrow: one is the endosteal microenvironment, which has been considered as the main HSC niche, while the other is the sinusoidal microenvironment, a zone around the endothelial cell network within the bone marrow. The *endosteum* is a thin layer of *connective tissue* which lines the inner surface of the bony trabeculae within the *medullary cavity* of long *bones*.

The microenvironment responds to the cellular density, local tissue hypoxia and systemic hypoxemia, inflammatory signals, and other stress response factors. The microscopic spaces within the microenvironment provide an important recess or niche within the marrow that nurtures HSCs and their progenies for highly regulated homeostatic hematopoiesis. The bone marrow microenvironment is relatively radioresistant and can reconstitute after ablative radiation therapy or chemotherapy.

Multipotent mesenchymal stromal cells (MSC) fibroblasts and adipose cells play important roles in the microenvironment of the bone marrow by providing hematopoietic growth factors and a nurturing space (niche) for hematopoiesis to take place. In addition, T cells also support and regulate hematopoiesis by providing specific cytokines and chemokines.

VII. Regulation of hematopoiesis

The bone marrow microenvironment provides one level of regulation of hematopoiesis. Another form of regulation is cell-to-cell contact mediated by cell adhesion molecules, such as integrins. Integrins are cell-surface molecules that impact cell-to-cell and cell-to-stromal adhesion and bi-directional signaling that stimulate hematopoietic progenitors towards lineage-specific differentiation. Additionally, circulating and locally produced cytokines provide important lineage-specific stimuli.

Early progenitor-stimulating cytokines include stem cell factor (SCF), thrombopoietin, IL-6, IL 3, and FLT3 ligand. These cytokines stimulate HSC to begin the proliferation process.

G-CSF and GM-CSF provide stimulation for myelopoiesis. G-CSF is used in clinical medicine to elevate neutrophil counts in patients receiving chemotherapy or who have developed neutropenia. M-CSF (macrophage colony-stimulating factor) stimulates macrophage proliferation. These hematopoietic growth factors are made by lymphocytes.

Erythropoietin stimulates erythroid differentiation, resulting in the production of mature RBCs. Erythropoietin is made in the kidney as a result of sensing hypoxemia by the periglomerular cells (see Chapter 3). Renal failure is associated with anemia because of the reduced concentrations of erythropoietin produced. Clinically, genetically engineered erythropoietin is effective in resolving the anemia in patients with renal disease.

Thrombopoietin as well as erythropoietin stimulate the production of megakaryocytes and their terminal differentiation and fragmentation into platelets. Anemia, a disease with decreased RBC number, stimulates the production of erythropoietin from the kidney, thrombocytopenia stimulates thrombopoietin production from the liver, and neutropenia results in increased G-CSF. These cytokines act as an autocrine regulatory loop for blood cells. Along with other hematopoietic growth factors, they are critical for hematopoiesis maintenance.

VIII. Abnormal hematopoiesis

1. Cytopenias

Cytopenias, or low blood cell numbers, represent a severe disruption of hematopoiesis. Under normal homeostasis, hematopoiesis would be maintained through all types of stress with induction of proliferation and stimulation of progenitor pools by cytokines. Over-production likewise would result in a feedback loop leading to reduced blood cell production. Cytopenias may occur when an abnormal immune response destroys progenitor cells or peripheral blood cells. Reduced cell numbers also may occur when there is specific decreased production of the cell lineage or multiple cell lineages due to a primary defect in the progenitor or a toxin (e.g., medication) interfering with cell production.

Common examples include immune thrombocytopenia as a result of the immunoglobulins targeting early megakaryocytes and platelets (see Chapter 14). The etiology is the production of auto-antibodies from a dysregulated B and T-cell population either idiopathic, after viral infection, or associated with lymphoma or chronic lymphocytic leukemia. Drug exposure can also cause idiopathic immune-mediated thrombocytopenia. Granulocytopenia can be caused by an antibody response to drugs with cross-reactivity towards drug metabolite bound to the surface of myelocytes or granulocytes. Likewise, anemia can be caused by antibodies against RBCs (see Chapter 8). These antibodies are autoimmune, producing a positive Coombs test (positive test to detect antibodies on RBCs also referred to as the direct antiglobulin test). Some RBC antibodies are produced during drug treatment, viral infection, or blood cell exposure during pregnancy. Other common causes of cytopenias include acute viral infections that may destroy progenitor cells. Specific examples include parvovirus infection targeting of RBC progenitors, HIV infection which targets lymphocytes or CMV which attacks leukocytes. Additional causes of cytopenias include rapid tissue margination or sequestration of cells in response to infection or exhaustion of the production pools due to rapid destruction. Blood loss or bleeding, or the cessation of production of cells during an acute illness due to a tumor necrosis factor (TNF)-alpha-mediated stress response may also result in low cell numbers. The anemia of chronic disease appears to be a chronic response of the marrow to inflammation by the cytokine hepcidin (see Chapter 5) and results in an anemia that resolves when the chronic disease dissipates.

Finally, chemotherapy and radiation therapy are common causes of iatrogenic cytopenias in cancer patients and those receiving these treatments for autoimmune diseases. These agents destroy the proliferative potential of HSCs resulting in loss of differentiation of lineage-specific cells. Over time, the remaining HSC pool usually recovers and hematopoiesis is restored and cell lineages repopulate.

In the presence of cytopenias, cytokines may be useful as therapeutic agents. Erythropoietin is given to promote erythropoiesis and is especially useful in renal failure because of the reduced levels of erythropoietin produced. G-CSF is given to promote granulopoiesis, either after chemotherapy, due to marrow failure, or during acute infection. Romiplostim, an injectable peptide thrombopoietin analog, or eltrombopag, an oral thrombopoietin mimic by targeting the TPO receptor, are given to promote platelet production in chronic idiopathic immune thrombocytopenic purpura. Presently, there is no clinically useful cytokine as yet available to stimulate lymphopoiesis.

2. Marrow failure states

Acquired marrow failure may result from damage to the microenvironment, HSC, or from cells that are responsible for producing the critical chemokines and cytokines that regulate hematopoiesis. They may also result from mutations in the HSC that renders them ineffective in cell proliferation. Such a situation could result from an exogenous stimulus including a viral infection, be the result of an autoantibody directed against a HSC, or represent genomic instability of the stem cell lineage, resulting in loss of hematopoietic function. Aplastic anemia, myelodysplastic syndrome, and paroxysmal nocturnal hemoglobinurea are examples of marrow failure states (Chapters 8, 18 and 19).

3. Leukemias

All leukemias arise from HSCs and their early progenies. Acute leukemias are characterized by cells that fail to differentiate. Specific chromosomal abnormalities giving rise to altered gene expression are commonly observed in acute leukemias. Most leukemias have many additional mutations that appear to convert the cell with the chromosomal translocation into a leukemic state, e.g., increased cell numbers due to a failure to differentiate, lack of programmed cell death, or increased proliferation. Leukemia-initiating cells or leukemia-sustaining cells are a minor population within the leukemic cell population. These cells share many features of HSC, but seem to be the more resilient with the greatest proliferative potential and the greatest resistance to common chemotherapeutic agents. The relationship between the leukemia-initiating cell and the onset of the chromosomal and other genetic changes is not clear. Treatment of leukemias tends to target a proliferative fraction with cell cycle specific and other DNA damaging agents.

IX. Conclusions

In this chapter, we present general concepts involving hematopoiesis. HSCs are the most studied adult stem cells. However, there are still large numbers of questions which remain to be answered. For example, what are the unique surface markers for a homogenous population of HSC? Only by identifying a more homogenous population can we accurately reveal their unique phenotype.

CHAPTER 3

3 Red Blood Cell Biochemistry and Physiology

Kevin T. McDonagh

University of Kentucky College of Medicine, Lexington, KY, USA

Understanding the factors that regulate RBC growth and development and the genetic and biochemical basis of RBC physiology is critical for an informed approach to the diagnosis and treatment of anemia.

I. Red blood cell development

A. Early development

Red blood cells (RBC) are normally produced in the *bone marrow*. The process of RBC development is called *erythropoiesis*. RBC are derived from *pluripotent hematopoietic stem cells* (*HSCs*), and share a common precursor (or *progenitor cell*) with other *myeloid lineage cells* including megakaryocytes, granulocytes, monocytes/macrophages, eosinophils, and basophils. HSC arise from developing vasculature early in embryological development. Thus, inherited or acquired abnormalities in hematopoietic stem cells or myeloid progenitor cells may be associated with functional or quantitative defects in multiple types of blood cells.

B. Regulation of growth

The growth and maturation of RBCs from the HSC and myeloid progenitor cells is regulated by a complex interplay between genetically defined developmental programs and external signals generated by remote and/or neighboring cells.

1. **Hematopoietic growth factors** are an important class of external signals used to regulate hematopoiesis. Multiple subtypes have been identified and characterized.
2. **Erythropoietin** (EPO) is the most important growth factor regulating erythropoiesis.
   (a) EPO is produced in the *kidney* by peritubular cells that sense tissue oxygen content. When oxygen delivery to the kidney falls (due to

Concise Guide to Hematology, First Edition. Edited by Alvin H. Schmaier, Hillard M. Lazarus.
© 2012 Blackwell Publishing Ltd. Published 2012 by Blackwell Publishing Ltd.

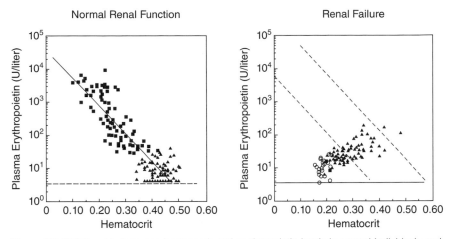

Figure 3.1 Relationship between hematocrit and erythropoietin levels in normal individuals and patients with renal failure. On the left, the triangles denote normal donors and the squares are patients with various anemias, excluding patients with renal failure, rheumatoid arthritis, and solid tumors. On the right, the open circles represent renal patients without kidneys; triangles represent patient with kidneys. (Reprinted with permission from Erslev A.J, Erythropoietin. N Engl J Med 1991;324:1339–44.)

anemia, hypoxemia, impaired blood flow, or other causes) these renal peritubular cells rapidly increase synthesis and release of EPO.
- The normal rise in EPO associated with anemia may be blunted or absent in patients with renal disease.
- As a result, renal disease is frequently associated with anemia and is a common indication for treatment with recombinant EPO.

(b) In response to EPO, erythroid precursors in the bone marrow are stimulated to divide and mature, resulting in increased production and release of RBC from the bone marrow.

(c) There is normally an inverse relationship between the hematocrit and plasma EPO levels (Figure 3.1). In individuals with a normal hematocrit, EPO levels are very low or undetectable. As the hematocrit progressively declines, EPO levels increase logarithmically.

C. Stages of development

1. The development stages of red blood cells are presented in Chapter 2, showing that as the erythron matures in mammals, in contrast to birds, the nucleus is extruded permitting greater deformability.

2. At the time of release from the bone marrow, the erythrocyte has not assumed the biconcave disc shape of the mature RBC. This young erythrocyte is anucleate, larger than a mature RBC and has a spherical shape characterized by the absence of central pallor.

(a) On a Wright stained peripheral blood smear, these cells have a faint bluish coloration in the cytoplasm (*polychromatophilia*) that reflects staining of residual messenger RNA directing the synthesis of hemo-globin. These cells may also contain punctate blue staining, referred to as *basophilic stippling*, which represents staining of precipitated ribosomes. Basophilic stippling is usually seen when there is abnormal heme or globin synthesis as seen in the microcytic anemias (see Chapter 4). It can also be seen when there is abnormal bone function as in the myelodysplastic syndromes (see Chapter 18).

(b) When stained with a supravital dye such as new methylene blue, the RNA and polyribosomes in these cells aggregate and are identified as *reticulocytes.*

3. Reticulocytes develop into fully mature RBC (smaller cells with central pallor and lacking polychromatophilia) within 1 or 2 days following release into the circulation from the bone marrow. Thus, reticulocytes are the youngest erythrocytes normally identified in the peripheral blood. An elevation in the number of reticulocytes present in the circulation is an indication that RBC production is increased, usually in response to the loss of RBC from bleeding or *hemolysis* (i.e., shortened RBC survival).

II. Hemoglobin: structure and function

A. Structure

1. **Hemoglobin (Hb)** is the major protein contained in mature RBCs. A hemo-globin molecule is composed of four *globin* chains. Each globin chain is bound to a *heme* moiety containing *iron*. Two of the globin chains are derived from the *alpha-globin* (α-globin) locus on chromosome 16, and the remaining two globin chains are derived from the *beta-globin* (β-globin) locus on chromosome 11 (Figure 3.2).

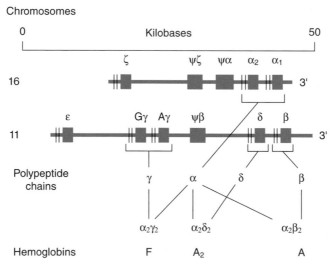

Figure 3.2 Chromosome locations of human hemoglobin. (Reproduced with permission from Harrison's Principles of Internal Medicine, Fauci, Anthony et al, © 2008 The McGraw-Hill Companies, Inc.)

2. **Different globin chains** are expressed during embryonic, fetal and postnatal/adult stages of development. Hemoglobin molecules containing different globin chains can be distinguished from one another by electrophoresis or liquid chromatography.
    (a) Fetal hemoglobin (*Hb F*) contains two α-globin chains and two gamma-globin (γ-globin) chains. Hb F is the major hemoglobin present during the later stages of fetal development because of greater oxygen-carrying capacity.
    (b) Around the time of birth, expression of γ-globin is suppressed.
    (c) Beta-globin (β-globin) is the major beta-like globin chain expressed after birth and in adults, although small amounts of γ-globin and delta-globin (δ-globin) are also produced.
    (d) *Hemoglobin A* is composed of two α-globin chains and two β-globin chains ($\alpha_2\beta_2$), and normally represents greater than 95% of the hemoglobin present in adult RBCs.
    (e) *Hemoglobin A2* ($\alpha2\delta2$) and Hb F ($\alpha2\gamma2$) are also normally found at low levels in normal adult RBCs.
3. **Genetic mutations** in the α-globin or β-globin locus may result in the expression of an abnormal hemoglobin (*hemoglobinopathy*) with a different amino acid composition and aberrant migration pattern on electrophoresis. The variant hemoglobin may be functionally normal, or may have physical and/or physiologic properties that differ from a normal hemoglobin molecule.
4. **A second category of genetic mutations in the globin loci (thalassemia)** is characterized by a quantitative reduction in the synthesis of α-globin or β-globin chains, and a net reduction in the formation of hemoglobin.

B. Function

1. The major physiologic role of hemoglobin is transport of oxygen from the lungs to the tissues. Oxygen binds to hemoglobin with high affinity in the oxygen rich environment of the alveolar capillary bed, and dissociates from hemoglobin in the relatively oxygen poor environment of the tissue capillary bed. The loading and unloading of oxygen from hemoglobin is facilitated by conformational changes in the hemoglobin molecule that alter its affinity for oxygen (*cooperativity*).
2. Hemoglobin oxygenation is classically depicted by an *oxyhemoglobin dissociation* curve, where the oxygen saturation of hemoglobin is measured as a function of the partial pressure of oxygen (Figure 3.3). A convenient measure of the oxygen affinity of hemoglobin is the partial pressure of oxygen where hemoglobin is 50% saturated (P_{50}). The P_{50} of hemoglobin varies as a function of temperature, pH, and the intracellular concentration of 2,3-diphosphoglycerate (2,3-DPG).
    (a) Acidosis (decreased pH) and elevations in RBC 2,3-DPG content stabilize the deoxyhemoglobin conformation, resulting in decreased affinity for oxygen, an increase in the P_{50}, and a right shift in the oxyhemoglobin dissociation curve.

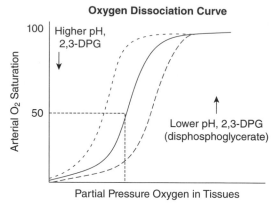

Figure 3.3 Red blood cell oxyhemoglobin dissociation curve.

(b) Physiologic changes in the oxyhemoglobin dissociation curve occur as adaptive responses to anemia and/or hypoxia. Intraerythrocyte 2,3-DPG levels are increased in individuals with chronic hypoxia or anemia and in individuals living at high altitude. The increase in 2,3-DPG levels results in a right-shift of the oxyhemoglobin dissociation curve, and the release of a greater proportion of hemoglobin-bound oxygen in tissue capillary beds.

III. Red blood cell membrane

A. The mature red blood cell

A mature red blood cell assumes the shape of a *biconcave disc*. When viewed from above on a peripheral blood smear, it displays an area of central pallor that corresponds to the region where the upper and lower membrane surfaces of the RBC are in close proximity. The unique morphology of the red blood cell is adapted for transit through narrow capillary beds and splenic sinusoids.

1. Young, healthy red cells are highly deformable, yet rapidly return to their native shape after exiting a capillary bed.
2. Red cells become more rigid and less deformable as they age, which contributes to their senescence and elimination from the circulation in the spleen. The average life span of a red blood cell is 120 days.

B. The "skeleton" of the red blood cell

This is formed by a network of structural proteins that tether the membrane lipid bilayer to the cell (Figure 3.4). Key structural proteins located in the RBC cytoskeleton include *spectrin*, *ankyrin*, and *band 3*. Congenital deficiencies in the function and/or quantity of these proteins are associated with abnormalities in RBC shape (*spherocytosis* or *elliptocytosis*) and shortened RBC survival (*hemolysis*).

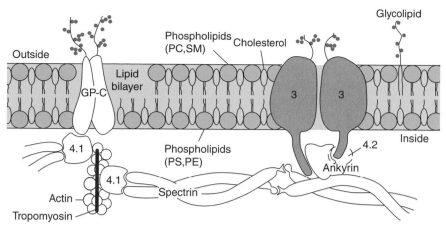

Figure 3.4 The red blood cell cytoskeleton. GP-C, glycophorin C; PC, phosphatidylcholine; PE, phosphatidylethanolamine; PS, phosphatidylserine; SM, sphingomyelin. (Reproduced with permission from Harrison's Principles of Internal Medicine, Fauci, Anthony et al, © 2008 The McGraw-Hill Companies, Inc.)

C. The volume and ionic content of the RBC

The volume and ionic content are actively regulated by energy dependent pumps that traverse the membrane. These pumps depend on a constant source of *adenosine triphosphate (ATP)*, which is generated by *glycolysis* within the red cell. Defects in the production of ATP are associated with loss of cell volume, increased red cell rigidity, and decreased red cell survival.

IV. Metabolic pathways in red blood cells

The RBC has a relatively simple pattern of metabolic pathways (Figure 3.5).

A. Embden–Meyerhof pathway (anaerobic glycolysis)

The anaerobic glycolytic pathway is the major source of ATP production in the RBC. It generates the ATP necessary to power the ionic pumps that regulate cellular ion content and hydration status. Congenital defects in the glycolytic pathway, which are rare, are associated with a wide range of clinical disorders (e.g., myopathy, mental retardation, neuropsychiatric abnormalities and hemolysis of variable severity).

1. The hemolysis associated with defects in glycolysis is referred to as *congenital non-spherocytic hemolytic anemias* because the RBC morphology is minimally altered. The common biochemical consequence for the RBC is *ATP deficiency*, leading to abnormalities in Na^+, K^+, Ca^{2+}, and water homeostasis. The RBC are typically more rigid than normal cells, and susceptible to retention and destruction in the spleen. The most common enzyme defect of glycolysis is pyruvate kinase deficiency.

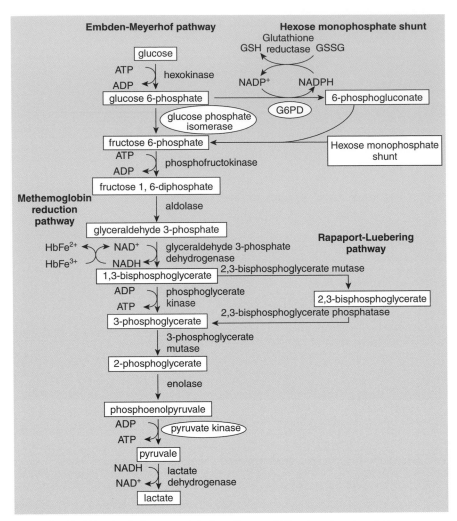

Figure 3.5 Red blood cell glucose metabolic pathways. ADP, adenosine phosphate; ATP, adenosine triphosphate; G6PD, glucose-6-phosphate dehydrogenase; GSH, glutathione; GSSG, oxidized glutathione; HbFe^{2+}, ferrous hemoglobin; HbFe^{3+}, ferric hemoglobin; NAD, nicotinamide adenine dinucleotide; NADH, reduced nicotinamide adenine dinucleotide; NADP, nicotinamide adenine dinucleotide phosphate; NADPH, reduced nicotinamide adenine dinucleotide phosphate. (Reproduced with permission from Harrison's Principles of Internal Medicine, Braunwald, Eugene et al, © 2002 The McGraw-Hill Companies, Inc.)

2. A subset of glycolytic enzyme defects (*Rapaport–Luebering pathway*) may also lead to reductions in RBC 2,3-DPG concentrations, causing a left shift in the oxyhemoglobin dissociation curve (increased affinity), and further impairing oxygen delivery to the tissues.

B. Hexose monophosphate shunt

A small portion of glucose metabolism proceeds through the hexose mono-phosphate shunt. The RBC is designed to transport high concentrations of oxygen, an extremely reactive molecule with the potential to do chemical damage to core components of the RBC. The RBC has elaborate defense mechanisms to protect itself from *oxidative damage*. *Glutathione* is a critical molecule necessary to detoxify *hydrogen peroxide*, the primary chemical inter-mediate involved in oxidative damage. Glutathione is maintained in a reduced state by the hexose monophosphate shunt. This pathway can also indirectly contribute to glycolysis and ATP production.

C. Methemoglobin reduction pathway

The methemoglobin reduction pathway maintains hemoglobin iron in the ferrous (Fe^{2+}) state. Defects in the pathway lead to hemolytic disorders sec-ondary to unstable hemoglobin.

V. Summary

Red blood cells are derived from precursor cells in the bone marrow. The major physiologic function of RBC is oxygen transport. Oxygen status has important direct effects on RBC production by the bone marrow and the biochemical properties of hemoglobin. The metabolic pathways of the RBC are streamlined to provide a simple, reliable source of ATP from glycolysis and maintain a steady pool of reducing substrates to protect RBC components from oxidative damage.

Further reading

Steinberg MH, Benz EJ, Adewoye AH, Ebert BL. Pathobiology of the human erythrocyte and its hemoglobins. In: Hoffman R, Benz EJ Jr, Shattil SJ, Furie B, Silberstein LE, McGlave P, Heslop H., eds. Hematology: Basic Principles and Practice, Philadelphia: Churchill Liv-ingstone Elsevier, 2009:427–38.

4 Anemia: Clinical Approach

Peter W. Marks

Yale University School of Medicine, New Haven, CT, USA

I. Definition of anemia

The oxygen carrying capacity of red blood cells is provided by hemoglobin. Anemia is present when this value in blood falls below age and gender appropriate normal values, which are defined by values two standard deviations below the mean for normal individuals of similar age and gender (i.e., outside the 95% confidence interval for the population). The volume of red blood cells reported as a percentage of the total volume of blood present is the hematocrit. This value is commonly used as an alternative method for defining anemia. In most cases the two values relate to one another roughly by a factor of three (hemoglobin $\times$ 3 $\approx$ hematocrit).

The hemoglobin value in children is lower than that of adults. During puberty, an increase in hemoglobin occurs in males due to androgenic steroids. The normal range for hemoglobin in males is therefore higher than for females (Table 4.1). In maturity, the difference between men and women decreases. In particular, over the two decades after 70 years of age, men's hemoglobin levels drop by about 1 g/dL. Thus, the mean hemoglobin concentration for a 90-year-old man is about 14.1 g/dL compared to about 13.8 g/dL for a 90-year-old woman.

II. Major broad causes of anemia

- Acute blood loss.
- Inadequate production of red blood cells.
- Destruction of red blood cells.

A. Acute blood loss

Loss of blood acutely may not be associated with an immediate decline in hemoglobin concentration, since this loss consists of an equivalent proportion

Table 4.1 Normal range for red blood cell parameters		
Parameter		Adult normal range
Red blood cell number (RBC)	Male	4.5–5.9×10^{12}/L
	Female	4.0–5.0×10^{12}/L
Hemoglobin (Hgb or Hb)	Male	13.5–17.5 g/dL
	Female	12–16 g/dL
Hematocrit (Hct)	Male	41–53%
	Female	36–46%
Mean corpuscular volume (MCV = Hct/RBC)		80–100 fL
Mean corpuscular hemoglobin (MCH = Hgb/RBC)		26–34 pg
Mean corpuscular hemoglobin concentration (MCHC = Hgb/Hct)		31–37 g/dL
Red cell distribution width (RDW = (SD* of MCV/MCV) × 100)		11–15%

*SD, standard deviation.

of cellular elements and plasma. However, after volume repletion a decrease in the hemoglobin concentration or hematocrit proportional to the amount of blood lost may be observed.

B. Inadequate production

There are a number of entities commonly associated with an inadequate production of red blood cells. Some of these affect other cell lineages as well.

- **Iron deficiency anemia** is the most common cause of anemia globally. With rare exception iron deficiency anemia in adults results from chronic blood loss. In women, menstrual blood loss may explain its development (and it is present in about 5% of menstruating females in the United States). In men, the identification of iron deficiency anemia should always provoke a search for blood loss. Even in younger women, consideration of gastrointestinal blood loss may merit consideration, depending on individual circumstance (see Chapter 4).
- **Anemia of inflammation (also known as the anemia of chronic disease)** is commonly encountered in association with a variety of conditions, including serious infections, rheumatologic disease, and malignancy. In this condition the iron regulatory protein hepcidin decreases the ability of the reticuloendothelial system to release stored iron. The lack of bioavailable iron essentially mimics the situation with iron deficiency anemia from blood loss. When combined with the suppressive effect of certain cytokines on red blood cell production, this circumstance leads to a mild to moderate anemia that may share some morphologic features with iron deficiency.
- **Anemia of renal disease** results from erythropoietin deficiency. The synthesis of this hormone is regulated by the oxygen tension in the periglomerular cells of the kidney. Hypoxia drives the synthesis of erythropoietin and its release into the bloodstream, which stimulates the maturation and development of erythrocyte precursors in the bone marrow. These activities

result in an increase in red blood cell mass, bringing additional oxygen to the kidney, and ultimately completing the feedback loop by down-regulating production of erythropoietin. A reduction in renal function is generally accompanied by a reduction of erythropoietin production.

- **Endocrine anemias** result from deficiencies or excess of hormones that contribute to blood cell development. To provide a few examples, hypothyroidism may be associated with a mild to moderate anemia sometimes associated with macrocytosis; adrenal cortical insufficiency may be accompanied by a normocytic anemia; and decreased levels of serum testosterone may lead to a mild anemia in males.

- **Pure red cell aplasia** in children may be the result of heritable disorders, such as congenital hypoplastic anemia (Diamond–Blackfan anemia), or may be the apparent result of infection with a virus (e.g., parvovirus B19) or an immunologic phenomenon (e.g., as seen in systemic lupus erythematosis). In contrast to aplastic anemia, in which two or more cell lineages are affected, pure red cell aplasia is characterized by preservation of the white blood cell count and platelet count.

- **Bone marrow replacement** is also known by the term myelophthisis. In this case, the blood forming bone marrow space is taken over by cells or material that should not be there. Causes of bone marrow replacement include hematologic malignancies such as leukemia or lymphoma, metastatic cancer (most commonly breast or prostate), infection with fungi or other microorganisms, and fibrosis such as that which may occur in conjunction with primary myelofibrosis.

- **Folate and vitamin-B_{12} deficiency** are two types of megaloblastic anemia and lead to maturation abnormalities in all three cell lineages. These disorders share in the common pathophysiology of impaired synthesis of DNA. Folate deficiency is generally related to inadequate dietary intake or to increased requirements due to red blood cell hemolysis. The situation for vitamin-B_{12} (also called cobalamin) is more complex. Vitamin-B_{12} is released from food in the acidic environment of the stomach and binds to the intrinsic factor that is secreted by the parietal cells in the stomach. The intrinsic factor-vitamin-B_{12} complex then travels to the terminal ileum where it is absorbed. Vitamin-B_{12} deficiency may result from several different causes including inadequate stomach acidity, pernicious anemia (an autoimmune phenomena destroying the parietal cells that synthesize intrinsic factor), structural lesions in the terminal ileum due to conditions such as Crohn's disease, and from surgical resection of portions of the GI tract. Inadequate dietary intake is generally only observed in vegans (see Chapter 6).

- **Sideroblastic anemias** represent an uncommon group of hereditary and acquired disorders in which iron is not effectively used in hemoglobin synthesis leading to iron accumulation in the mitochondria of red blood cell precursors. The deposition of iron in mitochondria leads to the morphologic entity of ringed sideroblasts in the bone marrow when it is stained for iron. Exactly as the name implies, ringed sideroblasts are cells in which iron-laden mitochondria encircle at least one-third of the circumference of the erythroblast nucleus. Usually at least five iron-laden mitochrondria need to be seen encircling the nucleus to make diagnostic criteria. Hereditary forms of sideroblastic anemia are rare and may be X-linked, autosomal dominant or recessive. Acquired forms may occur after exposure to drugs (e.g., cyclosporine, vincristine) or toxins (ethanol).

C. Destruction

Normally red blood cells circulate for about 100 to 120 days before they are cleared by the reticuloendothelial system. Premature red blood cell destruction may result from intrinsic defects within hemoglobin, cytoskeletal proteins, or enzymes. It may also result from defects extrinsic to the erythrocyte, including mechanical forces and antibody or complement-mediated red cell breakdown.

- **Hemoglobinopathies** include alpha and beta thalassemia, disorders in which there is insufficient production of one of the globin chains, and the structural mutations. Alpha or beta thalassemia traits (loss of two alpha genes, or one beta gene) are common causes of microcytosis associated with little or no anemia. Microcytosis occurs in thalassemia because the deficiency in hemoglobin stimulates additional cell divisions of erythrocyte precursors in order to try to preserve the hemoglobin concentration. Thalassemia trait is particularly common in individuals from Africa, Asia, and the Mediterranean Basin. Among the most commonly encountered structural mutations is a glutamine to valine substitution at position 6 of the beta globin gene. This change results in the production of hemoglobin S, which tends to polymerize in its deoxygenated state. Heterozygotes with one copy of hemoglobin S (sickle cell trait) are relatively protected against infection with the malaria parasite. This structural mutation provides a survival advantage; it is the selective pressure leading to persistence of this mutation. Homozygotes with two copies of hemoglobin S have sickle cell anemia, a serious life-defining hematologic disorder. Many other structural mutations exist and can result in changes in the properties of hemoglobin, such as reducing its solubility (e.g., hemoglobin C and hemoglobin D), decreasing its stability, or changing its oxygen affinity (see Chapter 7).
- **Red blood cell membrane defects** result from a variety of different defects affecting the red blood cell cytoskeleton or the membrane itself. Maintenance of the normal biconcave shape requires intact cytoskeletal architecture. Defects in any of the proteins involved, including ankyrin, spectrin, and band 3, among others, can lead to changes that reduce the resiliency of red blood cells as they pass through the narrow passageways in the spleen and other portions of the circulation. This initially leads to the formation of spherocytes, and ultimately results in hemolysis. The resulting disorder, hereditary spherocytosis, is most common in individuals of northern European descent. Liver disease is the most common cause of an acquired red cell membrane defect. Abnormalities in the lipid composition

of the red blood cell membrane result in cells that are abnormally stiff and unable to rebound from deformities arising from transit of the circulation. Paroxysmal nocturnal hemoglobinuria (PNH) represents a rare type of acquired membrane defect that is derived from a stem cell defect leading to the reduction or absence of phosphatidylinositolglyan-linked membrane proteins. The lack of one such erythrocyte phosphatidylinositolglyan-linked membrane protein, decay accelerating factor, is associated with the hemolysis of red blood cells through the unopposed constitutive activation of components of the complement cascade (see Chapter 7).

- **Red blood cell enzyme defects** are potentially the most common red cell abnormalities globally. Glucose-6-phosphate dehydrogenase (G-6-PD) is the enzyme required for function of the hexose monophosphate shunt in the red blood cell. This pathway provides the red blood cell with reduction capacity against oxidant stress. The gene encoding G-6-PD is on the X chromosome. Mutations in G-6-PD are very common, and have been preserved in populations because of their relative protection against infection with the malaria parasite, like sickle cell anemia. The two most common mutations cause a reduction in cell enzyme activity in the aging erythrocyte (A-variant) or result in absent function throughout the red cell life span (Mediterranean variant). Those carrying mutations in G-6-PD (especially males since this is an X-linked trait) have red cells that are susceptible to hemolysis under conditions of oxidant stress. Common causes of oxidant stress include medications such as antimalarials, dapsone, and sulfamethoxazole (see Chapter 7).

- **Mechanical causes of hemolysis** may result from microscopic or macroscopic forces. Microangiopathic hemolytic anemias include disseminated intravascular coagulation (DIC), thrombotic thrombocytopenic purpura (TTP), and hemolytic uremic syndrome (HUS). In these conditions abnormalities in the microvasculature result in shearing of the red blood cell and the formation of red cell fragments called schistocytes. Certain uncommon infections, such as those with clostridia or bartonella species can also be associated with the production of toxins that lead to red blood cell destruction through what is essentially mechanical disruption of the membrane. Accelerated or malignant hypertension and vasculities are additional etiologies producing mechanical destructional of red blood cells. Malfunctioning mechanical valves, perivalvular leaks, as well as long distance running can all result in the mechanical destruction of red blood cells by trauma.

- **Autoimmune hemolytic anemia** results from the formation of antibodies that bind to the red blood cell and either fix complement resulting in its destruction in the circulation (intravascular hemolysis) and/or result in clearance in the reticuloendothelial system and spleen (extravascular hemolysis). Warm autoantibodies are often idiopathic, but may be associated with hematologic malignancies such as chronic lymphoid leukemia or rheumatologic disorders such as systemic lupus erythematosus. Similarly,

cold autoantibodies may be idiopathic or associated with lymphoproliferative or rheumatologic disorders. Transient cold agglutinins may be associated with infectious mononucleosis and infection with mycoplasma (see Chapter 8).
• **Alloimmune hemolytic anemia** results from exposure of an individual to foreign red blood cells. In children and adults this most commonly results from blood transfusion in which there are mismatched minor antigens.

III. Symptoms and signs of anemia

The signs and symptoms of anemia correlate with reduction in the oxygen carrying capacity of blood and the ability of the affected individual to compensate for this defect. Rapid loss of an even moderate amount of blood may be associated with shock and collapse of the circulatory system. Blood loss that occurs gradually over time is often reasonably well-tolerated until relatively more severe, as adaptive changes can help compensate for the anemia. The corollary to this is that individuals with anemia that has developed gradually often do not require, and in fact can be harmed, by aggressive intervention with transfusions (e.g., pulmonary edema may develop with overaggressive transfusion).

The most common symptom of anemia that patients tend to report is fatigue. Decreased exercise tolerance and dyspnea on exertion may be noted by individuals as the extent of the anemia worsens. Certain types of anemia, such as iron deficiency anemia may be associated with pica, the dietary intake of non-food substances. When anemia is associated with a microangiopathy, bruising or bleeding may be reported.

Signs of anemia may include conjunctival pallor and a pale complexion. Tachycardia and/or systolic flow murmurs may be present if the degree of anemia is pronounced. Iron deficiency anemia may be associated with cracking of the edges of the lips (angular chelitis) and with spooning of the nails (koilonychia). Right upper quadrant pain may develop as a result of cholecystitis due to the formation of calcium bilirubin gallstones in the presence of hemolysis. Splenomegaly may result from chronic hemolysis leading essentially to hypertrophy of the reticuloendothelial system or from extramedullary hematopoeisis (the presence of maturing hematopoietic precursors outside of the bone marrow), which may be associated with some myeloproliferative disorders.

IV. Laboratory diagnosis

A systematic approach to the diagnosis of anemia is essential in order to minimize unnecessary diagnostic testing and to arrive expediently at the correct diagnosis. Despite the availability of sophisticated diagnostic testing, careful consideration of the information provided by the different parameters included in the complete blood count (CBC) and review of a well-prepared peripheral blood smear often provide a great wealth of diagnostic information.

Table 4.2 MCV and RDW in the categorization of anemia			
	Low MCV	*Normal MCV*	*High MCV*
Normal RDW	Chronic disease Thalassemia trait	Acute blood loss Inflammation Renal disease	Aplastic anemia Chronic liver disease Various medications
High RDW	Iron deficiency Sickle β-thalassemia	Early iron deficiency Early B_{12} deficiency Early folate efficiency Sickle cell anemia SC disease Chronic liver disease Myelodysplasia	B_{12} deficiency Folate deficiency Immune hemolysis Chronic liver disease Myelodysplasia

The CBC includes a variety of red blood cell indices. These calculated values are very important to classify anemia and guides one toward the differential diagnosis of anemic patient (Table 4.1).

When evaluating anemia, the two red blood cell indices that provide the greatest diagnostic information are the mean corpuscular volume (MCV) and red cell distribution width (RDW). MCV, which is calculated by the ratio of hematocrit (HCT) to red blood cell count (RBC), denotes red blood cell size in femtoliters (10^{-15} L). It may be small (microcytic), normal (normocytic), or large (macrocytic) depending on where it falls relative to the normal range. The red cell distribution width, which is actually the coefficient of variation of the mean erythrocyte size [(standard deviation of MCV/MCV) × 100], is either normal or elevated. When the MCV and RDW are used in combination, the various types of anemia tend to fall in one of the six possible categories, although overlap obviously exists (Table 4.2).

A. Reticulocyte count
The reticulocyte count measures the production and release of newly formed red blood cells. It should be obtained along with the CBC and peripheral blood smear in the evaluation of anemia, as it provides complementary information. The reticulocyte count is obtained by supravital staining of red cells with dyes that bind to nucleic acid (e.g., new methylene blue or ethidium bromide) in order to identify the newly released erythrocytes. These cells normally contain residual RNA for about the first day that they are present in the circulation. Since the normal lifespan of red blood cells is 100 to 120 days, it follows that in the absence of anemia the reticulocyte count is about 1%, which corresponds to an absolute reticulocyte count of 25,000 to 50,000/μL.

When the reticulocyte count is reported as a percentage it must be corrected for the degree of anemia. Since the same number of reticulocytes diluted in

Table 4.3 The reticulocyte count and causes of anemia	
Reticulocytes <100,000/μL or Reticulocyte Index <2%	Reticulocytes ≥100,000/μL or Reticulocyte Index ≥2%
Hypoproliferative anemias Iron deficiency anemia Anemia of acute inflammation Anemia of renal disease Endocrine anemias Pure red cell aplasia Bone marrow replacement	**Appropriate response to blood loss** **Hemolytic anemias** Hemoglobinopathies Membrane defects Enzyme defects Mechanical causes Autoimmune hemolytic anemia Alloimmune hemolytic anemia
Maturation defects Folate deficiency B$_{12}$ deficiency Sideroblastic anemia	

half the number of red blood cells will double the apparent percentage present, the following correction must be applied:

Reticulocyte count (%) × Patient's hematocrit/Normal hematocrit for age
  = Corrected reticulocyte count (%) or Reticulocyte index

In the presence of anemia, the absolute reticulocyte count should be at least 100,000/μL. This value corresponds to a reticulocyte index of at least 2%, and represents an appropriate response to blood loss or to red blood cell destruction (hemolysis). Alternatively, a decreased reticulocyte count indicates the presence of a hypoproliferative process or a red blood cell maturation abnormality. Anemias can be classified alone as to whether they are associated with an elevated reticulocyte count (Table 4.3) or this parameter can be combined with the MCV (Table 4.4).

B. Peripheral blood smear

The wealth of information provided by the CBC and reticulocyte count noted above is greatly complimented by review of the peripheral blood smear. Sometimes this may be all that is required in order to reach a diagnosis, and often carefully looking at the peripheral blood smear significantly narrows down the diagnostic entities under consideration.

A normal red blood cell is about the size of a lymphocyte nucleus (about 8 μM). The area of central pallor occupies about one-third of the overall diameter (Atlas Figure 1). Hypochromic cells have too much, and hyperchromic too little central pallor. *Anisocytosis* is the term used to describe variation in cell size; *poikilocytosis* describes variation in cell shape, and anisopoikilocytosis defines the two combined (Atlas Figure 23). Terminology describing the

Table 4.4 MCV and reticulocyte count scheme for classification of anemia			
	MCV 80–100		
MCV <80	**Low reticulocytes**	**High reticulocytes**	**MCV >100**
Iron deficiency	Anemia of acute	Acute blood loss	B$_{12}$ deficiency
Thalassemias	inflammation	Hemolytic anemias	Folate
Anemia of acute	Renal disease	Hemoglobinopathies	deficiency
inflammation	Endocrine anemias	Enzyme defects	Liver disease
Sideroblastic anemias	Aplastic anemia	Mechanical anemias	Thyroid
Lead poisoning	Pure red cell aplasia	Autoimmune	disease
	Bone marrow failure	hemolytic anemias	
	Leukemia	Alloimmune	
	Myelodysplasic	hemolytic anemias	
	syndromes		
	Myeloproliferative		
	syndromes		

more common morphologic abnormalities of the red blood cell and their associated features are listed in Table 4.5.

Integration of information from the CBC, reticulocyte count, and peripheral smear

Because the MCV, RDW, reticulocyte count, and peripheral smear all provide complementary information, integration of these parameters leads to the correct diagnosis or provide significant insight as to the differential diagnosis (Figure 4.1). For example, an anemia presenting with a low MCV and high RDW in which the reticulocyte count is low is almost always iron deficiency anemia. The finding of hypochromic, microcytic cells along with wide variation in cell shape and size makes the diagnosis very likely. Iron studies and a ferritin level can then be obtained. At the other end of the spectrum, a newly occurring anemia that presents with a high MCV and high RDW in which the reticulocyte count is high is most likely to be associated with autoimmune hemolysis. A finding of spherocytes on examination of the peripheral blood smear would be highly suggestive of this diagnosis and would provoke further laboratory investigation such as obtaining a direct antiglobulin test.

Table 4.5 Morphologic features of the erythrocyte

Normal erythrocyte 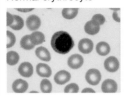	Biconcave disk about 8μM in diameter (about the size of the nucleus of a normal lymphocyte) Area of central pallor about ⅓ of the overall diameter
Spherocytes 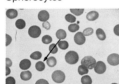	Loss of central pallor of the RBC DDx: immune hemolysis, hereditary spherocytosis
Schistocytes 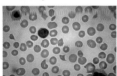	RBC fragmentation DDx: DIC, TTP, HUS, mechanical hemolysis
Bite cells 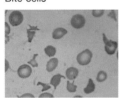	Bites taken out of the RBC membrane DDx: hemolysis w/G-6-PD deficiency, unstable hemoglobins
Burr cells (echinocytes) 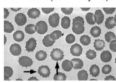	Undulations of the RBC surface on blood smear DDx: uremia
Spur cells (acanthocytes) 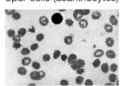	Spikes off of the RBC surface with loss of central pallor DDx: liver disease, abetalipoproteinemia

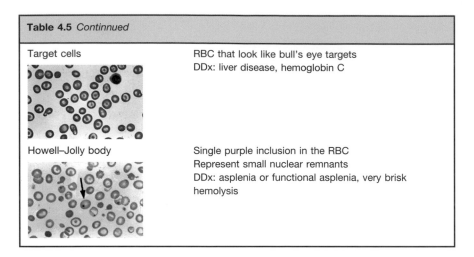

Table 4.5 *Continnued*	
Target cells	RBC that look like bull's eye targets DDx: liver disease, hemoglobin C
Howell–Jolly body	Single purple inclusion in the RBC Represent small nuclear remnants DDx: asplenia or functional asplenia, very brisk hemolysis

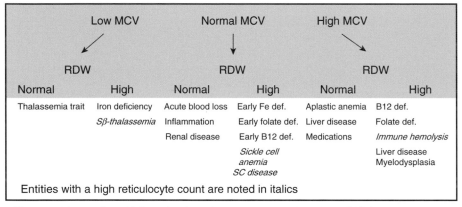

Low MCV		Normal MCV		High MCV	
RDW		RDW		RDW	
Normal	High	Normal	High	Normal	High
Thalassemia trait	Iron deficiency	Acute blood loss	Early Fe def.	Aplastic anemia	B12 def.
	Sβ-thalassemia	Inflammation	Early folate def.	Liver disease	Folate def.
		Renal disease	Early B12 def.	Medications	*Immune hemolysis*
			Sickle cell anemia		Liver disease
			SC disease		Myelodysplasia
Entities with a high reticulocyte count are noted in italics					

Figure 4.1 Integration of information from the mean corpuscular volume (MCV) and red cell distribution width (RDW).

VII. Summary

Anemia is the most commonly encountered hematologic abnormality in clinical practice. Careful consideration of the information provided by the complete blood count and reticulocyte count in conjunction with review of the peripheral blood smear often provides significant insight into the differential diagnosis, and by guiding further testing expedites appropriate diagnosis with a minimum number of tests.

Further reading

Andrews N. Forging a field: the golden age of iron biology. Blood 2008;112:219–30.
Bain BJ. Diagnosis from the blood smear. New Engl J Med 2005;353:498–507.
Packman CH. Hemolytic anemia due to warm autoantibodies. Blood Rev 2008;22:17–31.
Weiss G, Goodnough LT. Anemia of chronic disease. New Engl J Med 2005;10:1011–23.

5 | Iron Deficiency

Alice Ma

University of North Carolina, Chapel Hill, NC, USA

I. Introduction

Iron deficiency occurs when the intake and absorption of iron are insufficient to replenish the body's loss. When total body iron stores are depleted, the hemoglobin levels fall. This chapter will cover iron metabolism, the epidemiology of iron deficiency, and iron deficiency anemia—pathophysiology, clinical manifestations, diagnosis, and treatment.

II. Iron metabolism

A. Iron distribution

(i) Normal iron content in adult males is approximately 50 mg/kg of iron, and females have 35 mg/kg (3–4 g for an adult).

(ii) Iron-containing compounds are essential and are found in all cells and also in plasma. Since ionized iron is toxic, virtually all iron is found either within the heme moiety of a heme-protein (i.e., hemoglobin, myoglobin) or bound to a protein (i.e., transferrin, ferritin, and hemosiderin).

   1. <0.2% is in the plasma in the form of *transferrin* (Tf), the major iron transport protein.
   2. 70% of iron is found in the form of heme proteins.
      (a) **Hemoglobin** comprises 67% of total body iron. Since 1 mL of red cells contains 1 mg of iron, the average adult male has about 2 g of iron in the red cell mass. Women have 1.5 g of iron in their red cells.
      (b) Myoglobin makes up 3% of total body iron.
      (c) Some other heme proteins such as cytochromes, catalases, peroxidase) make up <1% of total body iron.
   3. The majority of the rest of iron is storage iron, which exists in two forms: ferritin and hemosiderin.

Concise Guide to Hematology, First Edition. Edited by Alvin H. Schmaier, Hillard M. Lazarus.
© 2012 Blackwell Publishing Ltd. Published 2012 by Blackwell Publishing Ltd.

(a) **Ferritin** is the major storage form of iron and holds the iron available for future use. It is made of a protein shell that encloses an iron core containing 4500 iron atoms.

(b) **Hemosiderin** is composed of aggregates of ferritin molecules that have partially lost their protein shells. It is a more stable but less accessible and soluble form of storage iron.

B. Overview

(i) Iron is mainly used for hemoglobin synthesis. It is used over and over again, cycling between the liver and the bone marrow.

1. Iron is continuously circulating through plasma while bound to *transferrin*.

2. The majority of circulating iron derives from destruction of approximately 20 mL of red cells daily, which liberates 20 mg of iron (Figure 5.1).

3. A further 5 mg of iron is carried in the plasma derived from iron stores and GI absorption.

4. Plasma iron is rapidly removed, mainly by erythropoietic tissues in the bone marrow, but some portion also goes to other dividing cells and to the iron stores. This conservation mechanism is to be distinguished from bilirubin, formed from degraded hemoglobin from senescent RBC needs to be conjugated and excreted by the extrahepatic biliary system.

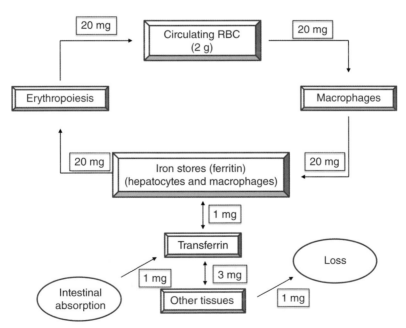

Figure 5.1 Iron kinetics *in vivo*. See text for description.

C. The iron cycle
(i) **Iron absorption**
1. Average iron in the Western diet is 7mg per 1000 kcal (10–15 mg/day). Only 10% is typically absorbed.
    (a) Heme iron is absorbed most efficiently:
       • Absorbed intact from gut, mainly in duodenum.
       • Accounts for 10–15% of non-vegetarian Western diet.
    (b) Non-heme iron is more poorly absorbed.
       • Ferric (Fe^{3+}) iron in food needs to be reduced to ferrous (Fe^{2+}) iron before absorption. The low pH environment in the proximal duodenum solubilizes food to liberate ferric iron that is reduced ferrous iron by a cytochrome b-like ferrireductase.
       • Non-heme iron can be bound to food phytates and phosphates which impair absorption (found in tea, egg yolks, grains).
       • Non-heme iron absorption is enhanced by formation of complexes with peptides from meat. Vitamin C also enhances absorption.
2. Extent of iron absorption is affected by iron stores. The more iron deficient the patient, the greater the iron absorption. Also, increased erythropoietic activity such as is found in hemolytic conditions, increases iron absorption.

(ii) **Cellular iron use**
1. Transferrin-bound iron is delivered to red cells and binds to specific transferrin receptors (TfRs).
2. Once Tf binds TfR, the complex is internalized. Iron is released into the cytosol, and Tf is sent back into plasma.
3. Fate of iron:
    (a) Most (80–90%) is used to make hemoglobin, myoglobin, and cytochromes.
    (b) Small amount is used for non-heme enzymes (e.g., ribonucleotide reductase).
    (c) Most of the remaining iron is stored as **ferritin**.

(iii) **Iron excretion**
1. There is no physiologic pathway for iron excretion.
2. Iron is lost from the body, only when cells are lost, especially epithelial cells from the GI tract, skin and renal tubules, and shedding decidua from menstrual cycles.

III. Iron depletion and iron deficiency

As iron stores become depleted, three phases occur sequentially:
(i) Initially, iron stores are depleted, but enough iron remains so that red cell production continues and hemoglobin values remain normal. Additionally, supply of iron to tissues remains normal. Ferritin levels are beginning to fall.

(ii) As iron levels continue to fall, tissues may become iron depleted, but there is still no anemia. At this level, ferritin levels are low, Tf levels are increased, Hb, MCV are within normal limits, but there may be a few hypochromic red cells.

(iii) Lastly, once iron stores are fully depleted, there is no longer sufficient iron to maintain red cell production, and anemia results. Cells become progressively hypochromic and microcytic. Other tissues may be affected by iron deficiency such as nails, tongue, etc.

IV. Prevalence of iron deficiency

(i) Iron deficiency anemia is the most common hematologic problem world-wide, affecting between 500 million to 2 billion individuals.

(ii) Most common in three populations:
   1. Infants and preschool children.
   2. Women of child-bearing years.
   3. Elderly.

V. Causes of iron deficiency

A. Causes of iron deficiency related to the GI tract

(i) GI blood loss must be considered in iron deficient men and post-menopausal women.

(ii) Colonoscopy, upper endoscopy are the beginning evaluation, and if negative, should prompt a capsule endoscopy. Common causes are listed in Box 5.1.

(iii) Iron malabsorption due to gastric bypass surgery for obesity (which removes parietal cells that produce HCl that contributes to the conversion

---

Box 5.1 Causes of GI blood loss

1. Esophagitis
2. Varices
3. Ulcers
4. Gastritis
5. Gastric antral vascular ectasia (GAVE syndrome, aka watermelon stomach)
6. Arteriovenous malformations
7. Polyps
8. Tumors
9. Inflammatory bowel disease
10. Parasitic infection
11. Meckel's diverticulum
12. Milk-induced enteropathy (in infants)

Box 5.2 Other causes of iron deficiency

Gynecologic

Lactation

Bladder neoplasms

Epistaxis

Blood donation

Hemoglobinuria

Self-induced bleeding (auto-phlebotomy)

Pulmonary hemosiderosis

Hereditary hemorrhagic telangiectasia

Runner's anemia

Iron loss through the urine in patients with chronic intravascular hemolysis

---

of food iron Fe^{3+} to Fe^{2+} form for optimal absorption and bypasses the duodenum—the major site of iron absorption) is an increasingly common condition.

(iv) Celiac sprue is an uncommon cause of iron deficiency.

(v) Non heme iron intake may be inadequate in vegetarians—especially since this form of iron is less-well absorbed than heme-iron found in meat. Iron deficiency is more common in vegans.

(vi) Other causes of iron deficiency (Box 5.2).

B. Causes of iron deficiency in infancy

(i) Inadequate iron stores at birth (usually due to iron deficiency in the mother). Prematurity also plays a role, since half of the infant's iron stores are deposited in the last month of fetal life. Fetal-maternal hemorrhage is a third mechanism.

(ii) Inadequate iron in the diet:

1. The growing child needs 0.5–1 mg of iron daily which cannot be supplied by breast milk alone.

2. Whole cow's milk increases intestinal blood loss in infants, and non-iron-fortified cow's milk formula increases the likelihood of developing iron deficiency anemia.

C. Causes of iron deficiency in women of child-bearing age

(i) **Iron loss through menstruation:**

1. Monthly blood loss in normal women ranges from 10–180 mL.

2. Maximum iron in a normal diet (20 mg daily) can replace the iron in 60 mL of monthly menstrual blood.

3. Thus, many women teeter on the brink of iron deficiency and need only slight changes in the diet or a single pregnancy to become frankly anemic.

(ii) **Iron loss in pregnancy and delivery:**
  1. With each pregnancy, a woman loses 500–700 mg of iron—250 mg to the fetus, and the remainder in the placenta and through hemorrhage.
  2. Pregnant women thus need additional iron intake of 20–30 mg/d.
  3. Further iron is required during lactation.

VI. Clinical presentation

(i) Patients may be asymptomatic or present with signs/symptoms of anemia, including fatigue, weakness, pallor, palpitations, lightheadedness, headaches, tinnitus, exertional dyspnea.
(ii) Some patients have signs or symptoms related to the underlying cause of their iron deficiency, e.g.:
  1. GI symptoms—abdominal pain from an ulcer, change in stools from a colon cancer.
  2. GYN symptoms—heavy menses, cramping from uterine fibroids.
(iii) There are some signs/symptoms related to the direct effects of iron deficiency on tissues:
  1. Glossitis (a smooth, waxy-appearing, red tongue, with atrophy of the papillae).
  2. Angular cheilitis (ulcerations or fissures at the corners of the mouth).
  3. Esophageal webs and strictures (a web of mucosa forms at the junction of the hypopharynx and esophagus and leads to dysphagia).
  4. Koilonychia (spooning of the nails, where the nails are concave instead of convex).
  5. Blue sclerae.
  6. Gastric atrophy.
  7. Pica (obsessive consumption of substances with no nutritional value, such as ice, starch, clay, paper).
  8. Restless leg syndrome—incidence higher in those with iron deficiency.
  9. Thrombocytosis—an elevated platelet count, for unexplained reasons.
  10. *In children, iron deficiency can lead to impaired psychomotor and mental development.*

VII. Laboratory diagnosis of iron deficiency

A. CBC
(i) First sign is an increasing RDW, followed by a decrease in the MCV.
(ii) Anemia develops last of all.

B. Peripheral blood smear (Figure 5.2, Atlas Figures 9 and 10)
This can show hypochromic, microcytic red blood cells with some aniso- and poikilocytosis. Target cells can also be seen in iron deficiency. The platelet count can be elevated as well.

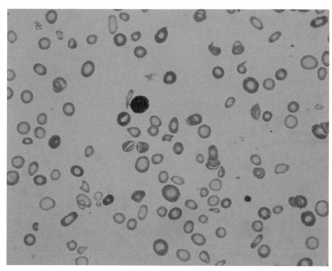

Figure 5.2 Blood smear from a 16-year-old male who presented with an Hgb of 6, MCV 55 and guaiac-positive stools. He was found to have gastric polyps and was diagnosed with familial adenomatous polyposis. Note the very microcytic, hypochromic red cells in relation to the small lymphocyte present in the center of the picture.

C. Iron studies

(i)   Serum iron levels fall, and TIBC increases *after* storage iron is depleted.

(ii) A transferrin saturation of <10% with an elevated TIBC is diagnostic of iron deficiency in an otherwise healthy person.

D. Serum ferritin

(i)   The serum ferritin reflects the total body storage of iron.

(ii) A serum ferritin of <12 is diagnostic of iron deficiency.

(iii) Serum ferritin is an "acute phase reactant" and will increase in the setting of inflammation, infection, malignancy, hemolysis, hepatitis, bone marrow or splenic infarctions.

E. Bone marrow biopsy

Bone marrow biopsy is the gold standard for diagnosing iron deficiency. It is essential to recognize the absence of intracellular iron in bone marrow normoblasts.

VIII. Treatment of iron deficiency

(i)   Treatment should be aimed at correcting the underlying cause.

(ii) Oral replacement is the treatment of choice:

    1.   Many forms, not all of which are equally tolerated by patients

2. Oral iron can cause GI upset (nausea and constipation) and it is wise to tell patients to take it with meals and to gradually increase the dose and frequency. Oral iron may also cause very dark and tarry stools.

3. Oral iron absorption can be impaired by certain foods and drink (tea, dairy, grains) and by proton pump inhibitors.

4. With adequate iron repletion, hemoglobin values should rise by approximately 1 g/dL per week. Failure to improve the hemoglobin should lead the clinician to suspect:
   (a) Ongoing hemorrhage.
   (b) Non-adherence to medical treatment.
   (c) Iron malabsorption.
   (d) Another contributing cause of anemia such as folate deficiency.
   (e) Incorrect initial diagnosis.

5. Once the hemoglobin normalizes, oral iron should be continued for a further 6 months to adequately replete the iron stores, or the patient risks early recurrence of anemia.

(iii) Parenteral iron:

1. Parenteral iron can be given if patient is intolerant of oral iron, or if there is iron malabsorption, or if there is considerable G.I. iron loss that cannot be maintained by oral replacement (e.g., bleeding small bowel angiodysplasia).

2. There is a significant risk of anaphylaxis and other infusion-related reactions. Several commercial preparations are available consisting of iron sucrose, iron dextran, or sodium ferric gluconate complex.

(iv) Blood transfusion:

1. Each unit of blood has 1 mg/mL of iron.
2. Each unit of blood will raise the hemoglobin value by about 1 g/dL.
3. In general, transfusion should be reserved for clinical signs or symptoms of cardiovascular compromise.

IX. The anemia of chronic disease

(i) This condition must be distinguished from iron deficiency anemia.

(ii) In inflammatory states, cytokines act to sequester iron away from the bloodstream. This is because certain microorganisms use iron as a growth factor.

(iii) These cytokines act to increase production of a peptide known as *hepcidin*.

(iv) Hepcidin actions:
   1. Decrease iron absorption from gut.
   2. Decrease iron export out of liver stores.
   3. Decrease transferrin levels and TIBC.

(v) Serum iron levels fall, but so do transferrin and TIBC.

(vi) Ferritin (which is an acute phase reactant) can be normal or elevated.

Box 5.3 Other microcytic anemias

Thalassemia (alpha or beta)
Other hemoglobinopathies (Hemoglobin Lepore, Hemoglobin C, Hemoglobin E)
Sideroblastic anemia (acquired or congenital):
  Congenital (X-linked)
  Acquired:
    myelodysplastic syndromes
    alcohol-induced
    lead poisoning
    vitamin-B_6 deficiency
    isoniazide
Anemia of chronic disease

X. Other microcytic conditions mimicking iron deficiency (Box 5.3)

(i)   Thalassemia.
(ii) Sideroblastic anemia.
(iii) Some hemoglobinopathies (e.g., Hgb E, C).
(iv) Acquired microcytic anemias: lead poisoning, B_6 deficiency, medication (isoniazid), alcohol, and myelodysplastic syndrome.

Further reading

Beutler E. Disorders of iron metabolism. In: Lichtman MA, Beutler E, Kipps TJ et al., eds. Williams Hematology, 7th edn. New York: McGraw Hill, 2006:511–553.

Cogswell ME, Looker AC, Pfeiffer CM, Cook JD, Lacher DA, Beard JL, Lynch SR, Grummer-Strawn LM, et al. Assessment of iron deficiency in US preschool children and nonpregnant females of childbearing age: National Health and Nutrition Examination Survey 2003–2006. Am J Clin Nutr 2009;89(5):1334–42.

Keel SB, Abkowitz JL. The microcytic red cell and the anemia of inflammation. N Engl J Med 2009;361(19):1904–6.

Killip S, Bennett JM, Chambers MD. Iron deficiency anemia. Am Fam Physician 2007;75(5):671–8.

Murray-Kolb LE, Beard JL. Iron deficiency and child and maternal health. Am J Clin Nutr 2009;89(3):946S–950S.

Parkes E. Nutritional management of patients after bariatric surgery. Am J Med Sci 2006;331(4):207–13.

6 | Vitamin-B$_{12}$ (Cobalamin) and Folate Deficiency

Aśok C. Antony

Indiana University School of Medicine, Indianapolis, IN, USA

A. General considerations

(i)   Folates and vitamin-B$_{12}$ participate in one-carbon metabolism (enzymatic reactions involving the transfer of one-carbon groups like methyl-, formyl-, methylene-, forminyl-, and formimino-) that are essential for pyrimidine and purine biosynthesis (including synthesis of three of four nucleotides of DNA).

(ii)   Defective DNA synthesis in rapidly-proliferating hematopoietic/gastrointestinal-epithelial/gonadal/fetal cells results in megaloblastic cells with DNA values that are "stuck" between 2n and 4n and therefore unable to divide, with adverse clinical consequences arising from affected hematopoietic/gastrointestinal-epithelial/gonadal/fetal cells.

(iii)   Megaloblastic cells have "nuclear-cytoplasmic dissociation" (large "immature" nucleus with a relatively mature cytoplasm) (Figure 6.1) (Atlas Figures 26, 28 and 29).

(iv)   Deficiency of either vitamin-B$_{12}$ or folates can present with megaloblastic anemia, but only deficiency of vitamin-B$_{12}$ can present with neuropsychiatric syndromes.

(v)   Correct vitamin replacement for either vitamin-B$_{12}$ or folate deficiency is essential.

B. Epidemiology

1. Vitamin-B$_{12}$ nutrition

(i)   Recommended daily allowance (RDA) vitamin-B$_{12}$:
(a) men/non-pregnant women = 2.4 micrograms.
(b) pregnant women = 2.6 micrograms; lactating women = 2.8 micrograms.

(ii)   Vitamin-B$_{12}$ solely produced in nature by microorganisms; main dietary cobalamin is animal-source foods:

Concise Guide to Hematology, First Edition. Edited by Alvin H. Schmaier, Hillard M. Lazarus.
© 2012 Blackwell Publishing Ltd. Published 2012 by Blackwell Publishing Ltd.

(a)   (b)

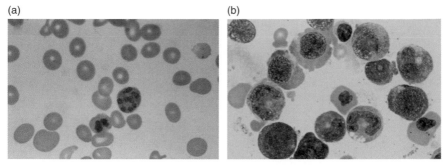

Figure 6.1 Characteristic features of megaloblastic anemia in peripheral blood and bone marrow. (a) The peripheral blood has oval macrocytes and marked hypersegmentation of polymorphonuclear neutrophils. (b) A bone marrow aspirate shows megaloblastic normoblasts that exhibit nuclear: cytoplasmic dissociation or asynchrony (nuclear maturation lagging behind cytoplasmic maturation). Megaloblastic changes in the leukocyte series are shown by the "giant metamyelocyte". The orthochromatic normoblasts do not have pyknotic nuclei. (Reproduced with permission from Antony AC. Megaloblastic anemias, Chapter 170. In: Goldman L, Ausiello D, eds. Cecil Medicine, 23rd edn. Saunders-Elsevier, 2008:1231–41.)

       (a) Meat >10 micrograms/100 g.
       (b) Fish, milk products, egg yolk 1–10 micrograms/100 g.
       (c) Nonvegetarian Western diets (5–7 micrograms/day).
       (d) Nonvegetarians (e.g., poverty-imposed near-vegetarians) with low animal source food intake are at risk.
       (e) Lacto-ovo-vegetarians consume <0.5 microgram/day and vegans <0.1 microgram/day.
(iii)   Vitamin-B$_{12}$ exceptionally well-stored (total stores = 2000–5000 micrograms vitamin-B$_{12}$); 50% liver.
(iv)   Daily loss = 1 microgram, so change in dietary vitamin-B$_{12}$ intake takes 5–10 years to manifest clinically.
(v)   Daily turnover (5–10 micrograms vitamin-B$_{12}$/day) via efficient enterohepatic circulation with 75% reabsorption, so interruption (e.g., ileal resection) results in greater fecal losses; clinical presentation ~3–4 years.
(vi)   Vitamin-B$_{12}$ resists high-temperature cooking but unstable to light.

2. Folates nutrition
(i)   RDA folate:
       (a) Adult men/non-pregnant women = 400 micrograms.
       (b) Pregnant women = 600 micrograms for fetus and maternal tissues; lactating women = 500 micrograms.
       (c) Folates synthesized by microorganisms, green-leafy vegetables/beans/fruit and animal-source foods.
(ii)   Balanced Western diet prevents folate deficiency, but still inadequate for fetal folate requirements (hence need for food fortification—see Tables 6.1 and 6.2).

Table 6.1 Beneficial effects of folic acid and B_{12} therapy on non-hematopoietic systems

1. **Using folic acid, vitamin-B_{12}, pyridoxine supplementation**
   - Reduced hip fracture*
   - Reduced the progression of carotid intima media thickness*
     (surrogate marker of early subclinical arteriosclerosis)
   - Reduction in age-related macular degeneration*
2. **Using folic acid supplementation**
   - Reduction in stroke*
   - Reduction in rate of cognitive decline among healthy elderly*
   - Reduction in age-related (sensorineural) hearing loss*
   - Reduction in recurrence of neural-tube defects*
3. **Beneficial effects of folic acid fortification of food (population-based studies)**
   - Reduction in neural-tube defects
     (anencephaly, spina bifida, encephalocele, meningocele, iniencephaly)
   - Reduction in cleft lip with/without cleft palate
   - Reduction in severe congenital heart disease
     (endocardial cushion defects, conotruncal defects)
   - Reduction in congenital pyloric stenosis, stenosis of pelvico-ureteric junction, limb-reduction defects, omphalocele
   - Reduction in stroke mortality
   - Decreased risk of low-birth weight and small-for-gestational-age babies

*Therapy is directed to lower homocysteine. (Signifies Paper with Randomized Controlled Trial Data; GRADE A; see "Further reading for Table 6.1")

Further reading for Table 6.1

De Wals P, Tairou F, Van Allen MI, et al. Reduction in neural-tube defects after folic acid fortification in Canada. N Engl J Med 2007;357:135–42.

Ionescu-Ittu R, Marelli AJ, Mackie AS, Pilote L. Prevalence of severe congenital heart disease after folic acid fortification of grain products: time trend analysis in Quebec, Canada. BMJ 2009;338:1673.

Khan U, Crossley C, Kalra L, et al. Homocysteine and its relationship to stroke subtypes in a UK black population: the south London ethnicity and stroke study. Stroke 2008;39:2943–9.

Spence JD. Homocysteine-lowering therapy: a role in stroke prevention? Lancet Neurol 2007;6:830–8.

Timmermans S, Jaddoe VW, Hofman A, Steegers-Theunissen RP, Steegers EA. Peri-conception folic acid supplementation, fetal growth and the risks of low birth weight and preterm birth: the Generation R Study. Br J Nutr 2009;102:777–85.

Wilcox AJ, Lie RT, Solvoll K, et al. Folic acid supplements and risk of facial clefts: national population based case-control study. BMJ 2007;334:464.

Yang Q, Botto LD, Erickson JD, et al. Improvement in stroke mortality in Canada and the United States, 1990 to 2002. Circulation 2006;113:1335–43.

Table 6.2 Prophylaxis with vitamin-B$_{12}$ or folate

A. Prophylaxis with vitamin-B$_{12}$:
  (a) Infants of vitamin-B$_{12}$-deficient mothers
  (b) Vegetarians, poverty-imposed near-vegetarians (fortified-food/beverages, or 5–10 micrograms vitamin-B$_{12}$/day orally)
  (c) Post-gastrectomy (1 mg/day orally lifelong, with iron)
  (d) Malabsorption of vitamin-B$_{12}$ from any mechanism (see Table 6.3) (1–2 mg vitamin-B$_{12}$/day orally)

B. Periconceptional supplementation of folate*:
  (a) All normal women (400 micrograms folic acid/day) of childbearing age
  (b) Women with prior neural-tube defect baby (need higher doses = 4 mg folic acid/day)
  (c) Women in childbearing-age taking anticonvulsants (dilantin/phenobarbital/carbamazepine) (1 mg folic-acid/day).

C. Folate supplementation given routinely*
  (a) Premature infants
  (b) Lactating mothers
  (c) Chronic hemolysis/myeloproliferative diseases (1 mg/day)
  (d) To reduce toxicity of methotrexate (rheumatoid arthritis/psoriasis) (1 mg/day)

*Note: If folate is given to a patient with vitamin-B$_{12}$ deficiency, the patient can develop progressive neurologic damage.

(iii) In developing countries folate intake often <½ to ⅓ of RDA.

(iv) Folates break down upon prolonged cooking (>15 minutes destroys 50–95% folate).

C. Vitamin-B$_{12}$ physiology

The complex mechanism involved in escorting small amounts of [precious] food vitamin-B$_{12}$ through the intestine (Figure 6.2) ensures maximal absorption. Main pathology is related to poor intake versus malabsorption.

1. Normal absorption and transport

(i) Two coenzyme forms (deoxyadenosylcobalamin or methylcobalamin) in food must be released from bound proteins via peptic digestion at low-gastric pH prior to absorption.

(ii) When released, vitamin-B$_{12}$ first binds salivary/gastric R-protein (haptocorrin).

(iii) After R-proteins digested by pancreatic proteases, vitamin-B$_{12}$ transferred to gastric Intrinsic-Factor.

(iv) Intrinsic-Factor–vitamin-B$_{12}$ complex binds Intrinsic-Factor–vitamin-B$_{12}$ receptors (a.k.a. Cubam receptors) on ileal mucosal cells—("Cubam" because receptor is composed of *cub*ulin-plus-*am*nionless proteins).

(v) Within enterocytes, vitamin-B$_{12}$ transferred to Transcobalamin-II and released into blood.

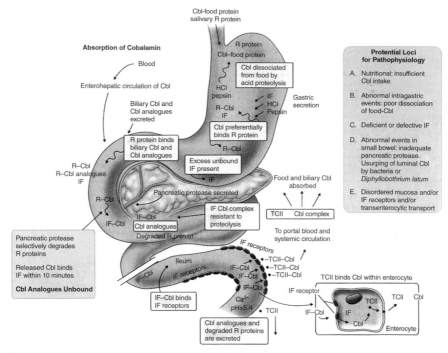

Figure 6.2 Components and mechanism of vitamin-B$_{12}$ absorption with an indication of the locus for malabsorption. See text for details. IF, Intrinsic-Factor; TCII, transvitamin-B$_{12}$ II. (Reproduced with permission from Antony AC. Megaloblastic anemias. In: Hoffman R, Benz EJ Jr, Shattil SJ et al., eds. Hematology: Basic Principles and Practice, 5th edn. Philadelphia: Elsevier, Churchill Livingstone, 2009:491–524.)

(vi)   Transcobalamin-II–vitamin-B$_{12}$ complex then binds to Transcobalamin-II receptors and internalized by receptor-mediated endocytosis.

(vii) Transcobalamin-I binds and stores ~75% vitamin-B$_{12}$ in blood.

(viii) Transcobalamin-III "mops-up" vitamin-B$_{12}$ analogs for hepatobiliary-to-fecal excretion.

2. Normal cellular processing

(i)   >95% intracellular vitamin-B$_{12}$ bound to deoxyadenosylcobalamin or methylcobalamin.

(ii)   Mitochondrial deoxyadenosylcobalamin is the coenzyme for methylmalonyl-CoA mutase (converts methylmalonyl-CoA to succinyl-CoA so products of propionate metabolism (methylmalonyl-CoA) are easily metabolized).

(iii) Cytoplasmic methylcobalamin is the coenzyme for methionine synthase (catalyzes transfer of methyl groups from methylcobalamin to homo-cysteine forming methionine; during reaction, methyl-group of 5-methyl-tetrahydrofolate (methyl-THF) donated to regenerate methycobalamin thereby forming THF that is essential to sustain one-carbon metabolism within cells).

(iv)   When methionine is adenylated to *S*-adenosylmethionine, it can donate its methyl group for biologic methylation reactions involving >80 proteins, phospholipids, neurotransmitters, RNA, and DNA.

D. Pathogenesis of vitamin-B$_{12}$ deficiency (Table 6.3)

(i)   **Nutritional vitamin-B$_{12}$ deficiency:** Vegetarianism and poverty-imposed near-vegetarianism commonest cause of nutritional vitamin-B$_{12}$ insufficiency worldwide in all age groups.

(ii)   **Inadequate dissociation of vitamin-B$_{12}$ from food protein:** Failure to release dietary vitamin-B$_{12}$ from food protein (food vitamin-B$_{12}$-malabsorption) in 30–50% elderly with low vitamin-B$_{12}$ status (~10-fold more common than pernicious anemia)

(iii)   **Absent intrinsic-factor secretion:**

(a)   Total gastrectomy, pernicious anemia.

(b)   Partial gastrectomy predisposes to multifactorial vitamin-B$_{12}$ deficiency (decreased Intrinsic-Factor, hypochlorhydria, bacterial overgrowth of vitamin-B$_{12}$-consuming organisms).

(c)   Pernicious anemia – autoimmune destruction of gastric fundus/body leads to gastric atrophy, absent Intrinsic-Factor and achlorhydria which lead to vitamin-B$_{12}$-malabsorption and then deficiency.

- Anti-Intrinsic-Factor antibodies (highly specific for pernicious anemia) ~60% serum; ~75% gastric juice.
- Average age for pernicious anemia ~60-years but all ages and races affected (S. California study: ~2% >60 years had undiagnosed subclinical pernicious anemia; but ~4%. white/African-American women had pernicious anemia).
- ~30% have positive family history.
- Positive associations with autoimmune diseases (Graves', Hashimoto's, vitiligo, Addison's, hypoparathyroidism, myasthenia gravis, Type-1-diabetes, hypogammaglobulinemia).

(iv)   **Abnormal events precluding absorption of vitamin-B$_{12}$**

(a)   Massive gastric hypersecretion (gastrinoma/Zollinger–Ellison syndrome) inactivates pancreatic protease and interferes with ileal absorption at luminal pH<5.4.

(b)   Overgrowth by vitamin-B$_{12}$-consuming bacteria or fish-tapeworms can usurp vitamin-B$_{12}$ before it binds Intrinsic-Factor.

(c)   Jejunal Adult fish-tapeworms *Diphyllobothrium latum* enter as plerocercoid larvae embedded in *sushi* (so *sushi* = Trojan Fish!); (Note:-fish-tapeworms are 10 meters long; 10^6 eggs released/worm/day; worm-lifespan = 20 years!; http://en.wikipedia.org/wiki/File:D_latum_LifeCycle.gif)

Table 6.3 Classification of vitamin-B_{12} and folate deficiency

1. **VITAMIN-B_{12} DEFICIENCY**
   A. **Nutritional vitamin-B_{12} deficiency** *(insufficient vitamin-B_{12} intake)*
      (i) vegetarians, poverty-imposed near-vegetarians
      (ii) breast-fed infants of mothers with pernicious anemia
   B. **Abnormal intragastric events** *(inadequate proteolysis of food vitamin-B_{12})*
      (i) atrophic gastritis with hypochlorhydria
      (ii) proton-pump inhibitors, H2 blockers
   C. **Loss/atrophy of gastric oxyntic mucosa** *(deficient Intrinsic-Factor molecules)*
      (i) total or partial gastrectomy or caustic destruction (lye)
      (ii) Adult and juvenile pernicious anemia
   D. **Abnormal events in the small bowel lumen**
      (a) Inadequate pancreatic protease *(R-protein–vitamin-B_{12} not degraded, vitamin-B_{12} not transferred to Intrinsic-Factor)*
         (i) Insufficient pancreatic protease—pancreatic insufficiency
         (ii) Inactivation of pancreatic protease—Zollinger–Ellison syndrome
      (b) Usurping of luminal vitamin-B_{12} *(inadequate binding of vitamin-B_{12} to Intrinsic-Factor)*
         (i) By bacteria—stasis syndromes (blind loops, pouches of diverticulosis, strictures, fistulas, anastomosis), impaired bowel motility (scleroderma), hypogammaglobulinemia
         (ii) By *Diphyllobothrium latum* (fish-tapeworm)
   E. **Disorders of ileal mucosa/Intrinsic-Factor-vitamin-B_{12} receptors** *(Intrinsic-Factor–vitamin-B_{12} not bound to Intrinsic-Factor–vitamin-B_{12} receptors [a.k.a., Cubam receptors]*
      (i) Diminished or absent cubam receptors—ileal bypass/resection/fistula
      (ii) Abnormal mucosal architecture/function—tropical/nontropical sprue, Crohn's disease, tuberculous ileitis, amyloidosis
      (iii) Cubam receptor defects—Imerslund–Gräsbeck syndrome, hereditary megaloblastic anemia
      (iv) Drug-effects—metformin, cholestyramine, colchicine, neomycin
   F. **Disorders of plasma vitamin-B_{12} transport** *(TCII-vitamin-B_{12} not delivered to TCII receptors)*—congenital TCII deficiency, defective binding of TCII-vitamin-B_{12} to TCII receptors (rare)
   G. **Metabolic disorders** *(vitamin-B_{12} not used by cell)*—Inborn enzyme errors (rare)
   H. **Acquired disorders:** *(vitamin-B_{12} functionally inactivated by irreversible oxidation)*—nitrous oxide (N_2O) inhalation
2. **FOLATE DEFICIENCY**
   A. **Nutritional causes**
      (1) Decreased dietary intake—poverty and famine, institutionalized individuals (psychiatric/nursing homes)/chronic debilitating disease, prolonged feeding of infants with goat's milk, special slimming diets or food fads *(folate-rich foods not consumed)*, cultural/ethnic cooking techniques *(food folate destroyed)*
      (2) Decreased diet and increased requirements
         (a) Physiologic—pregnancy and lactation, prematurity, hyperemesis gravidarum, infancy
         (b) Pathologic
            (i) *Intrinsic hematologic diseases* involving hemolysis with compensatory erythropoiesis, abnormal hematopoiesis, or bone marrow infiltration with malignant disease
            (ii) *Dermatologic disease*—psoriasis

Table 6.3 *Continnued*

    B. **Folate malabsorption**
    (1) With normal intestinal mucosa
        (a) Drugs: sulfasalazine, pyrimethamine, proton-pump inhibitors *(via inhibition of the proton-coupled folate transporters)*
        (b) Hereditary folate malabsorption *(mutations in proton-coupled folate transporters)* (rare)
    (2) With mucosal abnormalities—tropical and nontropical sprue, regional enteritis
    C. **Inadequate cellular utilization**
    (1) Defective CSF folate transport—cerebral folate deficiency *(auto-antibodies to folate receptors)*
    (2) Hereditary enzyme deficiencies involving folate (rare)
    D. **Drugs (multiple effects on folate metabolism)**—Folate antagonists (methotrexate), alcohol, sulfasalazine, triamterene, pyrimethamine, trimethoprim-sulfamethoxazole, diphenylhydantoin, barbiturates
3. **MISCELLANEOUS MEGALOBLASTIC ANEMIAS NOT CAUSED BY VITAMIN-B$_{12}$ OR FOLATE DEFICIENCY**
    A. **Congenital disorders of DNA synthesis, Orotic aciduria, Lesch-Nyhan syndrome, Congenital dyserythropoietic anemia**
    B. **Acquired disorders of DNA synthesis**
    (i) Deficiency—thiamine-responsive megaloblastic anemia *(thiamine transporter 1 mutation)*
    (ii) Malignancy—erythroleukemia
    (iii) All antineoplastic drugs that inhibit DNA synthesis *(antinucleosides used against human immunodeficiency and other viruses)*, toxic—alcohol

(v) Disorders of the intrinsic factor receptors or mucosa
    (a) Terminal 2-feet of ileum has greatest density of cubam receptors, so removal/bypass/dysfunction leads to severe vitamin-B$_{12}$-malabsorption.
    (b) Metformin interferes with vitamin-B$_{12}$ absorption in $\frac{1}{3}$; reversed by calcium (1.2 g/day).

(vi) Acquired vitamin-B$_{12}$ deficiency:
    (a) Nitrous-oxide (N$_2$O) irreversibly inactivates vitamin-B$_{12}$ molecule leading to intracellular functional folate deficiency; reversed by intravenous 5-formyl-THF (leucovorin).
    (b) Patients with marginal vitamin-B$_{12}$ stores at risk during prolonged surgery with N$_2$O anesthesia.
    (c) Chronic intermittent N$_2$O exposure presents with neuromyelopathic manifestations.

E. Folate physiology

(i) Normal folate absorption
    (a) ~50% food-folate (polyglutamylated) bioavailable after hydrolysis to monoglutamates.

(b) ~85% folic acid (in fortified-food/supplements) bioavailable.

(c) Luminal surface proton-coupled folate-transporter protein (duodenum/jejunum) facilitates folate transport into enterocytes, then released into plasma as methyl-THF.

(d) Serum folate level determined by dietary folate intake and an efficient enterohepatic circulation.

(ii) **Normal folate transport:** Rapid cellular uptake of methyl-THF/folic acid by two mechanisms.

(a) High-affinity surface folate receptors bind and internalize physiologically-relevant methyl-THF, folic acid, and some newer antifolates with high-affinity. After folate receptor-mediated endocytosis, proton-coupled folate transporter exports folate from acidified endosomes into cytoplasm of cells, across placenta to fetus, and across choroid plexus into CSF.

(b) Reduced folate carriers have low-affinity but high-capacity for methyl-THF, methotrexate and folinic acid (folic acid uptake is poor).

(c) Passive diffusion across all membranes operates at supraphysiologic folate concentrations.

(iii) **Intracellular metabolism and vitamin-B_{12}-folate interactions:**

(a) Methyl-THF must be converted to THF (via methionine synthase) so THF can be polyglutamated and retained for one-carbon metabolism. Vitamin-B_{12} is a cofactor for this reaction.

(b) THF converted to 10-formyl-THF for *de novo* biosynthesis of purines, and to methylene-THF.

(c) With inactivation of methionine synthase during vitamin-B_{12} deficiency, methyl-THF is not polyglutamylated, therefore leaks out of cell, resulting in intracellular THF deficiency.

(d) Methylene-THF used by thymidylate synthase to synthesize thymidine and DNA, or after conversion to methyl-THF (via methylene-THF-reductase) for methionine synthase.

(e) Vitamin-B_{12} deficiency can respond to replacement with folic acid because it can be converted to THF (via dihydrofolate reductase); alternatively, 5-formyl-THF (folinic acid) bypasses methionine synthase and can be converted to methylene-THF for DNA synthesis.

(f) When methionine synthase is inhibited during either vitamin-B_{12} or folate deficiency, there is a build-up of the thiol amino acid, homocysteine, which can have multiple deleterious effects on the body through a variety of molecular and biochemical pathways. This explains the observed beneficial effects noted following therapy with supplemental vitamin-B_{12} and/or folate deficiency to lower hyperhomocysteinemia (Table 6.1).

(iv) **Renal conservation**

(a) Folate receptors on proximal renal tubular cells bind and return luminal folate back to blood.

F. Pathogenesis of folate deficiency (key points) (Table 6.3)

(i) Folate deficiency arises from *decreased supply* (reduced intake, absorption, transport, or utilization) or *increased requirements* (from metabolic consumption, destruction, or excretion).
(ii) One individual may have multiple causes for folate deficiency.

1. Nutritional causes (decreased Intake or Increased requirements)

(i) Factors predisposing to reduced stores: poverty, seasonal reduction in folate-rich food, cultural/ethnic destructive cooking techniques/diets intrinsically poor in folates, anorexia (chronic illness), hemolysis (malaria), exfoliative skin diseases, alcoholism, pregnancy/lactation.
(ii) Body stores of folate adequate for ~4 months only.
(iii) Nutritional folate insufficiency (poor dietary intake) commonest cause worldwide in all age groups, with women and children in developing countries at highest risk.
(iv) Food-fortification with folic acid has almost entirely eliminated folate deficiency in USA, but socially isolated/infirm individuals subsisting on imbalanced diets still at-risk.

2. Pregnancy and infancy

(i) Short interpregnancy intervals and twin pregnancies predispose to folate deficiency.
(ii) Inadequate maternal folate predisposes to premature, low birthweight infants and predominantly midline fetal developmental abnormalities (neural-tube defects/cleft-lip/cleft-palate/endocardial-cushion defects), including early childhood behavioral abnormalities (Table 6.3).
(iii) Folate receptor auto-antibodies in some mothers linked to recurrent neural-tube defects.
(iv) Cerebral folate deficiency:
    (a) Caused by anti-folate receptor antibodies that bind to folate receptors on the choroid plexus and prevent folate transport into the cerebrospinal fluid.
    (b) These auto-antibodies to human folate receptors originally developed against closely-related folate-binding proteins found in cow's milk that share epitopes with human folate receptors.
    (c) Neonatal presentation (~6 months): agitation/insomnia, deceleration of head growth, psychomotor retardation, hypotonia/ataxia, spasticity, dyskinesias, epilepsy, and even autistic features.
    (d) Affected children respond to high-dose folinic acid *and* a bovine milk-free diet.
    (e) Similar auto-antibodies to folate receptors found in two autism spectrum disorders (Rett syndrome and infantile low-functioning autism with neurological abnormalities); some can respond

partially or completely to folinic acid. Rett syndrome—which occurs almost exclusively in girls and may be misdiagnosed as autism or cerebral palsy—is a disorder of the nervous system that is clinically silent until 6–18 months when it manifests itself by developmental reversals, especially in the areas of expressive language and hand use (https://health.google.com/health/ref/Rett+syndrome).

(v)   Hereditary folate malabsorption:
    (a) Mutation in proton-coupled folate transporter (intestine/choroid plexus).
    (b) Presents with megaloblastic anemia, chronic diarrhea, neurologic abnormalities (seizures/mental retardation).
    (c) Responds to high-dose parenteral folinic acid.

3. Tropical and nontropical (celiac) sprue

(i)   Tropical sprue responds to ~4–6 month course oral folic acid (5 mg/day) plus tetracycline 250 mg QID in ~60% of patients.
(ii) Chronic tropical sprue (>3 years) associated with vitamin-B_{12} malabsorption-plus-iron/pyridoxine/thiamine deficiencies.

4. Drugs

(i)   Trimethoprim, pyrimethamine, or methotrexate inhibit dihydrofolate reductase.
(ii)   Sulfasalazine inhibits proton-coupled folate transporters and induces Heinz-body hemolytic anemia.
(iii) pyrimethamine/proton-pump inhibitors inhibits proton-coupled folate transporters.
(iv)   Oral contraceptives increase folate catabolism.
(v)   Anticonvulsants reduce absorption and induce microsomal liver enzymes.
(vi)   Antineoplastics and antiretroviral antinucleosides (azidothymidine) perturb DNA synthesis independently of folate/vitamin-B_{12}.

G. Clinical presentations of folate/vitamin-B_{12} deficiency (Tables 6.1 and 6.2)

(i)   Vitamin-B_{12} deficiency develops insidiously whereas folate-deficient patients are usually poorly-nourished with multiple vitamin deficiencies.
(ii)   The underlying condition that predisposed to folate deficiency will have occurred ~6-months previously, and can dominate the clinical picture.
(iii) In developing countries nutritional vitamin-B_{12} deficiency can manifest as florid pancytopenia, mild hepatosplenomegaly, fever, and thrombo-cytopenia, with neuropsychiatric manifestations developing later.
(iv)   Among the affluent in developing/developed countries, vitamin-B_{12}-related neuropsychiatric disease may be found with only mild to

moderate anemia (~25–50% have normal hematocrit/MCV; inverse correlation between hematocrit and neurologic disease)

(v) Megaloblastosis with intramedullary hemolysis gives pallor and jaundice (lemon-tint icterus).

H. Spectrum of clinical presentations of folate/vitamin-B$_{12}$ deficiency (Tables 6.1 and 6.3)

(i) Clinical findings may be dominated by the underlying condition that caused deficiency of vitamin-B$_{12}$ or folate (Table 6.3).

(ii) Folate- and vitamin-B$_{12}$ deficiency can present with following "systems" abnormalities:
  (a) Hematologic pancytopenia with megaloblastic bone marrow.
  (b) Cardiopulmonary congestive heart failure secondary to anemia.
  (c) Gastrointestinal glossitis with a smooth (depapillated), beefy-red tongue.
  (d) Dermatologic hyperpigmentation of the skin and premature graying.
  (e) Reproductive infertility, sterility, megaloblastic cervical epithelium mimicking dysplasia.
  (f) Psychiatric with a flat affect.
  (g) Neurological presentations suggest associated vitamin-B$_{12}$ deficiency or additional systemic disease (e.g., alcoholism with folate+thiamine deficiency).

(iii) Vitamin-B$_{12}$ deficiency can present with either:
  (a) Dominant hematologic manifestations (like folate deficiency).
  (b) Neurological disease: widespread, patchy demyelination expressed clinically as cerebral abnormalities and subacute combined degeneration of the spinal cord.
  (c) Dorsal columns (thoracic segments) with contiguous involvement of corticospinal, spinothalamic, spinocerebellar tracts, and peripheral neuropathy.
  (d) Paresthesias are early findings with loss of position sense in index-toes (before great-toe); diminished vibration sense (256 cps tuning-fork); positive Romberg/Lhermitte signs; later bladder-bowel incontinence, cranial nerve paresis, dementia/psychoses/mood disturbances.

(iv) Patients with chronic hyperhomocysteinemia (longstanding vitamin-B$_{12}$/folate deficiency) may present with:
  (a) Occlusive vascular disease (small vessel cerebrovascular disease-related strokes, end-stage renal failure, thromboangiitis obliterans, aortic atherosclerosis, arterial and venous thromboembolism).
  (b) Occlusive placental vascular disease-related pregnancy complications (preeclampsia, placental abruption/infarctions, early recurrent-miscarriage) or poor pregnancy outcomes (preterm

delivery, neural-tube defects, congenital heart defects, and intrauterine growth retardation).

(c) Osteopenia with fractures.

(v) Clinical conditions benefitted by vitamin supplementation (Table 6.1) imply that patients with longstanding untreated deficiencies can present with:

(a) Hip fractures and age-related macular degeneration.

(b) Strokes.

(c) Poor cognitive function in adults.

(d) Reduced low-frequency hearing in older adults.

(vi) Children of mothers with low vitamin-B_{12}/folate during pregnancy can present with:

(a) Reduced neurocognitive performance (low-maternal vitamin-B_{12}), or

(b) Behavioral abnormalities (hyperactivity/inattention, peer problems in childhood) (low-maternal folate).

I. Diagnostic approach to the patient

There are three sequential steps:

(i) **recognize** underlying megaloblastic anemia (Figures 6.1 and 6.3) or potential vitamin-B_{12}-related neurological presentation.

(ii) **distinguish** whether folate, vitamin-B_{12}, or both deficiencies resulted in clinical picture (Table 6.4).

(iii) **identify the underlying disease** and likely mechanism causing deficiency (see Table 6.3 for identity of usual suspects).

J. Laboratory tests (Figure 6.1 and Table 6.4)

1. Megaloblastosis

The complete blood count (pancytopenia varying degree):

(i) Anemia–macrocytic anemia with steadily increasing MCV over time (hemoglobin ~5 g/dL sometimes).

(ii) Reticulocytopenia.

(iii) Neutropenia and thrombocytopenia (rarely neutrophils <1000/μL or platelets <50,000/μL.

(iv) Intramedullary hemolysis (increased serum LDH and bilirubin; decreased haptoglobin).

2. Peripheral smear (Figure 6.1)

(i) Macro-ovalocytes (~14 micrometer) (Atlas Figure 26).

(ii) Hypersegmented-polymorphonuclear neutrophils (5% with 5-lobes or 1% with 6-lobes) (Atlas Figure 29).

(iii) Megathrombocytes.

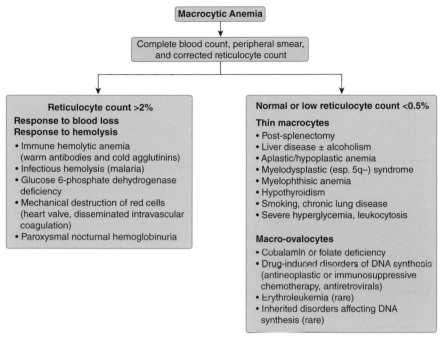

Figure 6.3 Algorithm for evaluation of a patient with macrocytosis*. (Reproduced with permission from Antony AC. Megaloblastic Anemias, Chapter 170. In: Goldman L, Ausiello D, eds. Cecil Medicine, 23rd edn. Saunders-Elsevier, 2008:1231–41.)
*Thin macrocytes have >⅓ central pallor; although deficiencies of vitamin-B$_{12}$ and folate are only two of the myriad of causes of macrocytosis, they become increasingly more likely as the MCV increases beyond 105 fL.

(iv)   Nucleated-RBC (rare).

(v)   Megaloblastic anemia can be masked by associated iron deficiency/ thalassemia (clue: look for hypersegmented-polymorphonuclear leukocytes in smear).

3. Vitamin-B$_{12}$ and folate levels (Table 6.4)

(i)   Suggestive clinical information improves pretest probability of results of serum vitamin-B$_{12}$/folate levels.

(ii)   Therefore these tests only useful to confirm a high index of suspicion that patient has either folate/vitamin-B$_{12}$ deficiency.

(iii)   If folate/vitamin-B$_{12}$ test results are borderline normal or ambiguous, proceed to use metabolite levels (Table 6.4).

4. Metabolite levels—serum homocysteine and methylmalonic acid (MMA) (Table 6.4)

(i)   Gold standards for confirming vitamin-B$_{12}$ deficiency.

Table 6.4 Stepwise approach to the diagnosis of vitamin-B_{12} and folate deficiencies***

Megaloblastic anemia *or* neurologic-psychiatric manifestations consistent with vitamin-B_{12} deficiency

plus
Test results on serum vitamin-B_{12} and serum folate

Vitamin-B_{12}* (pg/mL)	Folate† (ng/mL)	Provisional diagnosis	Proceed with metabolites?‡
>300	>4	Vitamin-B_{12}/folate deficiency is unlikely	No
<200	>4	*Consistent* with vitamin-B_{12} deficiency	No
200–300	>4	*Rule out* vitamin-B_{12} deficiency	Yes
>300	<2	*Consistent* with folate deficiency	No
<200	<2	*Consistent* with (i) combined vitamin-B_{12} *plus* folate deficiency or (ii) isolated folate deficiency	Yes
>300	2–4	*Consistent* with (i) folate deficiency or (ii) an anemia unrelated to vitamin deficiency	Yes

TEST RESULTS ON METABOLITES: SERUM METHYLMALONIC ACID AND TOTAL HOMOCYSTEINE

Methylmalonic acid (Normal = 70–270 nanoM)	Total homocysteine (Normal = 5–14 microM)	Diagnosis
Increased	Increased	Vitamin-B_{12} deficiency confirmed; folate deficiency still possible (i.e., combined vitamin-B_{12} plus folate deficiency possible)
Normal	Increased	Folate deficiency is likely; <5% may have vitamin-B_{12} deficiency
Normal	Normal	Vitamin-B_{12} and folate deficiencies are excluded

*Serum vitamin-B_{12} levels: abnormally low, less than 200 picograms/mL; clinically relevant low-normal range, 200 to 300 picograms/mL.
†Serum folate levels: abnormally low, less than 2 nanograms/mL; clinically relevant low-normal range, 2 to 4 nanograms/mL.
‡Any frozen-over sample from serum folate/vitamin-B_{12} determination can be subjected to metabolite tests.
***(Reproduced with permission from Antony AC. Megaloblastic anemias. In: Hoffman R, Benz EJ Jr, Shattil SJ, et al. (eds). Hematology: Basic Principles and Practice, 4th edn. Philadelphia: Churchill Livingstone, 2005, pp. 519–556.)

(ii)   Serum homocysteine and MMA rises proportionate to severity of deficiency (Table 6.4).

(iii) Serum MMA elevated in >95% with clinically confirmed vitamin-B_{12} deficiency (median ~3500 nanomolar).

(iv) Serum homocysteine elevated in both vitamin-B_{12} deficiency (median ~70-micromolar) and folate deficiency (median 50-micromolar).

(v)   Both homocysteine and MMA rise with dehydration or renal failure; colonic bacteria that contribute propionic acid can elevate MMA (metronidazole reduces this contribution)

(vi)   Increase in both metabolites cannot differentiate between pure vitamin-B$_{12}$ deficiency versus combined vitamin-B$_{12}$-plus-folate deficiency.

(vii)   Elevated metabolites return to normal in a week with appropriate vitamin replacement.

5. Bone marrow examination for rapid diagnosis (1 hour) of megaloblastosis

(i)   Trilinear hyperplasia with (ineffective) megaloblastic hematopoiesis.

(ii)   Megaloblastic orthochromatic megaloblasts containing finely-stippled, reticular, immature non-pyknotic nuclei (which contrasts with clumped chromatin of orthochromatic normoblasts) and hemoglobinized cytoplasm (Atlas Figure 28).

(iii)   Megaloblastic leukopoiesis pathognomonic giant (20–30 micrometer) metamyelocytes, hypersegmented-polymorphonuclear leukocytes.

(iv)   Megaloblastic megakaryocytes with complex hypersegmentation.

K. Determining the cause of vitamin deficiency

(i)   Previously, Schilling test helped determine the locus and mechanism of vitamin-B$_{12}$-malabsorption; however, this test is not currently available in the USA. So we are forced to rely heavily on history/physical examination and judicious use of confirmatory laboratory tests:

(a) Serum anti-Intrinsic-Factor antibodies are present ~60% with pernicious anemia. (Since anti-parietal cell antibodies are not sufficiently sensitive for the diagnosis of pernicious anemia, the author does not use or recommend this test.)

(b) Stool for ova.

(c) Serum IgA anti-tissue transglutaminase antibodies, lipase, gastrin.

(d) Intestinal biopsy.

(e) Radiographic contrast studies (stasis/strictures/fistulas).

(ii)   For young patients (gastric juice Intrinsic-Factor/achlorhydria, DNA for mutations in cubam receptor/proton-coupled folate transporters, or serum anti-folate receptor antibodies).

L. Treatment

(i)   In decompensated patient, draw blood for folate/vitamin-B$_{12}$/metabolite levels (consider urgent confirmatory bone marrow) and transfuse patient with one-unit packed-red cells SLOWLY under aggressive diuretic coverage to avoid acute pulmonary edema

(ii)   Administer full-doses folate and vitamin-B_{12} stat (1 mg folate and 1 mg vitamin-B_{12} parenterally).

M. Drug dosage

(i)   Rapid replenishment scheme for vitamin-B_{12}: 1 mg IM/SC cyanocobalamin/day (week-1), 1 mg twice-weekly (week 2), 1 mg/wk for 4 weeks, then 1 mg/month for life.

(ii)   Alternatively, after rapid replenishment of vitamin-B_{12} stores in first month, 2 mg vitamin-B_{12} tablets orally daily (1% absorbed daily via passive diffusion).

(iii)   Patients with food-vitamin-B_{12}-malabsorption require minimum 1 mg vitamin-B_{12}/day orally.

(iv)   Vegetarians/poverty-imposed near-vegetarians: Rapidly replenish stores with oral 2 mg/day vitamin-B_{12} for 3 months, then daily 5–10 micrograms/day (tablets or vitamin-B_{12}-fortified foods) lifelong.

(v)   Subclinical vitamin-B_{12} deficiency: course is unpredictable. So two options: either watch-and-wait until symptoms, *or* treat preemptively for 6 months with oral vitamin-B_{12} 2 mg/day (and reassess); latter approach (the author's preference) avoids potential for subtle (often clinically-unrecognized) cognitive dysfunction.

(vi)   Oral folate (folic acid) 1–5 mg/day sufficient replacement.

N. Prognosis

(i)   General response to vitamin-B_{12} replacement is dramatic improvement in sense of well-being, alertness, good appetite, resolution of sore tongue.

(ii)   Megaloblastic hematopoiesis reverts to normal within 12 hours, resolves by 48 hours.

(iii)   Hypersegmented-polymorphonuclear neutrophils remain in peripheral blood smear ~14 days.

(iv)   Reticulocyte count peaks days 5–8.

(v)   Complete blood count normalizes by 3 months.

(vi)   Most neurologic abnormalities improve in ~90% of patients with documented subacute combined degeneration, and most signs/symptoms <3 months are reversible.

O. Causes of incomplete response

(i)   Wrong diagnosis.

(ii)   Underlying untreated iron/thyroid deficiency.

(iii)   Infection (parvovirus-B19).

(iv)   Uremia.

(v)   Patient on drug that perturbs DNA (antiretroviral/antimetabolites, etc.).

P. Prophylaxis of vitamin-B$_{12}$ and folate deficiency (Tables 6.1 and 6.2)

Further reading

Antony AC. Vegetarianism and vitamin B-12 (cobalamin) deficiency. Am J Clin Nutr 2003;78:3–6.

Antony AC. In utero physiology: role of folic acid in nutrient delivery and fetal development. Am J Clin Nutr 2007;85:598S–603S.

Carmel R. How I treat cobalamin (vitamin B$_{12}$) deficiency. Blood 2008;112:2214–21.

Drake BF, Colditz GA. Assessing cancer prevention studies—a matter of time. JAMA 2009;302: 2152–3. *And* Bayston R, Russell A, Wald NJ et al. Folic acid fortification and cancer risk. Lancet 2007;370:2004 and 2007;371:1335–6.

Ramaekers VT, Blau N, Sequeira JM, et al. Folate receptor autoimmunity and cerebral folate deficiency in low-functioning autism with neurological deficits. Neuropediatrics 2007;38:276–81.

Schorah C, Smithells D. Folic acid and the prevention of neural tube defects. Birth Defects Res A Clin Mol Teratol 2009;85:254–9. *And* Czeizel AE. Periconceptional folic acid and multivitamin supplementation for the prevention of neural tube defects and other congenital abnormalities. Birth Defects Res A Clin Mol Teratol 2009;85:260–68.

Zhao R, Min SH, Qiu A, et al. The spectrum of mutations in the PCFT gene, coding for an intestinal folate transporter, that are the basis for hereditary folate malabsorption. Blood 2007;110:1147–52.

CHAPTER 7

7 Congenital Hemolytic Anemias

Archana M. Agarwal and Josef T. Prchal

University of Utah and ARUP Laboratories, Salt Lake City, UT, USA

I. Introduction

Congenital hemolytic anemias result from intrinsic defects of the red blood cells (RBCs) which lead to either a quantitative decrease or qualitative abnormalities of the RBCs. They are divided into three broad categories: membrane defects, enzymatic defects, and hemoglobinopathies. The clinical presentation ranges from asymptomatic to life threatening anemia.

II. General diagnostic approach to congenital hemolytic anemias

Careful clinical and genetic history, physical examination and specialized laboratory studies are required to define the underlying disease process. The history should explore the chronicity of the problem, ethnic and racial background, family history, underlying or associated medical condition(s), and medications. Hemolysis leading to jaundice and pigment gall stones is a common finding. Splenomegaly is also often present.

A. Laboratory studies
1. Reticulocyte index (see Chapter 4) is increased (usually more than 2%), consistent with adequate marrow response.
2. Increased unconjugated (indirect) bilirubin may be present. Decreased haptoglobin and increased serum lactate dehydogenase are seen with intravascular hemolysis.
3. Peripheral smear: Many different forms of RBCs (Table 7.1) can be seen. These abnormal forms of RBCs are not specific for a disease but give an important clue about the diagnosis.

Table 7.1 RBC morphology associated with hemolytic anemias			
Morphology	*Description*	*Cause*	*Disease states*
Spherocytes	Spherical cells with dense hemoglobin and absent central pallor	Loss of membrane	Hereditary spherocytosis, autoimmune hemolytic anemia
Target cells	Target like appearance with dark center	Increased ratio of RBC surface area to volume	Thalassemias, liver disease, iron deficiency, Hb C trait and disease
Schistocytes	Distorted, fragmented cells	Traumatic disruption of membrane	Microangiopathic hemolytic anemia (DIC, TTP, HUS)
Sickle cells	Sickle-shaped, tapered at both ends	Polymerization of hemoglobin S	Sickle cell disease
Elliptocytes	Elliptical cell	Abnormal cytoskeletal proteins	Hereditary elliptocytosis

Table 7.2 Features of membrane disorders	
Hereditary spherocytosis	Mixed inheritance pattern
	Defects in RBC structural proteins that play role in vertical interaction with lipid bilayer
	Marked heterogeneity in underlying mutations
	Marked clinical heterogeneity
	Splencectomy is curative
Hereditary elliptocytosis	Autosomal dominant inheritance pattern
	Defects in RBC structural proteins that mediate *horizontal* interaction in the RBC cytoskeleton
	Marked clinical heterogeneity
	No therapy is needed for most individuals

III. Red blood cell membrane disorders

Common features of membrane disorders are listed in Table 7.2.

A. Hereditary spherocytosis

1. **Overview:** Hereditary spherocytosis (HS) is a common congenital hemolytic anemia, particularly in northern European ancestry. The inheritance pattern is autosomal dominant in 75% of cases, while 25% are sporadic or occur due to autosomal recessive inheritance. The basic defect in HS is loss of RBC membrane surface area due to defects in several RBC structural proteins that mediate *vertical* interactions with the lipid bilayer (Figure 7.1). HS is associated with spectrin deficiency which occurs most commonly due to mutations in the ankyrin gene.

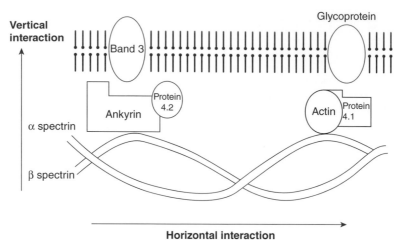

Figure 7.1 Schematic diagram showing assembly of major erythrocytic membrane proteins.

2. **Pathophysiology:** Structural protein deficiency results in the spontaneous release of spectrin from the membrane and leads to formation of spherocytes. The rigidity of spherocytes leads to trapping of erythrocytes in the spleen, where the RBCs lose additional membrane and become microspherocytes. Ultimately, after many trips through the splenic circulation, microspherocytes are trapped and destroyed. The anemia may be compensated by an increase in the production of new RBCs.

3. **Clinical presentation:** Clinical manifestations are variable, reflecting the heterogeneity of the molecular defects that underlie the disease. They range from no anemia to severe transfusion-dependent anemia. Members of a given kindred will often exhibit a similar pattern. Clinical presentation may include:
   (a) No clinical signs or symptoms.
   (b) Jaundice, often with concomitant viral infection.
   (c) Formation of pigment gallstones (from the high turnover of heme); complications of gallstones include cholecystitis, biliary obstruction, and cholangitis.
   (d) Mild to moderate splenomegaly.
   (e) Leg ulcers (in patients with severe HS).

4. **Laboratory evaluation:**
   (a) Spherocytes are seen on the peripheral blood smear.
   (b) The **osmotic fragility test**, a laboratory test used in the diagnosis of HS, is sensitive but not specific. The test measures the *in vitro* lysis of RBCs suspended in solutions of decreasing osmolarity. Spherocytes are characterized by membrane loss and less redundancy to withstand hypotonicity, and thus rupture in hypotonic solutions.

(c) Spherocytes formed by any mechanism (e.g., HS, autoimmune hemolytic anemia) will yield a positive result. At least 1–2% spherocytes must be present on the blood smear for the osmotic fragility test to be sensitive enough to be abnormal.
5. **Treatment:** Most RBC destruction occurs in the spleen, so splenectomy will either cure or ameliorate anemia. Splenectomy is recommended only for patients with symptomatic anemia. After splenectomy, spherocytes are present on the peripheral blood smear, but RBC survival is markedly improved.

B. Hereditary eliptocytosis
1. **Overview:**
   (a) Hereditary elliptocytosis (HE) is associated with an autosomal dominant inheritance pattern and is not associated with anemia in most cases. HE results from defects in RBC structural proteins that mediate *horizontal* interaction in the RBC cytoskeleton.
   (b) In most patients, the molecular defect resides in the α or β spectrin gene and interferes with the normal polymerization of spectrin molecules. In addition, mutation of genes encoding protein 4.1 and glycophorin C can also generate the elliptocytic phenotype.
   (c) Compound heterozygosity for qualitative mutations that cause HE and quantitative mutations of α spectrin gene are associated with a severe hemolytic disorder called hereditary pyropoikilocytosis.
   (d) Southeast Asian ovalocytosis, also known as *Melanesian elliptocytosis*, is widespread in certain ethnic groups of Malaysia, Papua New Guinea, Philippines, and Indonesia and is caused by a band 3 gene mutation.
2. **Clinical presentation:** The clinical features and natural history of HE are similar to those of HS, including marked variability in the severity of hemolysis depending on the specific mutation; however, unlike in HS, most subjects with HE are asymptomatic.
3. **Laboratory evaluation:** Elliptocytes are seen on the peripheral blood smear (Figure 7.2). The elliptical shape results from deformation of the RBC as it traverses the microcirculation, with failure to revert to the normal biconcave disk morphology.
4. **Treatment:** For most individuals, no therapy is needed. In those with severe hemolysis, splenectomy may ameliorate but does not cure the hemolytic anemia. In rare cases with severe hemolysis, occasional red blood cell transfusions may be required.

IV. Metabolic enzyme disorders

A. Overview
Specific enzyme deficiencies have been identified in the glycolytic pathway and hexose monophosphate shunt. RBCs are uniquely susceptible to enzymopathies because they are unable to synthesize additional protein after

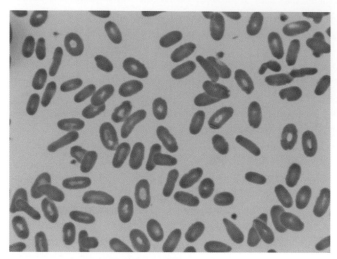

Figure 7.2 Blood film showing elliptocytes (100×).

Box 7.1 Features of glucose 6-phosphatase deficiency

X-lined inheritance pattern

Common in males of African, Mediterranean, South East Asian, and Asian Indian descent

Self-limited hemolysis precipitated by stress and oxidative injuries (characteristic of all common endemic variants)

Intra and extravascular hemolysis

---

being released into the circulation. Only three enzyme defects, glucose 6-phosphate dehydrogenase (G6PD) deficiency, pyruvate kinase (PK) deficiency, and pyrimidine 5′ nucleotidase (P5N) deficiency occur with any significant frequency.

B. Glucose-6-phosphatase dehydrogenase deficiency (Box 7.1)

1. Epidemiology:

(a) G6PD deficiency is the most common human enzymopathy, affecting nearly 10% of the world's population (more than 400 million people). The geographic distribution of G6PD deficiency coincides with the distribution of tropical malaria. The malaria hypothesis proposes that the high prevalence of certain hereditary disorders (e.g., G6PD deficiency, α and β thalassemia trait, and sickle cell trait) in malaria-endemic regions is due to slower growth of the malarial parasite in these defective erythrocytes, thus providing survival advantage to the subjects harboring these mutations.

(b) G6PD deficiency follows a typical X-linked recessive inheritance pattern. Males are most commonly affected as they either have normal gene expression or are deficient of the gene, as they have only one X-chromosome.

(c) Heterozygous females have a mosaic distribution of cells, with variable proportions of deficient and normal cells. The deficient cells are prone to the same degree of hemolysis as those of similarly affected hemizygous males.

2. **Pathophysiology:**

(a) G6PD, a pivotal enzyme in the hexose monophosphate shunt, mediates the generation of reduced nicotinamide adenine dinucleotide phosphate (NADPH), which in turn reduces glutathione. Reduced glutathione is a major free radical scavenger in the RBC.

(b) G6PD deficiency may result in acute hemolysis when the RBC is exposed to oxidant stress.

(c) Precipitates of oxidized, denatured hemoglobin (Hb), also known as Heinz bodies cause membrane damage.

(d) Heinz bodies can be visualized on staining with a supravital stain like crystal violet.

(e) RBCs containing Heinz bodies are recognized and preferentially destroyed by the spleen. So-called "bite" erythrocytes, while alleged to be specific, have never been shown to indeed be pathognomonic for G6PD deficiency (see Table 4.5).

(f) Classically, oxidant stress is induced by exposure to a variety of chemicals or medications. Acute viral or bacterial infection, acidosis, and liver disease may also precipitate acute hemolysis. G6PD activity in RBCs that survive an acute hemolytic attack will be normal, so measurement of G6PD activity immediately after a hemolytic attack may yield a false-negative result.

(g) Similarly, screening for G6PD deficiency may be normal in heterozygous females who, nevertheless, would be subjects for oxidant-induced hemolysis. However, in both these instances, DNA-based tests for specific mutation or DNA sequencing for G6PD gene will result in an accurate diagnosis.

3. **Variants of G6PD deficiency:**

(a) More than 400 variants of G6PD have been described, although most are uncommon.

(b) Several distinct G6PD deficient variants are present with high gene frequencies among individuals of African, Mediterranean (notably Sardinians and Sephardic Jews), Southern Chinese, and Asian Indian ancestries.

(c) All these endemic variants are associated with episodes of acute, short-lasting hemolysis precipitated by oxidant stress. However, some rare, sporadic variants are associated with chronic hemolytic anemia.

C. Pyruvate kinase deficiency

1. Pyruvate kinase (PK) deficiency is the most common cause of congenital non-spherocytic chronic hemolytic anemia caused by an erythrocyte enzyme defect.
2. The heterozygote frequency in the white population is approximately 1%, while the prevalence of the PK deficiency is approximately 50 cases per million population in the white population.
3. PK deficiency is inherited as an autosomal recessive disorder.
4. The derangement of the metabolic pathway leads to hemolysis of variable severity but no specific morphological abnormalities.
5. PK deficiency results in a variable increase in 2,3-diphophoglycerate levels and a right shift in the oxyhemoglobin dissociation curve, resulting in decreased affinity of Hb for oxygen that facilitates oxygen delivery at the tissue level leading to higher tolerance to anemia.
6. Diagnosis of PK deficiency, or any glycolytic enzymopathy, is made by direct measurement of enzyme activity in RBCs.
7. Severe disease may require frequent red cell transfusion throughout infancy and into adulthood.
8. Splenectomy ameliorates the severity of hemolysis.

D. Pyrimidine 5´ nucleotidase deficiency

1. P5N deficiency is the second most common cause of congenital chronic hemolytic anemia caused by an erythrocyte enzyme defect.
2. It was first described in 1974, since than approximately 100 cases have been reported and many more cases remain undetected.
3. P5N is located in cytoplasm of RBCs and participates in catabolism of the pyrimidine nucleotides, that results from RNA degradation during erythroid maturation. The pyrimidine nucleotides can be toxic to the cells if gets accumulated.
4. P5N deficiency results in the accumulation of the toxic pyrimidines in the red cells, and cause RBC hemolysis.
5. P5N deficiency is inherited in an autosomal recessive fashion and is the only congenital hemolytic anemia due to a red cell enzyme deficiency that results in a specific, consistent morphological abnormality—basophilic stippling (see Atlas Figure 14).
6. Lead is a powerful inhibitor of P5N, and determination of lead levels should be included whenever a constellation of hemolytic anemia, P5N deficiency, and basophilic stippling is found.

V. Hemoglobinopathies

A. Overview

Some globin gene mutations may be associated with hemolysis. These abnormalities can be further subdivided into quantitative defects of Hb synthesis (e.g., the thalassemias) or qualitative defects of Hb (e.g., sickle cell anemia).

B. Thalassemias

1. **Overview:** The thalassemias are characterized by a globin chain imbalance. Normally, production of α and β globin chains within an RBC are identical. Mutations that partially or completely inactivate production of either α or β globin chains can result in α and β thalassemia, respectively. Most of these gene mutations are present in heterozygous states and are asymptomatic with or without hypochromic and microcytic erythrocytes.

2. **α Thalassemias:**
    (a) Pathophysiology:
        (i) These most commonly occur due to deletion of one or more of the four α globin genes (~ 95% α thalassemias).
        (ii) Deletion of one or two α genes is not associated with any symptoms. However, deletion of three or four α globin genes results in Hb H disease and hydrops fetalis, respectively (summarized in Table 7.3).
        (iii) Non-deletional mutations of the α globin gene may also cause α thalassemia. Some non-deletional mutations result in a mutant unstable α globin: an example is Hb Constant Spring (CS).
        (iv) Although individuals harboring a mutation of one or two α globin genes are asymptomatic, children of asymptomatic parents harboring one (–α / α α) and two (– –/ α α) α globin gene deletions, respectively, have a 25% probability of inheriting Hb H disease (– –/– α).
        (v) Hb H disease: This disease is characterized by accumulation of free β globin chains. In contrast to free α globin, which is toxic to

	Syndrome	Mechanism	Genotype	Clinical manifestations
Table 7.3 α Thalassemia syndromes				
1	Silent career	Loss of one or two of the four α globin genes	(–α/α α)	Clinically normal. Normal or slight decrease of MCV and Hb (~30% African–Americans)
2	Mild hematologic changes	Loss of two of the α globin genes	(– –/α α; –α/–α)	Mild anemia, reduced cell Hb and MCV
3	Hemoglobin H disease	Loss of three of the four α genes	(– –/–α)	Varying degree of lifelong hemolysis, β chain Accumulate and make tetramers (β 4 or Hb H).
4	Hydrops fetalis with Hb Barts	Loss of three of the four α genes	(–/–)	Incompatible with life. Free gamma chains make tetramers (Hb Bart). Severe tissue ischemia, heart failure and generalized edema (hydrops fetalis)

the RBC membrane, free β globin chains can form homo-tetramers known as Hb H (β4), and free γ chains form homo-tetramers known as Hb Barts (γ4). Because of its instability, Hb H eventually precipitates in older red cells and makes inclusion bodies which lead to red cell breakdown and chronic hemolysis. Compensatory extramedullary erythropoiesis in the liver and spleen may lead to hepatosplenomegaly.

(vi) Hydrops fetalis: An absence of an α globin chain *in utero* leads to an accumulation of γ globin chains and Hb Barts. It has a high oxygen affinity which leads to severe impairment of oxygen release. The resultant tissue hypoxia results in massive tissue edema (hydrops fetalis) and death *in utero*.

(b) Laboratory diagnosis of α thalassemia:

This disorder can be suspected by mild microcytosis with mild to minimal anemia and an elevated RBC count. Hb gel electrophoresis or high-performance liquid chromatography (HPLC) are not helpful in individuals with one or two α globin gene mutations, but can detect Hb H or Hb Bart in those individuals with three α gene mutations. Multiplex PCR assay, and in some laboratories, globin chain synthesis assays are used for detection of one or two α globin genes deletions.

3. β Thalassemias:

(a) Pathophysiology: β thalassemia most often results from single nucleotide changes resulting in alterations in promoter, initiation, splicing, or termination codons.

(i) There are two classes of β thalassemia: $β^0$, in which there is a complete absence of β globin chains, and β+, in which the production of β globin chain is diminished but not absent.

(ii) Subjects who are heterozygous for $β^0$ or β+ mutations have one normal β globin gene and are asymptomatic with mild microcytic anemia , also known as β thalassemia minor (Atlas Figure 12).

(iii) Subjects with homozygosity or double heterozygosity for $β^0$ mutations produce no β globin and have no Hb A and suffer from the most severe phenotype of β thalassemia, also known as β thalassemia major or Cooley's anemia (Atlas Figure 13).

(iv) There are subjects who are double heterozygous for β+ and $β^0$ mutations. These subjects have a deficiency, but not absence, of β globin and have a less severe phenotype (β thalassemia intermedia) than that of β thalassemia major.

(v) β thalassemia major: Anemia manifests after the first 6 months life when γ globin production switches to β globin production. Due to the absence of β globin chains, free α globin chains accumulate. Precipitation of α globin chains results in the breakdown of red cell precursors within the marrow (ineffective erythropoiesis) and breakdown of red cells (hemolysis). Thus, the degree of hemolysis and ineffective erythropoiesis is more severe in β thalassemia, leading to a more severe phenotype than in Hb H disease due to β chain accumulation seen in α-thalassemia. These subjects are transfusion dependent, which further exacerbates their iron overload, the most common cause of death in these subjects.

(vi) β thalassemia intermedia: Clinical manifestations of β thalassemia intermedia are less severe than those in thalassemia major, and these subjects may or may not be transfusion dependent.

(b) Laboratory diagnosis of β thalassemia is made by gel electrophoresis and HPLC, which invariably reveal increased Hb A2 (α 2 δ2). In severe forms, Hb A is either absent or diminished, depending upon whether it is β thalassemia major or intermedia respectively. β globin gene sequencing can identify the underlying β globin mutation.

C. Sickle cell disease

1. **Overview:** Sickle cell disease (SCD) is a chronic hemolytic anemia resulting from a point mutation in the β globin gene (Hb S). It is an autosomal recessive disease. SCD is used to describe all those condition in which sickling of RBCs occurs.

2. **Epidemiology:** Sickle cell disease is a common disorder of people from African descent; however, it is also seen in people of Mediterranean, South and Central American and East Indian ancestry. Approximately 8% of African-Americans have sickle cell trait (a heterozygous form of Hb S), whereas approximately 1 in 600 are affected by sickle cell disease.

3. **Pathophysiology:**

(a) The genetic defect in sickle cell disease is a point mutation in codon 6 of the β-globin gene (GTG for GAG) that results in the formation of hemoglobin S (Hb S).

(b) The mutation results in the substitution of a hydrophobic valine residue for a hydrophilic glutamic acid residue.

(c) Homozygosity for the Hb S mutation is the most common form of SCD disease and is also known as sickle cell anemia. However, SCD can also be caused by compound heterozygosity for Hb S and either a β-thalassemia mutation or one of several β-globin variants (e.g., Hb C, Hb Lepore and Hb E) that support Hb S polymerization.

(d) Hb S polymerizes on deoxygenation. Polymerization of Hb S occurs in microvascular beds, where hypoxia and acidosis induce Hb to release oxygen, increasing the intracellular concentration of the deoxygenated form of Hb S.

(e) Polymerization of Hb S induces deformation and rigidity of the RBC membrane and impairs the transit of SCD RBCs through the microvasculature. The polymerization of Hb S is reversible after return of the RBCs to the arterial circulation. After multiple cycles of Hb S polymerization, RBCs become irreversibly damaged and are trapped in microvascular beds, where they are lysed (intravascular hemolysis). Chronic hemolysis in SCD leads to the release of free Hb. Free Hb produces reactive oxygen species and is a potent scavenger of nitric oxide. Nitric oxide is responsible for vasodilation and inhibition of adhesion molecule expression. Decreased availability of nitric oxide is responsible for endothelial dysfunction and vasoconstriction, one of the causes of pulmonary and systemic hypertension in these patients.

(f) In patients with sickle cell trait (genotype AS), the concentration of Hb S (usually approximately 40% of total Hb) falls below the threshold necessary to initiate pathologic polymerization *in vivo*. These patients are hematologically normal, except at high altitudes or after extreme physical exercise.

4. **Clinical presentation:**

(a) Sickle cell disease is characterized by periodic episodes of acute vascular occlusion (painful crisis) that have their onset in the first or second year of life. Painful crisis may be precipitated by events that impair tissue oxygenation, perfusion, or acid-base status. Infection, especially pneumonia, and systemic dehydration are common precipitation events.

(b) Vascular occlusion may lead to severe impairment of organ perfusion, leading to bone necrosis, acute chest syndrome; defined as a new infiltrate on chest radiograph associated with fever or respiratory symptoms, stroke, and skin ulcers.

(c) Acute chest syndrome and pulmonary hypertension are the most common causes of death in SCD patients.

(d) In patients with the SS genotype, recurrent splenic infarction results in complete splenic involution at a young age, also known as autosplenectomy. However, failure of the spleen to infarct may result in a life-threatening acute complication, i.e., splenic sequestration crisis, which is generally seen only before 5 years of age. Evidence of impaired or absent splenic function is documented on the peripheral blood smear by the appearance of Howell-Jolly bodies. These are round, purple staining nuclear fragments of DNA in the red blood cell which are usually removed by the spleen (Atlas Figure 15).

(e) Patients with SS disease are especially susceptible to infection with encapsulated bacteria due to "autosplenectomy", hence pneumococcal vaccination and antibiotic prophylaxis are standard components of treatment of children.

(f) Patients with SC and HbS/β-thalassemia genotypes have a milder form of sickle cell disease than SS patients. In HbS/β-thalassemia this occurs because the net reduction in intracellular Hb concentration that accompanies thalassemia trait also reduces Hb S concentrations. Painful crisis is generally less frequent, though it may be severe in some individuals. Autosplenectomy is less likely to occur in these two genotypes. Thus, patients with SC and HbS/β-thalassemia are more prone to splenic sequestration crisis compared to patients with SCD. Patients with SC disease have a significant increased risk for retinal vascular damage (retinopathy), which may lead to blindness and aseptic necrosis of head of femur and humerus.

5. **Laboratory diagnosis:** The blood film in all SCD genotypes has sickle cell (see Atlas Figure 21). Hb S has an altered electrophoretic mobility and is detected on HPLC and confirmed by solubility assay. More detailed genetic analysis is advisable in all cases.
6. **Treatment of sickle cell disease:**
   (a) Treatment for patients with sickle cell disease is supportive. Hydration and pain medication are used to treat acute painful crisis.
   (b) Strokes can be prevented in SCD patients by exchange RBC transfusion. The aim is to decrease the Hb S concentration to 30%. Chronic RBC transfusion is also recommended for children at high risk for stroke as defined by transcranial Doppler ultrasound.
   (c) In young individuals with severe clinical diseases and a matched sibling donor, allogeneic hematopoietic cell transplantation can be curative.
   (d) Because increased levels of Hb F inhibit Hb S polymerization, medications that increase γ-globin synthesis may be useful in decreasing the frequency of acute painful crisis. Hydroxyurea, an orally-administered chemotherapeutic agent is approved for the treatment of patients with frequent painful crisis. It has been shown to increase Hb F and may also have a role in generation of nitric oxide which may play a partial role in reversal of pulmonary vasoconstriction, an inhibitor of ribonucleotide reductase, has been shown to increase Hb F levels and is approved for the treatment of patients with frequent painful crisis.
   (e) Penicillin prophylaxis should be given to the children of SCD to prevent infections.

VI. Unstable hemoglobins

A. Pathophysiology

Unstable Hbs are an important group of clinically significant Hb variants. Several different mechanisms lead to the generation of unstable variants, which result in a congenital hemolytic anemia with Heinz bodies in RBCs (see G6PD deficiency above). Variant Hbs are found only in the heterozygous state. The more unstable the variant, the lower the quantity.

B. Clinical presentation

Patients with unstable Hb variants have varying degrees of hemolytic anemia. These range from an asymptomatic hemolytic state to severe, life threatening hemolysis. Typically, hemolysis is exacerbated by increased oxidant stress such as infections or the use of oxidant drugs. Patients may have splenomegaly.

C. Laboratory diagnosis

The presence of an unstable variant in the hemolysate can be demonstrated by simple tests of stability. The most commonly used tests are heat denaturation and isopropanol precipitation.

D. Treatment

Splenectomy does not result in improvement; therapy is supportive only.

VII. Summary

Congenital hemolytic anemias result from heritable defects in the components of the RBC, metabolic pathways, or hemoglobin. Important clues to diagnosis are obtained from the family history and peripheral blood smear.

Further reading

Kaushansky K, Lichtman MA, Beutler E, Kipps TJ, Prchal J, Seligsohn U. Willam's Hematology, 8th edn. McGraw Hill Professional, 2010.

Steinberg MH, Forget BG, Higgs DR, Nagel RL. Disorders of Hemoglobin. Genetics, Pathophysiology, and Clinical Management, 2nd edn. New York: Cambridge University Press, 2009.

8   Acquired Hemolytic Anemias

Scott D. Gitlin

University of Michigan, Ann Arbor VA Health System, Ann Arbor, MI, USA

I. General principles

A. Hemolytic anemia

1. **Hemolysis:** Hemolysis refers to the shortened survival of erythrocytes (red blood cells; RBCs) in the blood circulation before the normal expected lifespan of the RBC has been reached. In this situation, RBCs are typically produced in the bone marrow but are destroyed after they enter the blood stream. When there is an increased rate of RBC destruction, the bone marrow is able to increase production in an attempt to compensate for the losses. Bone marrow has the capacity to increase RBC production 6–8 times normal, a process that involves an increase in erythropoietin production.

2. **Anemia:** Anemia is the term used to define when the amount of RBCs, measured as hemoglobin or hematocrit, is below the lower limit of the normal value for the population being examined. There are many potential causes of anemia which do not involve hemolysis. Likewise, due to the ability of a normal bone marrow to increase production in response to increased destruction of RBCs, hemolysis can occur in the absence of anemia when the bone marrow is able to compensate for the rate of RBC loss with an equivalent level of RBC production. Anemia occurs when RBC production cannot match the rate of RBC loss.

Hemolysis is due to both inherited abnormalities of RBCs and acquired causes introduced after birth (Box 8.1). Acquired mechanisms of hemolysis include those that involve the immune system, physical damage to RBCs, infectious agents which damage RBCs, and medications/drugs. In addition, there is an acquired genetic disease that results in the clonal proliferation of RBCs that have an inherent predisposition for hemolysis (i.e., paroxysmal nocturnal hemoglobinuria; PNH).

Concise Guide to Hematology, First Edition. Edited by Alvin H. Schmaier, Hillard M. Lazarus.
© 2012 Blackwell Publishing Ltd. Published 2012 by Blackwell Publishing Ltd.

> **Box 8.1 Etiologies of hemolysis**
>
> **Immune-mediated hemolysis**
> Warm antibody autoimmune hemolytic anemia (AIHA)
> Cold antibody AIHA
>   Cold agglutinin disease
> Donath–Landsteiner AIHA
>   Paroxysmal cold hemoglobinuria
>
> **Drug-induced hemolysis**
> Hapten mechanism
> Immune complex mechanism
> Autoantibody mechanism
> Immunogenic drug–RBC complex mechanism
>
> **Non-immune hemolysis**
> Fragmentation hemolysis (aka microangiopathic hemolysis)
> Hypersplenism
> Infection
> Liver disease
> Hypophosphatemia
> Severe burns
> Copper excess (Wilson's disease)
> Drug-induced oxidative damage
> Vitamin E deficiency
>
> **RBC transfusion-associated hemolysis**
> Acute hemolytic reactions
> Delayed hemolytic reactions
>
> **Paroxysmal nocturnal hemoglobinuria**

B. Classification of hemolysis

Hemolytic disorders can be classified by a number of different approaches. Each approach allows for a differential diagnosis to be developed and has its own unique features. There are many clinical and laboratory characteristics of the different causes of hemolysis that often are helpful in classifying them.

II. Origin of hemolysis

1. Congenital (i.e., inherited).
2. Acquired.
   (a) Can be further subclassified based on pathophysiology features.
   (b) All (except PNH) are the result of extrinsic features that affect RBC survival.

III. Location of where hemolysis occurs

1. **Extravascular:**
   (a) Tissue macrophages in the spleen (most common) or liver.
   (b) Laboratory features often include unconjugated hyperbilirubinemia (indirect bilirubin) and normal to slightly decreased haptoglobin (an α-globulin produced in the liver that binds free hemoglobin and is decreased in hemolysis and in severe liver disease).

2. **Intravascular:**
   (a) Within the blood circulation (blood vessels).
   (b) Laboratory features often include hemoglobinemia (i.e., pink plasma due to free hemoglobin in the blood), hemoglobinuria (i.e., free hemoglobin observed in voided urine), hemosiderinuria (i.e., water soluble hemosiderin in urine), and decreased serum haptoglobin.

A. Clinical characteristics

1. **Anemia (these are not specific for hemolysis):**
   (a) Fatigue.
   (b) Dyspnea.
   (c) Pallor.

2. **Symptoms and signs that may be related to hemolysis:**
   (a) Jaundice.
   (b) Gallstones (pigmented; bilirubin).
   (c) Splenomegaly.

3. **Extravascular:**
   (a) Often associated with jaundice, splenomegaly.

4. **Intravascular:**
   (a) Often associated with fever, chills, tachycardia, backache, renal failure.

B. Laboratory evaluation (Box 8.2)

1. **Complete blood count (CBC)** for hemoglobin determination and RBC indices:
   (a) Hemoglobin and hematocrit levels establish the extent of hemolysis in comparison with the bone marrow's ability to compensate.
   (b) Mean corpuscular volume (MCV) of the RBCs may be elevated due to presence of an increased number of reticulocytes. However, the presence of microspherocytes or fragmented RBCs (low MCV) may offset the larger MCV of reticulocytes to result in a "normal" range MCV.

2. **Reticulocyte count:**
   (a) Reticulocytes are young, less mature RBCs than the majority of normal circulating RBCs.
   (b) The number of reticulocytes present in the peripheral blood represents the level of bone marrow erythropoiesis and the rate of entry of RBCs into the peripheral blood.

Box 8.2 Diagnostic studies used for evaluation of hemolysis*

Complete blood count
  (hemoglobin/hematocrit)
Reticulocyte count
Serum lactate dehydrogenase (LDH)
Serum bilirubin—total and indirect
Direct antiglobulin (Coombs) test
Indirect antiglobulin (Coombs) test
Serum haptoglobin
Serum free hemoglobin
Urinalysis (hemoglobin, urobilinogen)
Urine hemosiderin
Cold agglutinins
Donath–Landsteiner antibody
Anti-nuclear antibodies
Peripheral blood smear
Flow cytometry
Bone marrow aspirate and biopsy

*All of the above assays are blood tests, unless indicated otherwise.

---

3. **Serum lactic dehydrogenase (LDH):**
   (a) May be elevated as a result of its release from destroyed RBCs.
4. **Serum free hemoglobin:**
   (a) Elevated in some cases of intravascular hemolysis.
   (b) Found early in the course of hemolysis. Free hemoglobin binds to haptoglobin for clearance out of the blood stream. Can also be identified if haptoglobin levels have been depleted.
   (c) Often associated with hemoglobinuria, if the conserving mechanisms like haptoglobin have been consumed.
5. **Direct antiglobulin test** (DAT; direct Coombs test) (Figure 8.1):
   (a) Detects the presence of IgG or C3 complement bound to the RBC membrane, the hallmark of many types of autoimmune (antibody)-mediated hemolytic anemias.
   (b) Antibody or C3 complement titer can be determined, but this does not necessarily correlate with the severity of the hemolysis.
6. **Indirect antiglobulin test** (indirect Coombs test) (Figure 8.1):
   (a) Detects the presence of antibodies directed against RBCs in the serum of patients with immune-mediated hemolysis. It is used to check blood for transfusion incompatibility.
   (b) Additional tests are needed to differentiate between autoantibodies and alloantibodies.

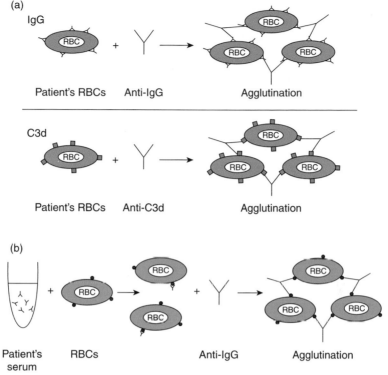

Figure 8.1 Direct and indirect antiglobulin (Coombs) tests. (a) The direct antiglobulin test (DAT) is performed by incubating the patient's washed red blood cells (RBCs) with a reagent that contains antibodies to IgG, C3 complement or both (nonspecific reagent). Agglutination of the RBCs indicates that there is either IgG or C3, respectively, bound to the RBC membrane. (b) The indirect antiglobulin test is performed by incubating a normal donor's washed RBCs with the patient's serum in the presence of a reagent that contains antibodies to IgG, C3 or both. Agglutination of the RBCs indicates the presence of an antibody, or complement, directed toward an RBC cell surface antigen in the patient's serum.

7. **Serum unconjugated** (i.e., indirect) bilirubin:
   (a) May be elevated as a result of its release from destroyed RBCs.
   (b) The body eliminates bilirubin via conjugation to glucuronic acid to make a water soluble form ("conjugated") that is excreted into the biliary system.
8. **Review of peripheral blood smear** (Figure 8.2):
   (a) Presence of polychromatophilic (blue-tinged) RBCs (i.e., reticulocytes) and nucleated RBCs demonstrate compensation by the bone marrow with release of RBC progenitors.
   (b) Morphologic features of RBCs may help identify hemolysis etiology:
       (i)   Microspherocytes (e.g., extravascular and intravascular hemolysis).
       (ii) Schistocytes and helmet cells (e.g., fragmentation in the intra-vascular compartment).
       (iii) RBC inclusions (e.g., infections).

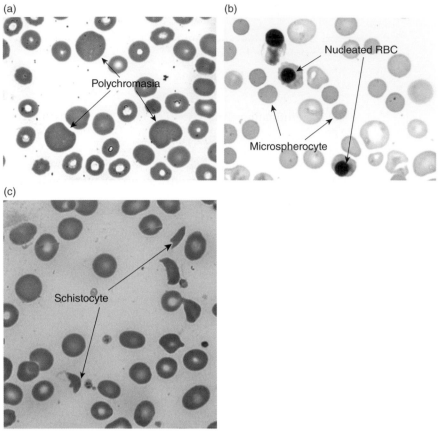

Figure 8.2 Peripheral blood smears with hemolytic anemias. (a) Autoimmune hemolytic anemia showing polychromasis which is a sign of reticulocytosis (AIHA); (b) Autoimmune hemolytic anemia (AIHA showing microspherocytes and nucleated RBCs. Spherocytes of varying sizes is a characteristic of warm antibody hemolytic anemias; (c) Fragmentation hemolysis with schistocytes as seen in a microangiopathic hemolytic anemia (MAHA).

9. **Plasma haptoglobin:**
   (a) Removed from the circulation after binding to free hemoglobin in the blood stream.
   (b) Typically decreased with intravascular hemolysis.
10. **Urine hemosiderin:**
    (a) The result of iron released from destroyed RBCs that deposit into renal epithelial (proximal tubule) cells before being excreted in the urine.
    (b) Typically found at least 2–3 days after an episode of hemolysis.
11. **Serum free hemoglobin:**
    (a) The result of hemoglobin being released from RBCs in the vasculature.

    (b) Typically elevated with intravascular hemolysis.

    (c) Will be found shortly after hemolysis begins or when the level of free hemoglobin is greater than the available haptoglobin to bind to it.

12. **Urinalysis** (hemoglobin, urobilinogen).

C. Special tests

1. **Cold agglutinins:**

    (a) Detects cold-agglutinating antibodies (i.e., IgM) in a patient's serum.

    (b) Patient's serum is incubated with normal RBCs at 4°C, then the extent of RBC agglutination (clumping or clustering of RBCs) present is "scored" usually based upon the dilution of serum necessary to detect the agglutinating antibodies. Agglutination occurs when an agglutinating antibody is present.

2. **Anti-nuclear antibodies:**

    (a) Evaluates for the presence of an underlying autoimmune disorder.

3. **Peripheral blood flow cytometry** for CD55 and CD59:

    (a) Blood cell antigens that are deficient or absent in PNH.

    (b) These epitopes are representative GPI (glycosylphosphatidylinositol)-linked proteins that normally protect cells from complement-mediated destruction.

4. **Bone marrow aspirate and biopsy:**

    (a) Rarely needed; when performed will show erythroid hyperplasia.

    (b) Evaluates the response of the bone marrow to the hemolysis.

    (c) Can be used to evaluate for bone marrow-infiltrating processes.

5. **Serum iron, TIBC, ferritin:**

    (a) Iron deficiency can occur when hemolysis is prolonged or chronic (e.g., PNH)

6. **Donath–Landsteiner antibody test:**

    (a) Typically IgG antibodies that bind to RBCs at cold temperatures, fixes complement and then destroys RBCs by complement-mediated lysis.

    (b) Present in paroxysmal cold hemoglobinuria seen in various infectious diseases.

IV. Immune-mediated hemolytic anemias

A. Disease types

1. **Warm antibody autoimmune hemolytic anemia (AIHA).**

2. **Cold antibody AIHA:**

    (a) Cold agglutinin disease.

3. **Donath–Landsteiner antibody-mediated:**

    (a) Paroxysmal cold hemoglobinuria.

B. Warm antibody AIHA

1. **Antibodies bind directly** to RBC cell surface antigens at 37°C, but fail to agglutinate RBCs.

2. **The antibody-bound RBC is removed** from the circulation primarily by splenic macrophages (reticuloendothelial system; RES). Fc portion of antibody binds to monocyte/macrophages in the splenic circulation and the antibody-RBC complex is removed from the circulation.
3. **Antibody: IgG.**
4. **Direct antiglobulin test:** positive for IgG.
5. **Peripheral blood smear: microspherocytes:**
   (a) Spherocyte: a small, more dense-appearing RBC without central pallor (Atlas Figures 16 and 17).
6. **Primary location of hemolysis:** spleen (extravascular).
7. **Associated underlying diseases:**
   (a) Idiopathic.
   (b) Lymphoproliferative diseases (e.g., chronic lymphocytic leukemia, non-Hodgkin lymphoma).
   (c) Connective tissue diseases (e.g., systemic lupus erythematosus).
   (d) Immune deficiency disorders (e.g., AIDS, common variable immunodeficiency).
   (e) Drugs (e.g., alpha-methyl dopa, an agent used in the treatment of hypertension).
8. **Clinical features:**
   (a) Jaundice.
   (b) Splenomegaly.
   (c) Symptoms/signs associated with underlying disease.
9. **Treatment:**
   (a) Folic acid (used for most forms of hemolysis to avoid deficiency that can occur during reticulocytosis).
   (b) Glucocorticoids.
   (c) Immune globulin (IVIg).
   (d) Splenectomy.
   (e) Rituximab.
   (f) Danazol.
   (g) Vinca alkaloids.
   (h) RBC transfusions (in emergency situations).

C. Cold agglutinin disease

1. Group of disorders in which an IgM autoantibody (i.e., cold agglutinin) that is directed against RBCs and preferentially binds to them at cold (4–18°C) temperatures.
2. After binding to the RBC membrane, the IgM autoantibody activates the complement cascade at the RBC membrane which leads to binding of C3b complement to the RBC membrane and eventual phagocytosis.
3. Severity of disease correlates with the antibody titer and its ability to activate complement.
4. Primary location of hemolysis: hepatic macrophages (extravascular).
5. Antibody: IgM; usually directed against the I/i antigen.
6. Direct antiglobulin test: positive for C3, but negative for IgG.

7. There are two forms of cold agglutinin disease:
   (a) **Chronic disorder:**
      (i) Older persons (5th to 8th decade).
      (ii) Often associated with an underlying B-lymphocyte neoplasm:
         • Chronic lymphocytic leukemia.
         • Lymphoma.
         • Waldenström's macroglobulinemia.
   (b) **Acute disorder:**
      (i) Younger persons than for the chronic disorder.
      (ii) Self-limited course.
      (iii) Associated with several infectious diseases.
         • *Mycoplasma pneumoniae* (anti-I).
         • Infectious mononucleosis (anti-i).
8. **Clinical features:**
   (a) Cold-induced acrocyanosis (i.e., blue coloration of fingertips, toes, nose, ear lobes, and ulcerations if cold exposure is severe and prolonged).
   (b) Jaundice.
   (c) Splenomegaly—very friable and can rupture on vigorous examination.
   (d) Symptoms/signs associated with underlying disease.
9. **Laboratory studies:**
   (a) Cold agglutinins (need to keep the blood sample warm after collection).
   (b) Elevated serum bilirubin and LDH.
   (c) Reticulocytosis.
   (d) DAT positive for C3 complement only.
   (e) Peripheral blood smear: RBC agglutination, polychromatophilia, spherocytes (Atlas Figure 20).
10. **Treatment:**
    (a) Folic acid.
    (b) Treat underlying condition, if recognized.
    (c) Corticosteroids, cyclophosphamide, rituximab, fludarabine.

D. Paroxysmal cold hemoglobinuria (PCH)
1. Rare disorder; 1% of autoimmune hemolytic anemias.
2. Occurs most frequently in children following a recent viral disorder. Also occurs in people with tertiary or congenital syphilis.
3. The result of a circulating IgG antibody that binds to RBCs at the P blood group system (tetraglycosylceramide-globoside) at cold temperatures that fixes C1 and C2 complement and then, upon warming to 37°C, completes the complement cascade leading to lysis.
4. **Clinical features:**
   (a) Symptoms occur following cold exposure.
   (b) Paroxysms of fever, back pain, leg pain, abdominal cramps, rigors.
   (c) Hemoglobinuria.
   (d) Renal failure.

5. **Laboratory studies:**
   (a) DAT negative; because antibody-coated cells have been lysed.
   (b) Donath–Landsteiner antibody positive:
       (i) Patient's serum is incubated with normal RBCs and fresh normal serum (source of complement) first at 4°C and then at 37°C. Lysis is then measured.
       (ii) Specificity for P blood group antigen.
6. **Treatment:**
   (a) Avoidance of cold temperatures.
   (b) Supportive care.

E. Drug-induced immune hemolytic anemias

There are four main mechanisms of drug-induced immune-mediated hemolysis that appear to be drug-specific (Figure 8.3):

1. **Hapten mechanism:**
   (a) Drug forms an antigenic complex with a RBC membrane protein that is recognized by an antibody. Binding of the antibody to this complex on the RBC membrane leads to destruction of the RBC. Hemolysis occurs only when the drug is present.
   (b) Laboratory studies:
       (i) DAT positive for IgG.
   (c) Examples: penicillins.
2. **Immune complex mechanism:**
   (a) The offending drug, or its metabolite, forms an antigenic complex with a plasma protein. An anti-drug antibody (usually IgM) binds to this antigenic complex to form an immune complex that adheres to RBCs and activates complement which leads to hemolysis.
   (b) Most common form of drug-induced hemolysis.
   (c) Laboratory studies:
       (i) DAT positive for C3.
   (d) Examples: quinidine, phenacetin.
3. **Autoantibody mechanism:**
   (a) An autoantibody (IgG) is induced by the offending drug. This autoantibody is usually directed against an Rh blood group antigen.
   (b) Laboratory studies:
       (i) DAT is positive for IgG.
       (ii) An antibody or a positive DAT can be present in the absence of hemolysis.
   (c) Examples: alpha-methyldopa, ibuprofen.
4. **Immunogenic drug-RBC complex (*in vivo* sensitization) mechanism:**
   (a) An antibody binds to the drug (or a metabolite) that is in an immunogenic complex that is formed by the drug (or a metabolite) associating with a specific RBC membrane antigen. The binding of the drug to the RBC antigen provides specificity for the anti-drug

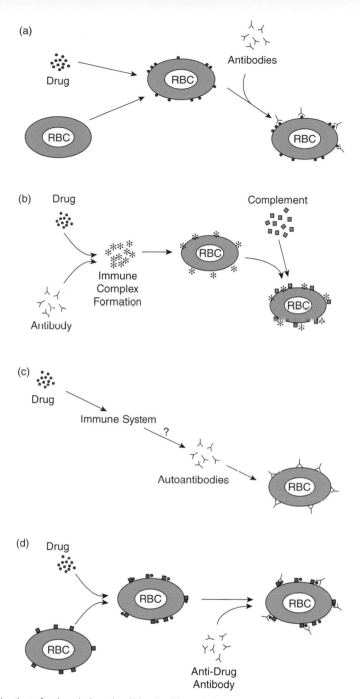

Figure 8.3 Mechanisms for drug-induced red blood cell hemolytic anemia. (a) Hapten mechanism of drug-induced immune hemolytic anemia. The implicated drug forms an antigenic complex with a protein on the RBC membrane. An antibody directed against the complex leads to destruction of that RBC. (b) Immune complex mechanism of drug-induced immune hemolytic anemia. An antigenic complex is formed by the offending drug or drug metabolite and a plasma protein. Formation of this complex leads to production of an antidrug antibody, forming an immune complex that adheres to RBCs, activates complement, and leads to destruction of the RBC. (c) Autoantibody mechanism of drug-induced immune hemolytic anemia. The offending drug induces the formation of an autoantibody that reacts against a protein on the RBC membrane, typically against an Rh blood group antigen. Interaction of this antibody with the RBC membrane destroys the RBC. (d) *In vivo* sensitization mechanism of drug-induced immune hemolytic anemia. The drug or metabolite forms an immunogenic drug–RBC complex in association with a specific RBC antigen. This drug–RBC antigen complex conveys specificity to an antidrug antibody that interacts with the drug on the RBC membrane, destroying the RBC.

antibody to bind to the drug (the antibody does not bind to the RBC antigen).
(b) The RBC antigens involved are often of the Rhesus (Rh) and I/i systems.
(c) DAT is often positive for C3.

V. Non-immune hemolytic anemias

A group of disorders that typically involve the effects of extrinsic factors on otherwise normal RBCs. Antibodies do not play a role in these mechanisms of hemolysis.

A. Fragmentation hemolysis

1. Also known as microangiopathic hemolytic anemia (MAHA).
2. Occurs when RBCs are exposed to mechanical trauma or shearing forces that disrupt the RBC membrane.
   (a) Damaged microvasculature:
   - (i)   Disseminated intravascular coagulation (DIC).
   - (ii)   Thrombotic thrombocytopenic purpura (TTP).
   - (iii) Hemolytic uremic syndrome (HUS).
   - (iv)   Atypical HUS.
   - (v)   Pre-eclampsia/eclampsia.
   - (vi)   HELLP (hemolysis [microangiopathic], elevated liver enzymes, and low platelets) syndrome.
   - (vii) Malignancy.
   - (viii) Vasculitis.
   - (ix)   Renal allograft rejection.
   - (x)   Malignant or accelerated hypertension.
   - (xi)   Atrioventricular malformations or shunts.
   - (xii) Prosthetic or calcific heart valves.
   - (xiii) Drugs (e.g., cyclosporine, cocaine).
3. **Laboratory features:**
   (a) Reticulocytosis.
   (b) Elevated serum LDH.
   (c) Findings consistent with an intravascular hemolysis.
   (d) Peripheral blood smear: fragmented RBCs (i.e., schistocytes, helmet cells, microspherocytes (Figure 8.2b; Atlas Figures 18 and 19).
4. **Treatment:**
   (a) Treat underlying disorder.
   (b) Folic acid, iron.
   (c) Supportive care.

B. Hypersplenism

1. Functional state of hyperactivity by the spleen, including its sequestration of blood cells and, subsequently, a shortened RBC lifespan. This condition

is usually associated with a shortened life span for white blood cells and platelets, as well. Hypersplenism is often, but not always, associated with splenomegaly. Increased RBC destruction and splenic sequestration of RBCs contribute to the development of anemia.

2. **Causes of hypersplenism:**
   (a) Vascular congestion:
       (i)   Portal hypertension; cirrhosis.
       (ii)   Right heart failure.
       (iii) Portal vein thrombosis.
       (iv)   Hepatic vein thrombosis (Budd–Chiari syndrome).
       (v)   Splenic vein thrombosis.
   (b) Neoplastic infiltration:
       (i)   Lymphomas.
       (ii)   Leukemias.
       (iii) Myeloproliferative disorders.
   (c) Infections:
       (i)   Bacteria.
       (ii)   Tuberculosis.
       (iii) Fungi.
       (iv)   Viruses.
       (v)   Parasites.
   (d) Inflammatory diseases:
       (i)   Rheumatoid arthritis.
       (ii)   Systemic lupus erythematosus.
   (e) Storage disorders:
       (i)   Gaucher disease.
       (ii)   Mucopolysaccharidoses.
   (f) Hemolytic processes:
       (i)   Congenital.
       (ii)   Acquired.
   (g) Non-malignant structural abnormalities:
       (i)   Cysts.
       (ii)   Hamartomas.
   (h) Sarcoidosis.
   (i) Amyloidosis.

3. **Therapy:**
   (a) Treat underlying cause of hypersplenism/splenomegaly.
   (b) Splenectomy reserved for cases of severe anemia.

C. Infection

1. Infectious agents can lead to hemolysis by several mechanisms that are organism specific:
   (a) Direct parasitization: organism either infects the RBC or attaches to the RBC membrane, leading to destruction (intravascular or extravascular):

(i)   Malaria.
(ii)   Babesiosis.
(iii) Bartonellosis.
(b) Immune mechanisms:
(i)   *Mycoplasma pneumoniae.*
(ii)   Mononucleosis.
(c) Induction of hypersplenism:
(i)   Schistosomiasis.
(ii)   Malaria.
(d) Alteration of RBC surface:
(i)   *Hemophilus influenzae.*
(e) Release of toxins, enzymes, etc.
(i)   *Clostridium.*
(ii)   *E. coli* 0192.

D. Other factors
1. Liver disease.
2. Hypophosphatemia.
3. Severe burns:
   (a) In part due to vascular injury associated with the burn.
4. Copper excess (Wilson's disease).
5. Drug-induced oxidative damage.
6. Vitamin E deficiency (in newborns).

VI. RBC transfusion-associated hemolysis

The transfusion of RBCs can lead to a variety of different types of reactions, including some that result in hemolysis. Only the reactions that involve hemolysis will be discussed here.

A. Acute hemolytic reactions
1. Typically occur within 24 hours of a RBC transfusion and has features of an intravascular hemolysis.
2. Results when a recipient antibody binds to donor RBCs and activates complement
3. Usually involves ABO incompatibility.
4. Can lead to renal failure, disseminated intravascular coagulation, and death.

A. Delayed hemolytic reactions
1. Occurs 1 day to several weeks after a RBC transfusion.
2. Typically presents as an extravascular hemolysis.
3. Usually the result of IgG antibodies directed against RBCs.
4. May be clinically silent.

VII. Paroxysmal nocturnal hemoglobinuria (PNH)

An acquired, clonal disorder of the hematopoietic stem cell that results from mutation of the *pig-A* gene, that encodes for the glycosylphosphatidylinositol (GPI) linker proteins, CD55 and CD59. These proteins bind (link) the hematopoietic cell (RBC, granulocytes, platelets) surface to other molecules that "protect" the cell from complement-mediated destruction.

1. **Clinical:**
   (a) Presentation in the second decade of life and older.
   (b) Aplastic anemia.
   (c) Myelodysplastic syndromes.
   (d) Acute myeloid leukemia.
   (e) Hemolysis.
   (f) Iron deficiency (due to hemoglobinuria and hemosiderinuria).
   (g) Venous thrombosis (30–40% of patients).
2. **Laboratory studies:**
   (a) Peripheral blood smear: normal RBC morphology.
   (b) Flow cytometry for CD55 and CD59 preferred study.
   (c) Ham's test (not used much any more):
      (i) Normal (fresh) serum has the pH lowered to 6.4 in order to activate complement.
      (ii) The patient's RBCs are added to the acidic serum.
      (iii) Lysis of the RBCs (sensitive to complement lysis) indicates a positive test.
   (d) Sucrose lysis test (not used much any more):
      (i) Normal (fresh) serum is incubated with an isotonic sucrose solution, which activates complement.
      (ii) The patient's RBCs are added to this sucrose-serum solution.
      (iii) Lysis of the RBCs (sensitive to complement lysis) indicates a positive test.
   (e) Leukocyte alkaline phosphatase (LAP) score: low.
3. Bone marrow aspiration and biopsy for recognition of complications from this stem cell disorder can demonstrate a hypercellular bone marrow in response to hemolysis or can demonstrate bone marrow failure, another manifestation of this disease.
4. **Treatment:**
   (a) RBC transfusions.
   (b) Folic acid.
   (c) Glucocorticoids.
   (d) Anabolic steroids.
   (e) Antithymocyte globulin.
   (f) Antibiotics.
   (g) Iron replacement.
   (h) Allogeneic hematopoietic stem cell transplant.

    (i) Eculizumab (anti-C5 antibody).

    (j) Anticoagulants (e.g., aspirin, warfarin, low molecular weight heparin).

VIII. Summary

Destruction of RBCs (hemolysis) can occur through a wide variety of mechanisms. Clinical features and laboratory studies can help identify the etiology of the hemolysis. The bone marrow's ability to increase RBC production in an attempt to compensate for the RBC losses often alleviates the immediate need to treat these diseases. However, when rates of RBC destruction are not adequately compensated by increased erythropoiesis, severe anemia that requires intervention can result. The primary goal of therapy is to alleviate significant symptoms and signs of the hemolysis and underlying disease. This supportive care often includes providing folic acid supplementation, monitoring for iron deficiency, and intervening with the hemolytic process as possible. Use of RBC transfusions should be reserved only for symptomatic, severe anemias, due to the possible risks that can occur if there is hemolysis of the transfused blood or if the transfused blood exacerbates the hemolytic processes present. Although hemolytic processes can be satisfactorily maintained for long periods of time, treatment of the underlying cause of the hemolysis is the preferred approach.

Further reading

Brodsky RA. Narrative Review. Paroxysmal nocturnal hemoglobinuria: The physiology of complement-related hemolytic anemia. Ann Intern Med 2008;148(8):587–95.

Friedberg RC, Johari VP. Autoimmune hemolytic anemia. In: Greer JP, Foerster J, Rodgers GM, et al., eds. Wintrobe's Clinical Hematology, 12th edn. Philadelphia: Lippincott Willams & Wilkins, 2009:956–77.

Hoffman PC. Immune hemolytic anemia—selected topics. Hematology 2009;2009:80–86.

Richards SJ, Hill A, Hillmen P. Recent advances in the diagnosis, monitoring, and management of patients with paroxysmal nocturnal hemoglobinuria. Cytometry Part B, Clin Cytom 2007;72B(5):291–8.

Valent P, Lechner K. Diagnosis and treatment of autoimmune haemolytic anaemias in adults: a clinical review. Wien Klin Wochenschr 2008;120(5–6):136–51.

Zarandona JM, Yazer MH. The role of the Coombs test in evaluating hemolysis in adults. Can Med Assoc J 2006;174(3):305–7.

CHAPTER 9

9   Overview of Hemostasis

Alvin H. Schmaier

Case Western Reserve University, University Hospitals Case Medical Center, Cleveland, OH, USA

I. The hemostatic system

A. Overview

Development of much of our understanding of the hemostasis and thrombo sis protection systems derived from translation of clinical observations seen in patients with unique biochemical and genetic processes. More recently mutant mice deleted of specific proteins in this system have additionally contributed to our understanding.

1. **Hemostasis,** the cessation of bleeding, occurs within the intravascular compartment lined with endothelium. Normal hemostasis and thrombosis (the occlusion of a blood vessel) is the sum of activity of two components: (i) a cellular part and (ii) a protein portion from the blood plasma or cells in the intravascular compartment. Some patients have normal blood coagulation proteins but abnormal hemostasis due to a platelet defect (e.g., Bernard–Soulier syndrome; see Chapter 13). Alternatively, other patients have normal platelet function, but abnormal hemostasis due to a blood coagulation protein defect (e.g., Hemophilia A—see Chapter 11).

2. **Components.** The cellular and protein components comprise the system and closely interact. The cellular components mostly consist of platelets and endothelium, but polymorphonuclear leukocytes and monocytes also contribute activating and regulating agents. Platelets, an anucleated cell fragment, provide an initial locus upon which hemostatic reactions occur. Vessel walls constitutively are anticoagulant surfaces which when injured become procoagulant. Monocytes and neutrophils contribute tissue factor initiating hemostasis and have potent clot lysing system. The protein components that contribute to hemostasis and thrombosis include 3 protein systems: the blood *coagulation* (clot forming), the *fibrinolytic* (clot lysing) and *anticoagulant* (regulating) protein systems. Each of the proteins in these three systems balances the activities of the others.

Concise Guide to Hematology, First Edition. Edited by Alvin H. Schmaier, Hillard M. Lazarus.
© 2012 Blackwell Publishing Ltd. Published 2012 by Blackwell Publishing Ltd.

3. **Regulation.** Physiologic hemostasis is a tightly regulated balance between the formation and dissolution of hemostatic plugs by the coagulation and fibrinolytic systems. Blood coagulation proteins circulate as zymogens or proenzymes and are unactivated. When a stimulus/injury occurs, the proenzymes of the system are activated to enzymes initiating a series of proteolytic reactions leading to thrombin formation, the main clotting enzyme. [Note: the convention in the coagulation protein field is to indicate a proenzyme (zymogen) as a roman numeral and its active, enzyme with the small letter "a" after the roman numeral]. The blood coagulation proteins become activated in a cascade. The *anticoagulation* proteins regulate the coagulation and fibrinolytic systems. The proteins of the anticoagulation system join those of the fibrinolytic system to prevent or counterbalance coagulation reactions. Thus, the hemostatic system is tightly modulated by a series of serine proteases (enzymes), their cofactors for activity, and serine protease inhibitors that regulate their function.

B. Process

A number of events are involved in hemostasis:

1. **Overview of the role of blood coagulation proteins in hemostasis:** When a vessel wall is injured several events occur simultaneously. Von Willebrand factor helps flowing platelets to adhere to the vessel wall. Collagen in the vessel wall, now exposed, allows platelets to adhere by their collagen receptors leading to activation. Platelet activation leads to thrombin formation on or about the platelet surface. Independently or simultaneously depending upon the circumstance, vessel injury leads to exposure of subendothelial tissue factor (TF) along with factor VIIa activates factor IX to factor IXa. Factor IXa activates factor X to factor Xa which leads to thrombin formation. Thrombin protolyses fibrinogen to form fibrin, which is the protein basis of a clot. Thrombin also recruits more platelets to the site of injury. It is recognized that *in vivo*, several pathways lead to thrombin formation. Similarly, when injured, endothelium too becomes a procoagulant surface. The procoagulant nature of endothelial cells is due to increased expression of TF and factor VIIa to initiate thrombin formation, increased synthesis of factor V to serve as a co-factor for more thrombin formation, inactivation of thrombomodulin for protein C activation, and increased plasminogen activator inhibitor expression with reduced tissue plasminogen activator.

2. **Overview of anticoagulation and fibrinolysis in hemostasis:** Circulation anticoagulants include antithrombin, tissue factor pathway inhibitor, and protein C. Under resting conditions, endothelial cells provide an anticoagulant surface. The anticoagulant nature of the endothelial cell membrane consists of a number of entities: antithrombin-that inhibits all coagulation enzymes (see below), thrombomodulin for protein C activation (see below); tissue plasminogen activator release that stimulates fibrin

clot lysis; nitric oxide and prostacyclin that stimulate vasodilation; and membrane-associated ectoADPases, CD39, that degrade ADP to limit platelet activation.

II. Coagulation protein system

A. Coagulation proteins (Table 9.1)

Blood coagulations proteins can be grouped into three categories:

1. **Phospholipid-bound proenzymes (zymogens)** make up the physiologically essential hemostatic system.
   (a) These proteins are vitamin K-dependent and are synthesized in the liver. Vitamin K is required for an essential γ-carboxylation reaction that takes place on each of these proteins' Gla residues located on their amino terminal ends, making them an α-carboxyglutamic acid. This carboxylation reaction allows these proteins to bind to lipid and cell membranes, where they are activated. Without this carboxylation reaction, these proteins do not function normally. Inhibition of this reaction is the basic mechanism on how the common oral anticoagulant warfarin works.
   (b) These proenzymes (zymogens) include factor X, factor IX, factor VII, and factor II (prothrombin). These proteins are essential for normal blood coagulation hemostasis and life. A complete deletion of factors VII, X, or II leads to lethal hemorrhage *in utero* or at the time of delivery. Factor IX deficiency is hemophilia B, one of the most severe bleeding states that survives gestation and delivery.
2. **Surface-bound proenzymes (zymogens)** are part of the plasma kallikrein/kinin system or "so-called" contact system.
   (a) Surface-bound proenzymes include factor XII (Hageman factor), prekallikrein (Fletcher factor), and factor XI. The terms Hageman and Fletcher factor were used to name these proteins based upon the first patients recognized with the protein deficiency. Factor XI deficiency is associated with clinical bleeding; factor XII or prekallikrein deficiency is not.

Table 9.1 Proteins of the plasma blood coagulation system

Phospholipid-bound zymogen of the vitamin k-dependent proteins	Surface-bound zymogens	Cofactors and substrates of the enzymes of the blood coagulation system
Factor VII	Factor XII	Tissue factor
Factor IX	Prekallikrein	Factor VIII
Factor X	Factor XI	Factor V
Factor II		Fibrinogen
		High M_r Kininogen*

*M_r, Molecular weight.

Factor XII levels, however, influence thrombosis (see Sections IV and V below). However *all* of these proteins influence the common blood coagulation screening test called the activated partial thromboplastin time. This test and its interpretation will be discussed in detail in Chapter 10.

(b) These protein zymogens are also known as the "contact system" because factor XII autoactivates when associated with a negatively charged surface (e.g., a glass tube *in vitro* or collagen, aggregated protein, RNA, or inorganic polyphosphate (polyP) released upon platelet activation *in vivo*). Autoactivation is the process when a coagulation protein binds to a surface, has a structural change, and changes from a proenzyme to an active enzyme. The molecular basis for this event has not yet been explained.

3. **Hemostatic cofactors and substrates** of the enzymes of the coagulation system facilitate the coagulation enzyme activity (see below in the next section).

(a) **Tissue Factor** (TF) is an essential cofactor for activated factor VIIa. It is found in most tissues and cells. Its synthesis is upregulated in inflammatory and injury states. Upregulation of TF results in the formation of complexes with factor VII that produces the initiation of hemostatic reactions. The absence of tissue factor is incompatible with successful mammalian gestation, i.e., intrauterine death.

(b) **Factor VIII** (antihemophilic factor) is a cofactor that greatly facilitates the ability of the enzyme factor IXa to activate factor X. Its absence is associated with the most severe clinically recognized bleeding disorder that survives gestation and delivery, hemophilia A.

(c) **Factor V** (proaccelerin) is a cofactor that facilitates the ability of the enzyme factor Xa to activate factor II. Its deficiency is associated with death from intrauterine hemorrhage or at delivery.

(d) **Fibrinogen** is the main substrate of thrombin (factor IIa). When fibrinogen is proteolyzed by thrombin, fibrin monomer is formed. Fibrin monomer associates end-to-end and side-to-side to become insoluble and cross-linked to form a fibrin mesh which is an actual clot (thrombus). Severe deficiencies of fibrinogen survive gestation and delivery.

The stability of the fibrin clot is created by an enzyme called *factor XIII*, a tissue transglutaminase that cross-links the strands of associating fibrin to make a stronger insoluble structure. Factor XIII is like mortar and stabilization rods in a brick wall.

(e) **High molecular weight kininogen** (Fitzgerald or Williams factor) is a cofactor for the activation of all the contact system proenzymes (zymogens), factor XII, prekallikrein, and factor XI. High molecular weight kininogen also is a substrate of the activated forms of the contact system enzymes to liberate a biologically active peptide called bradykinin. Bradykinin stimulates nitric oxide and prostacyclin formation in endothelial cells to produce vasodilation. Deficiency of high molecular weight kininogen is not associated with bleeding, but it delays induced arterial thrombosis.

B. Critical proteins in hemostatic reactions

The essential proteins of the blood coagulation system were identified by observation of patients and the first recognized defect was named for the patient (e.g., Stuart factor, factor X deficiency). Deficiencies in coagulation factors VIII and IX are the most severe bleeding disorders that occur in patients who survive gestation and birth. The rare patients who have congenital deficiencies of coagulation factors VII, X, V, and II usually do not have severe bleeding states because these individuals must have some small amounts of functional coagulation factor to have survived gestation and birth. Directly or indirectly, all of these proteins participate in two critically important assemblies, "tenase" and "prothrombinase" that are essential for kinetically fast blood coagulation protein activation for thrombin generation. The tenase and prothrombinase assembly are important because they are anticoagulant targets.

1. **Tenase assembly** (Figure 9.1) is the ability of activated factors VIII and IX to assemble on phospholipid surfaces or cell membranes to accelerate the activation of factor X to factor Xa. When all of these components are present, the rate of factor X activation by factor IXa (i.e., catalytic efficiency) is increased a billion-fold, 1×10^9 faster over the rate of factor IXa activation of factor X alone. This fast rate is what makes it physiologic and an important juncture point in the system.

2. **Prothrombinase assembly** (Figure 9.2) is the ability of factor Xa and thrombin-activated factor Va to assemble on phospholipid membranes or cell membranes to accelerate the activation of factor II (prothrombin) to factor IIa (thrombin). When all of these components are present, the rate of factor II activation by factor Xa is increased 400,000-fold over the rate of factor Xa activation of factor II alone.

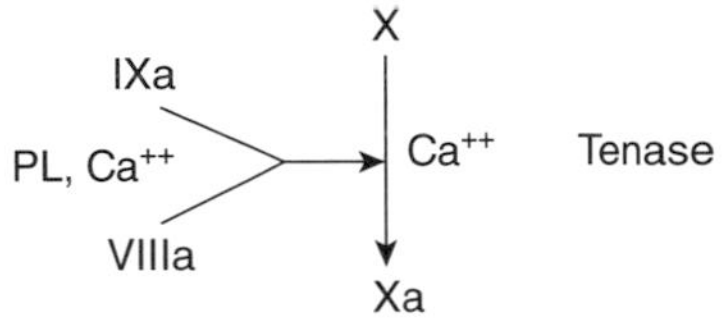

Figure 9.1 The tenase assembly for factor Xa formation.

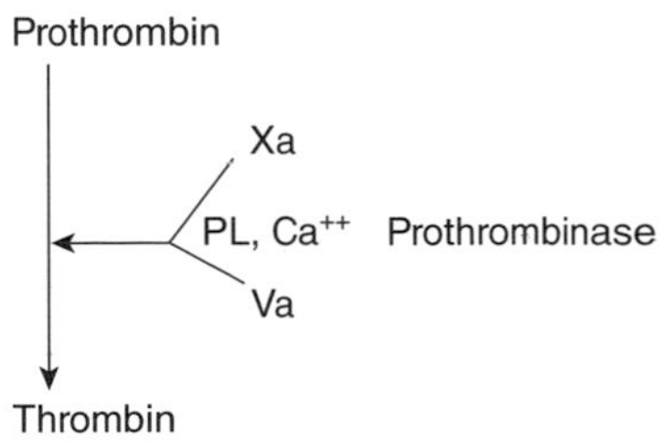

Figure 9.2 The prothrombinase assembly for thrombin generation.

3. **Thrombin generation** in a kinetically fast manner is the goal of these protein assemblies. In static *in vitro* systems, as little as 5–10 pM (10^{-12} M) tissue factor is sufficient to induce clot formation leading to a 1000–4000-fold amplification of the process that increases the concentration of thrombin to 10–20 nM (10^{-9} M), a concentration sufficient to initiate clot formation. The addition of 5 pM tissue factor results in an average clot time of ~5 min, a time sufficiently fast for physiologic hemostasis.

C. Summary of physiologic blood coagulation system

The assembly of blood coagulation proteins whose deficiency are associated with bleeding are shown in Figure 9.3. Blood coagulation leading to hemostasis initiated by the complex formation between tissue factor and factor

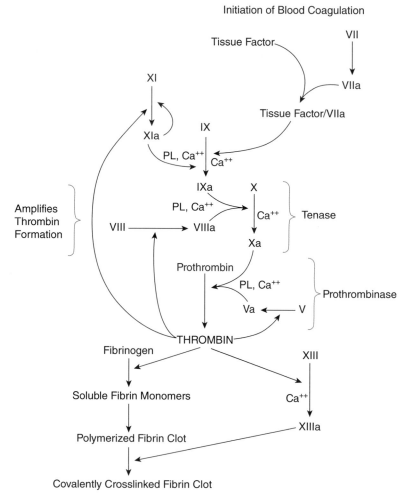

Figure 9.3 Blood coagulation system leading to hemostasis.

VII–VIIa. Tissue factor is expressed after injury upon exposure of subendothelium or is synthesized in monocytes, neutrophils, endothelium or platelets in inflammatory states. It has been proposed that there may be TF–VIIa complexes in cryptic microparticles circulating in plasma that are available to spring into action if a hemostatic insult occurs. Although factor VIIa directly activates X to Xa *in vitro* in the prothrombin time assay (see Chapter 10), under physiologic conditions this pathway is blocked by tissue factor pathway inhibitor (see below under Anticoagulation systems). Physiologic blood coagulation mostly occurs when sufficient tissue factor/VIIa is available to activate factor IX to IXa. Subsequently, IXa in the presence of VIIIa assembles to activate X to Xa in tenase (Figure 9.3). Formed Xa in the presence of Va leads to prothrombin activation to form thrombin in prothrombinase (Figure 9.3). Formed thrombin proceeds to proteolyze (chew-up) fibrinogen to form soluble fibrin monomers that polymerize to form a fibrin clot. Thrombin also activates factor XIII to XIIIa that cross-links polymerized fibrin monomers to form insoluble cross-linked fibrin, a clot. A clot, for example, is the soft bloody gel that hardens on a severely abraded knee. At times, the stimulus for thrombin formation can be great. Thrombin amplifies its own formation by feeding back to activate factor XI to factor XIa that activates more factor IX to re-initiate the cascade of proteolytic events just described. Please note there is no mention of the contact activation proteins, factor XII, prekallikrein, and high molecular weight kininogen in physiologic hemostasis. These proteins do not contribute to the cessation of bleeding.

III. The fibrinolytic system

One process limiting the extent of clot formation is the fibrinolytic protein system (Figure 9.4). It consists of the zymogen plasminogen and its naturally occurring activators. Plasminogen is activated to the main clot-lysing enzyme, plasmin, by the endogenous plasminogen activator tissue plasminogen activator (tPA), single-chain urokinase plasminogen activator (ScuPA), and two-chain urokinase plasminogen activator (tcuPA). These activators are found in the endothelium as well as in neutrophils and monocytes. Plasminogen activation is regulated by the inhibitor plasminogen activated inhibitor-1 (PAI-1). PAI-1 is mostly found in endothelium and cells; it is not a plasma protein. Formed plasmin degrades fibrinogen, soluble non-cross-linked fibrin, and cross-linked fibrin to liberate fibrin or fibrinogen degradation products (Figure 9.4). Plasmin degrades insoluble cross-linked fibrin clots to liberate D-dimer, i.e., a two D-domain protein fragments held together by a unique bond between them (Figure 9.4). Measurement of D-dimer indicates that thrombin-activated factor XIII has cross-linked fibrin to make insoluble cross-linked fibrin and plasmin has cleaved the insoluble cross-linked fibrin. The plasma serine protease inhibitor, alpha-2-antiplasmin, regulates plasmin activity. A defect of plasminogen is associated with thrombosis. An absence or defect in PAI-1 or alpha-2-antiplasmin is associated with a hyperfibrinolytic bleeding

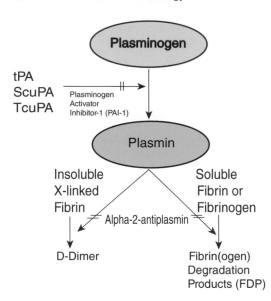

tPA
ScuPA
TcuPA

Figure 9.4 The fibrinolytic protein system.

state. Elevation of PAI-1 or alpha-2-antiplasmin is associated with increased risk for myocardial infarction and stroke.

IV. The anticoagulation system

A. Three anticoagulation systems

A second process limiting the activation of the blood coagulation system is the anticoagulation system. Three *anticoagulant systems* regulate activation of the *blood coagulation proteins* to inhibit clot formation. These systems are the protein C/protein S system, the plasma SERPIN serine protease inhibitor antithrombin and the Kunitz serine protease inhibitor tissue factor pathway inhibitor (TFPI). In Figure 9.5, these anticoagulation systems with red lines are drawn over the blood coagulation system in black lines.

1. **Protein C/protein S system.** When activated, *protein C*, a vitamin K-dependent protein, is an enzyme that functions as an inhibitor. Protein C is activated to its enzymatic form by thrombin when bound in a trimolecular complex with an endothelial cell receptor call thrombomodulin. Activated protein C makes a complex with protein S to function as an inhibitor by degrading active forms of factor Va, a cofactor for prothrombinase, and factor VIIIa, a cofactor for tenase (Figure 9.5). *Protein S*, a vitamin K-dependent protein, is not an enzyme. It serves as a receptor for activated protein C to perform its activities on cell membranes. Protein S levels are modulated by the complement inflammatory protein C4b-binding protein. Clinical deficiencies of protein C or S are associated with serious risk for thrombosis (see Chapter 15).

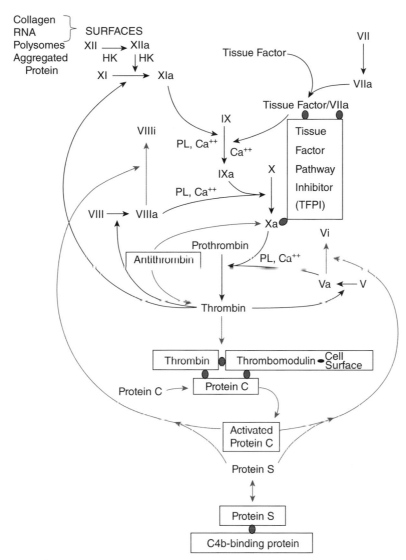

Figure 9.5 The anticoagulation protein system.

2. **Antithrombin anticoagulation system.** Antithrombin, a serine protease inhibitor (SERPIN), exerts its anticoagulant effect primarily by inhibiting factors IIa and Xa (Figure 9.5). It also inhibits each of the other hemostatic enzymes: factors VIIa, IXa, XIa, kallikrein, and XIIa (not shown in the figure). The presence of antithrombin is what gives heparin its anticoagulant properties. Heparin binds to antithrombin and makes the latter a better inhibitor by changing the conformation of its reactive region. The importance of antithrombin is indicated by the fact that in the mouse, a complete

deficiency results in fetal death. In the presence of heparin, antithrombin is a 1000-fold more effective inhibitor of factor IIa (thrombin). The clinical state of heterozygous deficiency of antithrombin is associated with venous thrombosis (see Chapter 15).

3. **Tissue factor pathway inhibitor (TFPI),** a Kunitz-type serine protease inhibitor, is the third anticoagulation system. It is most potent inhibitor of the factor VIIa/tissue complex. Under physiologic conditions, TFPI forms a quaternary complex with tissue factor–factor VIIa and factor Xa to prevents the FVIIa–TF complex from activating factor X directly (Figure 9.5). This fact directs FVIIa–TF to factor IX for activation. The importance of TFPI is indicated by the observation that in the mouse, a complete deficiency results in fetal death.

B. Additional anticoagulation proteins

Additional serine protease inhibitors regulate some of the blood coagulation enzymes. However, the significance of their clinical deficiency has not been defined. Heparin cofactor II is a thrombin inhibitor. Protein Z inhibitor in the presence of its cofactor protein Z is a factor Xa inhibitor. C1 esterase inhibitor (C1 inhibitor) along with alpha-1-antitrypsin and the amyloid β-protein precursor are potent inhibitors of factor XIa. The amyloid β-protein precursor also inhibits factors IXa, VIIa-tissue factor, and factor Xa, but not thrombin. It appears to be a cerebral anticoagulant, i.e., the major anticoagulant protein in brain.

V. Cohesive hypothesis for the initiation of the hemostatic system

It is challenging to have a cohesive understanding of the many parts contributing to normal hemostasis. In the present chapter, no detailed discussion was presented on the contribution of platelets to hemostasis (see Chapters 13 and 14). Furthermore, physiologic hemostasis or thrombosis is not a linear sequence or cascade of enzymatic reactions. It is an event occurring in the intravascular compartment in the presence of flowing blood which produces shear forces, an additional factor contributing to these events. With these caveats, a proposed model for *in vivo* hemostasis and thrombosis is presented (Figure 9.6). In the intravascular compartment, intact endothelium has a constitutive anticoagulant and antithrombotic nature by its secretion of nitric oxide, prostacyclin, tissue plasminogen activator (tPA) and the presence on its membrane of antithrombin, thrombomodulin, and an ADP-degrading enzyme called ECTO-ADPas (CD39).

At sites of developing injury, platelets under shear are slowed by adherence to von Willebrand factor (vWF) (see Chapter 11) and activated after their interaction with exposed collagen through the platelet receptor GPVI. Exposed collagen, aggregated protein, or extracellular RNA also has the

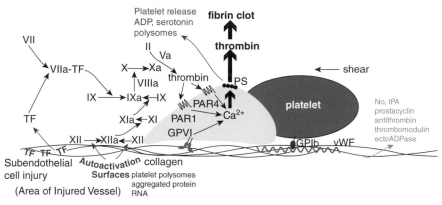

Figure 9.6 An overview hypothesis for hemostasis and thrombosis in the intravascular compartment with flowing blood.

ability to bind plasma factor XII (XII) to support its autoactivation to factor XIIa (XIIa). Factor XIIa formed in such a manner leads to a cascade of activation of blood coagulation protein leading to thrombin formation. This pathway is not essential for hemostasis but may be important for pathologic thrombosis. Simultaneously or alternatively, injured subendothelium results in the expression of tissue factor which complexes with factor VII/VIIa to activated factor IX and lead to thrombin formation. This latter mechanism for thrombin formation is essential for hemostasis and is an alternative process for thrombosis. Most probably, different stimuli lead to different mechanisms for thrombin formation. For example, a laser injury to a blood vessel results in tissue factor, factor VIIa, and thrombin formation before platelets adhere and aggregate. Alternatively, in vessels where collagen is exposed, simultaneous platelet adherence and activation with factor XII autoactivation lead to thrombin formation with no role for tissue factor and factor VIIa (Figure 9.6).

Formed thrombin by any mechanism leads to more fibrin clot and platelet activation through the platelet thrombin receptors, protease-activated receptors 1 and 4 (PAR1 and PAR4). These events additionally activate platelets and expose surface phospholipids like phosphatidyl serine (PS) which itself is a procoagulant, i.e., a thrombin generating surface. Activated platelets also release ADP and serotonin to recruit more platelets and polysomes, lipid material that can support factor XII activation (Figure 9.6). All of these processes occurring variably simultaneously contribute to bleeding cessation or hemostasis or, unchecked occlusive thrombosis. Even though these systems are interacting, overlapping, and redundant, they function in an elegant balance. The remarkable thing is that the absence of only one factor alters the balance that leads to a bleeding or thrombotic state.

Further reading

Furie, B, Furie BC. Molecular basis of blood coagulation. In: Hematology: Basic Principles and Practice. Hoffman R, Benz EJ, Shattil SJ, Furie B, Silberstein LE, McGlave P, Heslop H, eds. Philadelphia, PA: Churchill Livingstone, 2009:1819–36.

Schmaier AH, Miller JL. Coagulation and fibrinolysis. In: Henry's Clinical Diagnosis and Management by Laboratory Methods, 23rd edn. McPherson RA, Pincus MR, eds. Philadelphia, PA: Elsevier, 2011 (in press).

10 Approach to the Bleeding Patient

Alvin H. Schmaier

Case Western Reserve University, University Hospitals Case Medical Center, Cleveland, OH, USA

I. Introduction

This chapter aims to provide a simple diagnostic framework in which the physician can approach most patients with abnormal bleeding in a logical fashion to recognize the underlying cause. The diagnostic approach to bleeding disorders is based upon a full understanding of what the current screening assays for bleeding states measure.

II. Pathogenesis of bleeding disorders

When faced with a bleeding patient, the physician must use an analytical diagnostic approach to determine the etiology of the problem.

A. All bleeding states are caused by one of three defects

1. **Plasma protein defect** (i.e., a quantitative or functional defect in one or more plasma coagulation, fibrinolytic, or anticoagulant proteins).
2. **Platelet abnormality** (i.e., a quantitative deficiency or function defect in this hemostatic cell fragment—one of adherence, aggregation, spreading, and activation).
3. **Defect in platelet-endothelial cell interactions** (i.e., a defect in the adhesive interactions between platelets and the vessel wall).

B. Coagulation protein defects

Coagulation protein defects that lead to bleeding can be classified as follows:

1. **True protein deficiency.** Insufficient protein is present for its required function.

Concise Guide to Hematology, First Edition. Edited by Alvin H. Schmaier, Hillard M. Lazarus.
© 2012 Blackwell Publishing Ltd. Published 2012 by Blackwell Publishing Ltd.

Table 10.1 Clinical presentation of bleeding disorders		
	Hemophilioid state	*Purpura*
Bleeding source	Small artery	Capillary
Relation to trauma	Frequent	Rare
Presenting signs	Hematoma, ecchymosis	Ecchymosis, petechiae
Underlying cause	Factor deficiencies (e.g., VIII, IX, XI)	Platelet defects, von Willebrand disease
Bleeding time	Normal	Abnormal

2. **Inhibition of an active region of a protein.** The protein is present, but an inhibitor to its function arises. These inhibitors are usually immunoglobulins, but other forms of inhibitors can be present as well (e.g., a tumor secreting a heparin-like substance).
3. **Production of abnormal protein molecule.** The protein is present, but as a result of a mutation, missense, or deletion, an active portion of the protein is altered such that it cannot participate in its physiologic functions.
4. **Enhanced clearance of the protein.** The antigen–antibody complex is recognized as foreign. An antibody arises against the protein and resulting in the complex being removed from the circulation. The resultant increased clearance of the protein gives the appearance of a deficiency.

III. Clinical presentation of bleeding disorders

The clinical presentation of bleeding disorders is shown in Table 10.1.

IV. Coagulation cascade hypothesis

This 50-year-old theory of hemostasis still has merit in explaining the mechanisms for clot formation seen in the clinical screening tests below for coagulation reactions. It is *not* a complete model of physiologic hemostasis (see Chapter 9). In the coagulation cascade hypothesis, coagulation proteins are classified as members of the intrinsic system, the extrinsic system, or the common pathway (Figure 10.1).

A. Intrinsic system
1. Factor XII.
2. Prekallikrein (PK).
3. High molecular weight kininogen (HK).
4. Factor XI.
5. Factor VIII.
6. Factor IX.

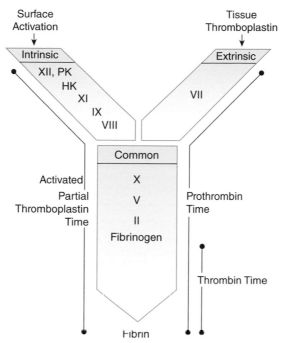

Figure 10.1 Plasma coagulation assays and the factors they measure. The plasma proteins involved in *in vitro* coagulation reactions can be classified into three systems; intrinsic, extrinsic or common. The screening tests for coagulation proteins [activated partial thromboplastin time (APTT), prothrombin time (PT), or thrombin time (TT)] measure one or more of the proteins involved in *in vitro* clot formation. Knowing what test(s) is abnormal pinpoints the likely protein defect that will give this result. HK, high-molecular weight kininogen; PK, prekallikrein.

B. Extrinsic system
1. Factor VII.
2. Tissue factor.

C. Common pathway
1. Factor X.
2. Factor V.
3. Factor II.
4. Factor I (fibrinogen).

V. Screening tests for bleeding disorders

Several screening tests are used to classify and diagnose bleeding disorders. When these assays are performed simultaneously on a sample of plasma, the results indicate almost all the diagnostic categories for a bleeding state.

A. Activated partial thromboplastin time (APTT)

To perform this common coagulation assay, a mixture of a negatively charged surface, phospholipids, and patient plasma is incubated for a few minutes. Plasma is made from whole blood anticoagulated with 3.2 g% sodium citrate (Chapter 1). Calcium chloride is added to overcome the calcium chelation of the sodium chloride, and the time required for clot formation is measured. The APTT assesses the coagulation proteins of the intrinsic system and the common pathway.

B. Prothrombin time (PT)

To perform this common coagulation assay, a preparation of tissue factor (usually recombinant, but can be isolated from animal tissues) and patient plasma are incubated for a few minutes. Afterward, calcium chloride is added and the time required for clot formation is measured. PT assesses the coagulation proteins of the extrinsic system and the common pathway.

C. Platelet count

This assay measures the number of platelets in a microliter of blood. It is used to exclude a quantitative platelet defect as the cause of a bleeding disorder.

D. Bleeding time

To perform this assay, the forearm is scratched using a special device and the time until bleeding stops is measured. It assesses platelet number or function. It is not commonly used today because it is technically not reproducible and requires experienced individuals to perform the assay.

E. Thrombin clotting time (TCT)

To perform this assay, purified thrombin is added to plasma to determine the time for clot formation. It is a direct measure of fibrinogen amount and/or function only.

VI. Interpretation of screening tests of the proteins in the coagulation system

Using the coagulation cascade hypothesis and its grouping of proteins, the screening tests for bleeding disorders can be used to measure specific coagulation proteins (Figure 10.1).

A. APTT

In the APTT, factor XII autoactivates by exposure to an artificial negatively charged surface. The APTT measures the proteins of the intrinsic system (factor XII, prekallikrein, high-molecular weight kininogen, factor XI, factor IX, and factor VIII) and the proteins of the common pathway (factors X, V, and II, and fibrinogen).

B. PT

The PT measures the extrinsic system of the coagulation, which consists of activated factor VII (factor VIIa), and tissue factor which is part of the reagent for the assay and the proteins of the common pathway (factors X, V, II, and fibrinogen).

C. Thrombin time

Thrombin time only measures the ability of fibrinogen to clot after proteolysis by the addition of exogenous thrombin.

VII. Differential diagnosis of an isolated prolonged activated partial thromboplastin time

The following approach can be used to evaluate patients who have an isolated prolonged APTT.

A. Disorders associated with bleeding

1. Congenital factor VIII deficiency or defect is sex-linked (i.e., carried on the X chromosome). Congenital factor VIII deficiency occurs only in males. Acquired factor VIII deficiency due to antibodies to the protein occurs in both males and females.
2. Factor IX deficiency or defect is sex-linked.
3. Factor XI deficiency is autosomal recessive.

B. Disorders not associated with bleeding

1. Factor XII deficiency is autosomal recessive and is the most common type. It gives very prolonged APTTs and is not associated with bleeding.
2. Prekallikrein (PK) deficiency is autosomal recessive. It gives a mildly prolonged APTT that corrects on own if the plasma sits at room temperature on bench for 1 hour. PK influences the rate of factor XII activation but is not essential for factor XII autoactivation.
3. High-molecular-weight kininogen (HK) deficiency is autosomal recessive and extremely rare. It gives a very prolonged APTT.
4. Lupus anticoagulants are antiphospholipid antibodies that interfere with coagulation reactions. These antibodies arise for many reasons and are not specific to illness, although they are often seen in patients who have connective tissue disorders (e.g., systemic lupus erythematosus [42%]). Usually, they do not interfere with the protein itself, but rather with the phospholipids reagents that are used in the coagulation assay. Thus calling these entities "anticoagulants" is a misnomer. Although these antibodies prolong coagulation protein assays, they are not associated with bleeding unless hypoprothrombinemia or thrombocytopenia is present. Paradoxically, they are often associated with thrombosis because they interfere with endothelial cell-based anticoagulation systems. When lupus anticoagulants prolong the APTT, it is a diagnosis made by exclusion of other

specific entities that are associated with bleeding (e.g., FVIII, FIX, and FXI deficiency). It is important to note that a lupus anticoagulant does not only prolong the APTT, it can at times prolong the PT. The diagnosis of a lupus anticoagulant is made by assays designed to detect an entity interfering with assay reagents and not coagulation factors. Currently, assays such as the dilute Russell viper venom time (DRVVT), tissue thromboplastin inhibition assay (TTI), dilute APTT, and kaolin clotting time are used. All these assays reduce the concentration of the reagents so that in the presence of the inhibitor, the defect is amplified in relation to a normal sample run simultaneously. Additionally one examines for antibodies to phospholipids such as anticardiolipin and anti-beta-2-glycoprotein I. If antibody titers are positive twice over 3 months, this observation is consistent with diagnosis.

VIII. Differential diagnosis of a prolonged prothrombin time only

An isolated PT prolongation usually indicates factor VII deficiency. Most of these patients usually have partial VII defects. Occasionally, isolated prolonged PT is seen in a patient who has dysfibrinogenemia (abnormal and/or deficient fibrinogen) or a deficiency in coagulation factors X, V, or II. These results are dependant upon the sensitivity of the tissue factor (thromboplastin) used in the reagents a clinical laboratory employs. In general, recombinant human tissue factor is the most sensitive reagent.

IX. Differential diagnosis of a prolonged activated partial thromboplastin time and prothrombin time

Usually, these abnormalities in the coagulation protein screening tests are not specific protein conditions, but rather acquired general medical conditions (see Chapter 12). These abnormalities may be caused by many reasons.

A. Medical causes

Medical causes include disseminated intravascular coagulation (see Chapter 12), liver disease, vitamin K deficiency, the use of therapeutic anticoagulants (e.g., heparin, warfarin, low-molecular-weight-heparin, fondaparinux, argatroban, bivalirudin, dabigatran), and massive transfusion with an anticoagulation effect from receiving too much acid-citrate-dextrose anticoagulant in the infused blood products.

B. Hypofibrinogenemia/dysfibrinogenemia

This occurs when a low and/or abnormal fibrinogen molecules do not participate properly in coagulation reactions. A normal blood coagulation time requires a plasma fibrinogen to be $\geq 100\,mg/dL$.

C. Rare cases

In rare cases, patients with low factors X, V, or II are seen and these patients will present with a prolonged APTT and PT.

X. Use the activated partial thromboplastin time and prothrombin time to monitor anticoagulation

A. APTT

The APTT is often used to monitor the extent of anticoagulant produced by unfractionated heparin, argatroban, and bivalirudin. Use of the APTT to monitor these anticoagulants is expedient but not ideal. The APTT should only be considered a general guide on the degree of anticoagulation in patients. The increase in the APTT in a patient on unfractionated heparin, argatroban, or bivalirudin is not literally related to the concentration of the anticoagulant. The APTT will prolong in a hyperbolic, not linear manner, as the anticoagulant concentration is used. Direct measurement of unfractionated heparin levels is determined by neutralization of factor Xa or IIa activity. Direct measurement of argatroban, bivalirudin or dabigatran levels, three agents that are direct thrombin inhibitors, is determined by neutralization of factor IIa activity.

B. PT

The prothrombin time is used to monitor the oral anticoagulant warfarin. When using the PT to monitor warfarin, the degree of anticoagulation is expressed as a value called the INR (International Normalized Ratio). The INR is determined by the ratio of the patient's PT to the mean PT performed in the laboratory on a population of normals (n ≥ 20). If a patient sample is normal, than the INR ~1.0. Therapeutic levels of warfarin usually have an INR between 2 and 3. This value is about 5–15% normal functional levels of the vitamin K-dependent coagulation factors II, VII, IX, and X.

XI. Differential diagnosis of a prolonged bleeding time and a normal platelet count

Defects in bleeding time in the presence of a normal platelet count signify abnormalities in the following:
1. **Von Willebrand factor** (von Willebrand disease; see Chapter 11).
2. **Platelet function** (see Chapters 12, 13).
3. **Rare connective tissue disorders**, including pseudoxanthoma elasticum, Ehlers–Danlos syndrome, and scurvy that is associated with collagen breakdown and perifollicular hemorrhage.

XII. Prolonged bleeding time as a result of platelet defects

This abnormality occurs when the number of platelets is decreased or when a true intrinsic defect in platelet function occurs.

1. **Quantitative decrease in platelet count.** As the platelet count decreases to less than 100,000/μL, the bleeding time becomes prolonged.
2. **True platelet function defect** (see Chapter 12).

XIII. Differential diagnosis of a bleeding state that is not associated with an abnormality in the screening tests

These entities are rare and mainly consist of abnormalities of the fibrinolytic system (e.g., defects in alpha-2-antiplasmin or plasminogen activator inhibitor) or abnormalities in factor XIII.

A. Factor XIII deficiency

Factor XIII deficiency may be congenital or acquired. Factor XIII is a thrombin-activated transglutaminase that cross-links fibrin monomers into polymers that produces the fibrin clot. Patients bleed excessively as a result of surgery or trauma. Middle-aged adults have a high incidence of spontaneous intracerebral hemorrhage.

B. Alpha-2-antiplasmin deficiency

Alpha-2-antiplasmin deficiency is the absence of the major serine protease inhibitor (serpin) of plasmin. These patients have a bleeding disorder that is caused by a hyperfibrinolytic state, which lyses any clots that are formed. Alpha-2-antiplasmin is a SERPIN inhibitor of plasmin. Alpha-2-antiplasmin deficiency can be acquired as result of consumption in disseminated intravascular coagulation (e.g., as seen in acute promyelocytic leukemia).

C. Plasminogen activator inhibitor-1 deficiency

Plasminogen activator inhibitor-1 deficiency is a deficiency in the major serpin inhibitor of plasminogen activators. This abnormality causes increased activation of plasminogen. A profibrinolytic state occurs as a result.

D. Alpha-1-antitrypsin PITTSBURGH

Alpha-1-antitrypsin PITTSBURGH is an abnormal serpin that changed alpha-1-antitrypsin into a very potent antithrombin. It causes a severe bleeding disorder because it has exceedingly tight binding and potent inhibition of the activity of thrombin. Thus, any thrombin that forms is rapidly neutralized, and as a result, no clotting can occur.

IX. Summary

The physician can recognize the underlying cause of most bleeding disorders that one may encounter in clinical practice by having a good understanding what the APTT, PT, platelet count, and bleeding time measure. It is of great clinical value to fully understand the results of these assays.

Further reading

Schmaier AH. Laboratory evaluation of hemostatic and thrombotic disorders. In: Hoffman R, Benz EJ, Shattil SJ et al., eds. Hematology: Basic Principles and Practice. Philadelphia, PA: Churchill Livingstone, 2009:1877–84.

Schmaier AH, Miller JL. Coagulation and fibrinolysis. In: McPherson RA, Pincus MR, eds. Henry's Clinical Diagnosis and Management by Laboratory Methods, 23rd edn. Philadelphia, PA: Elsevier, 2011 (in press).

11 Congenital Bleeding Disorders

Anjali A. Sharathkumar[1] and Steven W. Pipe[2]

[1]*Children's Memorial Hospital, Northwestern University, Feinberg School of Medicine, Chicago, IL, USA*
[2]*C.S. Mott Children's Hospital, University of Michigan, Ann Arbor, MI, USA*

I. Overview

- The clinical phenotype of congenital bleeding disorders can range widely dependent upon the type and severity of factor deficiency.
- Laboratory diagnosis of a coagulation factor deficiency is guided by the results of screening tests, including prothrombin time (PT), activated partial thromboplastin time (APTT), and thrombin time (TT) and confirmed with specific factor assays.
- Specific factor replacement therapy, prophylactically where appropriate, is the foundation of clinical care for these disorders.
- Patients with deficiencies of the contact pathway (factor XII, prekallikrein and high molecular weight kininogen) can have significant prolongation of the APTT without clinical symptoms of bleeding.

II. Hemophilia

Hemophilia is the most common inherited bleeding disorder. Conventionally, hemophilia refers to deficiencies of the coagulation proteins, factor VIII (FVIII) and factor IX (FIX).
- FVIII deficiency is known as hemophilia A or classic hemophilia.
- FIX deficiency is known as hemophilia B or Christmas disease.

A. Role of FVIII and FIX in hemostasis
- Both FVIII and FIX are synthesized in the liver. They participate in the intrinsic pathway of blood coagulation. The primary function of the intrinsic pathway is to amplify thrombin generation and facilitate formation of a strong fibrin clot at the site of vascular injury and arrest the bleeding (see Chapter 9).

Concise Guide to Hematology, First Edition. Edited by Alvin H. Schmaier, Hillard M. Lazarus.
© 2012 Blackwell Publishing Ltd. Published 2012 by Blackwell Publishing Ltd.

- FVIII circulates in plasma non-covalently bound to von Willebrand factor (VWF). Upon activation by thrombin, it dissociates from VWF and acts as a cofactor for FIXa to activate factor X (FX) to FXa. The assembly of FVIIIa, FIXa and FX on the phospholipid surface constitutes the intrinsic tenase complex. FXa generated from the intrinsic tenase complex is critical for amplifying the conversion of prothrombin to thrombin in the presence of its cofactor, factor Va, within the prothrombinase complex.
- Deficiency of FVIII or FIX leads to a significant reduction in thrombin generation resulting in reduced fibrin clot formation that manifests as severe bleeding even after minor trauma and an increased tendency to re-bleed during physiologic clot lysis.

B. Epidemiology
- **Incidence:** The incidence of hemophilia A is approximately 1 in 5000 live male births while the incidence of hemophilia B is 1 in 30,000 live male births.
- **Race:** Hemophilia has no racial predilection, and is present in all ethnic and racial groups.
- **Family history:** Although the majority (~70%) of cases of hemophilia are inherited, ~30% of cases arise from a spontaneous mutation, with no family history of hemophilia.

C. Genetics
- **Genetic locus:** The genes for both factor VIII (*F8*) and factor IX (*F9*) are located near the terminus of the long arm of the X-chromosome, Xq28 and Xq27.1 respectively. *F8* gene is 186 Kb and consists of 26 exons while *F9* spans 33 Kb and contains 8 exons.
- **Relationship between mutation type and the disease phenotype:** The type of mutations within the *F8* or *F9* gene predicts the disease severity. Typically deletions, insertions and nonsense mutations result in severe disease while missense mutations are more often found in mild to moderate disease.
- **Commonly encountered mutations:**
  - The majority of patients with hemophilia A have severe disease and 40% of patients with severe hemophilia A carry an intron 22 gene inversion. This condition is caused by an intra-chromosomal recombination between a 9.5 kb sequence within intron 22 of the *F8* gene and one of two closely related inversely oriented sequences located 5' to the *F8* gene. An additional inversion within intron 1 of the *F8* gene is found in 5% of patients with severe hemophilia A. Most laboratories carry out initial screening for intron 22 inversion in cases of severe hemophilia A.
  - The majority of patients with hemophilia B have mild disease with missense mutations occurring most commonly. Up to 25% of Caucasian patients have one of three founder mutations (Gly60Ser, Ile397Thr, and Thr296Met).
- **Mode of inheritance:** Hemophilia A and B are transmitted as X-linked recessive disorders, hence males are typically affected and females are

carriers of the disease. All the daughters of an affected male are "obligate carriers" of hemophilia while all his sons are unaffected. A carrier female has a 50% risk of transmitting her affected X-chromosome with each pregnancy; therefore half of her sons can be affected with hemophilia and half of her daughters can be carriers of hemophilia.

D. Clinical classification

Hemophilia is classified as mild, moderate and severe on the basis of the patient's residual FVIII and FIX blood concentrations ($1\,\text{IU}/\text{dL} = 1\%$).
- Severe hemophilia: <1%.
- Moderate hemophilia: ≥1 to 5%.
- Mild hemophilia: ≥6–40 %.

E. Bleeding manifestations

(i) **Overview**

The hallmark of hemophilia is hemarthroses (joint bleeds), but bleeding manifestations may include any of the following: prolonged bleeding post-circumcision, neonatal intracranial bleeding or cephalohematomas, muscle hematomas, prolonged bleeding/oozing or renewed bleeding after trauma or surgical procedures, unexplained GI bleeding or hematuria, recurrent epistaxis, and excessive bruising.
- Bleeding manifestations vary depending on the severity of the factor deficiency, type of hemophilia and the age at presentation. Patients with severe hemophilia may experience spontaneous bleeding while patients with moderate hemophilia bleed after trivial trauma. Without prophylactic therapy, patients with severe hemophilia typically experience 4–6 bleeding events per month or 20–30 events/year while patients with moderate hemophilia typically experience 4–6 bleeding events per year. Clinical spectrum ranges from musculoskeletal bleeding such as hemarthrosis and muscle bleeding to, rarely, bleeding within internal organs.
- Bleeding in mild hemophilia may only manifest with significant trauma or with surgery. Bleeding pattern is predominated by mucocutanous bleeding such as bruising, epistaxis and prolonged bleeding after minor trauma.
- In general, patients with hemophilia B have relatively milder bleeding tendency compared to hemophilia A for the same residual factor levels.
- The clinical symptoms of bleeding in female carriers of hemophilia depend upon the baseline factor levels. Although the majority are asymptomatic, some female carriers of hemophilia A and B have significant reduction of their FVIII and FIX through skewed lyonization of the normal X chromosome. Lyonization is a process by which one of the two copies of the X chromosomes in female mammals are inactivated so that only genes from the other active chromosome are expressed. Though typically random, disproportionate inactivation of the normal X chromosome within the

expressing cells of female carriers with hemophilia, can result in significantly reduced production of FVIII and FIX. These women are conventionally known as "symptomatic carriers" as they experience bleeding
symptoms. Specifically, symptoms of menorrhagia and post-partum
hemorrhage are common.

(ii) Hemarthrosis and hemophilic arthropathy

- Hemarthosis, bleeding within the joint space, can occur spontaneously or
  after a minor trauma. The frequency and age of onset of joint bleeding
  depends upon the severity of deficiency. In severe deficiency, joint bleeds
  typically begin between age 6 months and 6 years and can occur several
  times a month.
- Quite often, patients will have a tendency to repeated bleeds within a specific joint. This joint is known as a "target joint". Repeated bleeding into
  the same joint initiates synovitis and ultimately progression to hemophilic
  arthropathy.
- Hemophilic arthropathy typically has five stages:
  - **Stage I:** Soft tissue swelling and inflammation due to bleeding within
    and around the joint.
  - **Stage II:** Osteoporosis and epiphyseal overgrowth with an intact joint
    space and no bone cysts.
  - **Stage III:** Subchondral cyst formation and joint surface irregularities
    with preservation of joint space.
  - **Stage IV:** Subchondral cyst formation, prominent joint surface irregulari-
    ties and narrowing of joint space due to cartilage destruction.
  - **Stage V:** Loss of joint space and epiphyseal overgrowth.
- **Treatment:** Progression of hemophilic arthropathy leads to loss of range of
  motion and joint function. Prophylaxis treatment regimens can prevent the
  progression of hemophilic arthropathy by reducing the frequency of joint
  bleeds but does not necessarily reverse the joint damage. Surgical or radioactive synovectomy can be performed to reduce the bleeding tendency.
  Joint replacement surgeries may be required as adults.

(iii) Muscle and soft tissue bleeds

- Muscle bleeding is the second most frequent type of bleeding in patients
  with hemophilia. Intramuscular hemorrhages within a closed compartment
  such as the volar aspect of the wrist, deep palmer compartments of the
  hand, anterior or posterior tibial compartments, and inguinal region can
  cause significant morbidity due to compression of neurovascular bundles
  (compartment syndrome).
- **Treatment:** Besides treatment with factor concentrates (detailed below) to
  raise the factor levels to the hemostatic range, 30–50%, immediate surgical
  decompression may be necessary to release the pressure to prevent irreversible tissue damage (e.g., Volkmann's contracture due to compartment syndrome within the forearm).

Table 11.1 Characteristics of hemophilia and its management

	Hemophilia A	Hemophilia B
Underlying deficiency	Factor VIII deficiency	Factor IX deficiency
Subtypes according to severity	Severe: <1% Moderate: 1–5% Mild: ≥6–40%	Severe: <1% Moderate: 1–5% Mild: ≥6–40%
Therapy considerations		
Dose increment	1 Unit of exogenous FVIII will increase *in vivo* plasma FVIII levels by 2%	1 Unit of exogenous FIX will increase *in vivo* plasma FVIII levels by 0.8%
Dose calculation	Units required to raise blood levels (%) = 0.5 Units/kg × body weight (Kg) × desired increase (%)	Units required to raise blood levels (%) = 1.2 Units/kg × body weight (Kg) × desired increase (%)
Half-life of exogenously infused product	8–12 hours	~24 hours
Frequency of administration	8–12 hours	24 hours
Mode of administration	Intravenous bolus or continuous infusion	Intravenous bolus or continuous infusion
Prophylaxis therapy	20–40 IU/kg, q 2–3 times/ week	50–100 IU/kg, q 2 times/ week
Recommended dosing for bleeding diathesis		
Mild to moderate bleeding events (joint bleeding, cuts, minor trauma, minor surgery, soft-tissue bleeding)	30–50% correction × 1–7 days	30–50% correction × 1–7 days
Major bleeding events (CNS bleeding, any life-threatening bleeding)	100% correction until bleeding is controlled and 50–100% correction × 1–3 weeks followed by prophylaxis	100% correction until bleeding is controlled; 50–100% correction × 1–3 weeks followed by prophylaxis

(iv) Life-threatening bleeds

Bleeding into areas that can compress vital structures (e.g., central nervous system, upper airway) or that can lead to excessive blood loss (e.g., gastrointestinal or iliopsoas hemorrhage) can be life threatening and require prompt aggressive treatment with factor concentrates and possibly surgical management (Table 11.1).

F. Diagnosis of hemophilia

The diagnosis of hemophilia can be suspected based on personal history of the typical clinical phenotype of bleeding and family history of bleeding.

History of hemarthrosis and the X-linked inheritance pattern are important clues for the diagnosis of hemophilia. Special coagulation tests are mandatory to confirm the diagnosis.

(i) Special coagulation tests

- **Activated partial thromboplastin time (APTT):** Deficiency of FVIII and FIX prolongs the APTT. In severe hemophilia, the APTT is usually two to three times the upper limits of normal. In mild hemophilia, the APTT assay can be normal. Therefore in patients with a suspected bleeding disorder, specific factor assays should be performed to rule out FVIII or FIX deficiency.
- **Other screening tests of hemostasis:** Platelet count, prothrombin time, and thrombin time are normal in patients with hemophilia.

(ii) Genetic testing

- Genetic testing for families with hemophilia is rapidly becoming a part of routine clinical care.
- Testing for the commonly encountered mutations such as inversion 22 and inversion 1 is the recommended first step in evaluating a patient with hemophilia A. In the absence of a commonly encountered mutation, direct DNA based analysis of the *F8* and *F9* genes to identify the mutations within these genes may be performed.
- Identification of a mutation in a proband is particularly useful in carrier detection and prenatal diagnosis of hemophilia.
- In cases with borderline low factor VIII/IX levels (~40–50%), it is often prudent to confirm the diagnosis of mild hemophilia by performing genetic mutation analysis.

(iii) Special considerations in newborns

- Neither factor VIII nor factor IX crosses the placenta; thus, these patients can present with bleeding symptoms during the neonatal period.
- **Clinical symptoms:** Majority of bleeding symptoms in the newborn period are related either to trauma during labor and delivery (e.g., cephalo-hematoma or intracranial hemorrhage), or interventions and procedures, such as injections, heel stick and or circumcision.
- **Laboratory diagnosis:** Specific factor assays are required to confirm the diagnosis of hemophilia as the APTT assay may be prolonged in the newborn period due to deficiency of vitamin K dependent proteins.
  - **Hemophilia A:** FVIII concentrations are at adult levels in the newborns, therefore diagnosis of severe and moderate hemophilia A can be made in the newborn period. However, the diagnosis of mild hemophilia can be challenging as the FVIII levels are often increased in the newborn period in response to acute stress and maternal hormonal effects. Repeat testing after several months is recommended.
  - **Hemophilia B:** FIX is a vitamin K-dependent protein and the level of FIX could be physiologically low in the newborn period. Therefore, the

diagnosis of mild and moderate hemophilia B needs to be confirmed after the newborn period.

- Genetic testing can be an alternative to confirm the diagnosis provided the genetic mutation within the family is known.

(iv) Prenatal testing

Prenatal diagnosis of hemophilia in a male fetus can be offered to carrier females to provide additional information to guide pregnancy and delivery management. This is performed by either chorionic villous sampling at 10–12 weeks of gestation or amniocentesis at 15 to 16 weeks of gestation. These procedures however are associated with risk of bleeding (to both mother and fetus) and miscarriage.

G. Principles of management of hemophilia

(i) Factor replacement therapies

- Replacement of deficient coagulation factors by administration of exogenous factor concentrates is the primary treatment for patients with hemophilia. These clotting factor concentrates are either derived from plasma or recombinant technology.

  The commonly used treatment regimens fall into one of four categories:

  1. **Primary prophylaxis:** The regular and long-term administration of clotting factor concentrates in order to prevent bleeding. It is typically started before the age of 2 years and after no more than one joint bleed.

  2. **Secondary prophylaxis:** Regular continuous (long-term) treatment started after two or more joint bleeds or at an age >2 year.

  3. **Episodic prophylaxis:** Regular infusion of factor concentrates for a short period of time related to activity, follow up after an injury or a procedure.

  4. **On-demand therapy:** Infusion of factor concentrates during an episode of an acute bleed.

  The choice of treatment regimen depends upon:

  - Severity of hemophilia.
  - Frequency of bleeding.
  - Severity of the bleeding event.

  Primary prophylaxis is now considered the standard of care for patients with severe hemophilia and has been demonstrated to prevent joint bleeds and subsequent arthropathy.

- **Recommended treatment for acute bleeding**

  In the event of an acute bleeding episode, it is critical to raise the levels of FVIII or FIX to the hemostatic range. The intensity and duration of factor replacement therapy depends upon the severity of the bleeding (Table 11.1).

  - **Minor bleeding episodes:** it is recommended to raise the factor level up to 30 to 50%. Usually one or two doses are enough to control minor bleeding events.

▪ **Major bleeding episodes (e.g., CNS bleeds):** factor levels should be raised up to 80 to 100% until the bleeding is arrested. Subsequent maintenance of hemostatic levels will depend upon the severity of bleeding episode and its response to treatment and may be achieved by continued bolus injections or a continuous infusion. Table 11.1 illustrates the recommended dosing regimens for commonly encountered bleeding manifestations in patients with hemophilia.

(ii) Adjuvant therapies

Desmopressin (DDAVP) is a synthetic peptide that causes release of VWF from storage sites within endothelial cells. DDAVP also results in a parallel increase in plasma FVIII levels. This agent is particularly useful in patients with mild hemophilia and may obviate the need for factor replacement therapy with minor bleeds such as epistaxis or gum bleeding. Other adjuvant therapies such as antifibrinolytic medications (aminocaproic acid and tranexamic acid) and topical hemostatic agents (thrombin, fibrin sealant) may also be used even in severe hemophilia along with specific factor replacement therapy.

(iii) Inhibitors of coagulation factor VIII and factor IX

- **Definition:** Development of allo-antibodies against exogenously administered factor (FVIII or FIX) that interfere with their procoagulant function are conventionally known as "inhibitors".
- **Prevalence of inhibitors:** Up to 30% of patients with severe hemophilia A develop inhibitors to exogenously administered FVIII while 3–5% of patients with severe hemophilia B develop inhibitors against exogenously administered FIX.
- **Impact of inhibitors on coagulation:** These antibodies are typically directed against functional epitopes on FVIII or FIX; hence they neutralize the functional activity of exogenously administered clotting factor making the treatment ineffective.
- **Measurement of inhibitors:** The quantitative Bethesda assay is performed to assess the level of inhibitor (titer). One Bethesda unit (BU) is the amount of antibody that will neutralize 50% of FVIII or FIX in a 1:1 mixture of the patient's plasma and normal plasma (after 2 hour incubation at 37 degrees Celsius).
- **Clinical presentation of inhibitor:** Patients with inhibitors typically present with bleeding manifestations despite adequate prophylaxis, failure to achieve hemostasis with replacement therapy in the context of an acute bleed, or through routine screening.
- **Management of inhibitors:**
  ▪ **Treatment of an acute bleeding episode:** Includes the use of "bypassing agents" such as activated prothrombin complex concentrates (APCC) or recombinant factor VIIa (rVIIa). APCCs contain multiple activated serine protease molecules such as activated forms of factor X and prothrombin

to drive hemostasis without inhibition by FVIII or FIX inhibitors. Whereas, rVIIa is able to directly activate factor X and increase thrombin production on the surface of activated platelets in the absence of FVIII or FIX. Antifibrinolytics may also be used as adjunct therapy.

- **Eradication of inhibitors:** Immune tolerance induction regimens are used to eradicate the inhibitor. These regimens include frequent, often daily, infusions of high doses of factor concentrates with or without immunosuppressive agents. Patients with inhibitors should be treated at a specialized hemophilia treatment center.

Hemophilia treatment centers are federally recognized specialized clinics where a team of doctors, nurses, social workers, and physical therapists work together to deliver comprehensive care to people with bleeding disorders. These centers have been shown to significantly decrease the morbidity and mortality for patients with bleeding disorders and have particular expertise to manage hemophilia with inhibitors. The list of these centers is available on the Centers for Disease Control and Prevention website (http://www.cdc.gov/ncbddd/hbd/htc_list.htm).

III. Von Willebrand disease

A. Overview
Von Willebrand disease (VWD) is the most common inherited bleeding disorder with an autosomal dominant or recessive inheritance due to quantitative or qualitative deficiency of von Willebrand factor (VWF). Some reports suggest that VWD has a prevalence of about 1% in the general population, but the prevalence of clinically relevant cases is lower, ~100/million population.

B. Structure and function of VWF
- **Synthesis:** VWF is a large multimeric glycoprotein that is synthesized in megakaryocytes and endothelial cells. It is stored within specific storage granules, the α-granules of platelets and Weibel–Palade bodies within endothelial cells. VWF is an acute phase reactant and the levels of VWF increase with physiological or pathological stress such as exercise, emotional stress, pregnancy, infections and inflammatory conditions.
- **Structure:** The primary translation product contains a signal peptide of 22 amino acids, a propeptide of 741 residues and the basic VWF monomer of 2050 amino acids. Each mature monomer contains nine domains: three A domains (A1, A2, A3), one B domain, two C domains (C1, C2), and three D domains (D′, D3, D4) with a specific function; elements of note are:
  - the D′/D3 domain binds to FVIII, heparin
  - the A1 domain binds to platelet GPIb receptor, heparin, and collagen
  - the A3 domain binds to collagen.

Two monomers of VWF are initially dimerized through disulfide bond formation at their C-termini. The C-terminal dimers are then N-terminal multimerized into multimers of 0.6 kD to 20 million daltons. Unusually large VWF multimers that are synthesized and secreted by endothelial cells are processed into normal sized multimers in the plasma through the action of a novel VWF-cleaving metalloprotease, ADAMTS13, which cleaves VWF within its A2 domain. This cleavage event is believed to occur under conditions of high shear stress in parts of the circulation, which partially unfolds the VWF molecule exposing the cleavage site. This physiologic regulation protects against abnormal platelet-VWF aggregation in the microvasculature, as seen in TTP and HUS (see Chapter 14).

- **Function:** High-molecular-weight (HMW) VWF multimers mediate platelet adhesion at sites of vascular injury by binding to subendothelial matrix and to platelets. VWF also serves as a carrier protein for plasma coagulation factor, FVIII. Therefore, defects in VWF can cause bleeding with features typical of platelet dysfunction, or of mild to moderately severe hemophilia A, or of both.

C. Genetics of VWD

- The *VWF* gene spans 178 kilobases in the human genome, and is localized to the tip of the short arm of chromosome 12, at 12p13.3. In general, quantitative abnormalities of the *VWF* gene are due to promoter, frameshift nonsense mutations, and large deletions, whereas missense mutations typically result in qualitative defects. Mutations and polymorphisms in the *VWF* gene are currently being cataloged in an international database (www.shef.ac.uk/vwf/index.html).
- In several families, no mutations have been identified within the VWF gene implying the role of modifier genes in clinical expression of VWD. ABO blood type is shown to be an important modifier of VWF plasma levels; patients with "O" type have lower plasma levels of VWF while "AB" blood type is associated with the highest plasma levels of VWF.

D. Clinical presentation

- In general, VWD is a mild bleeding disorder. Unlike hemophilia, spontaneous bleeding symptoms and bleeding within the internal organs such as CNS or joints is extremely rare in patients with VWD (Table 11.2).
- The primary clinical presentation in patients with VWD is mucocutaneous bleeding such as:
  - superficial bruising
  - subcutaneous hematoma
  - epistaxis
  - gastrointestinal mucosal bleeding
  - menorrhagia
  - post-partum hemorrhage
  - bleeding after common surgical procedures such as wisdom tooth extraction or tonsillectomy and adenoidectomy.

Table 11.2 Clinical* characteristics of subtypes of Von Willebrand disease and related disorder

Features	Type 1	Type 2 A	Type 2 B	Type 2 N	Type 2 M	Type 3	PT-VWD
Population frequency	1–2%	Rare	Rare	Rare	Rare	1:250,000	Rare
Defect	Partial quantitative deficiency with normal structure & function of VWF	Quantitative and qualitative defect with loss of HMWM	↑ affinity of VWF to platelet membrane GP Ib/IX/V complex	↓ affinity of VWF for FVIII mimicking	Qualitative defect with retention of HMWM	Complete deficiency of VWF	↑ affinity of platelet membrane receptor GP Ib/IX/V complex to VWF
Pattern of bleeding	Mucocutaneous	Mucocutaneous	Mucocutaneous	Mucocutaneous, soft tissue, joint (rare)	Mucocutaneous	Mucocutaneous, soft tissue, joint	Mucocutaneous
Inheritance	AD	AD	AD	AR	AD	AR	?AD
Bleeding time and/or PFA-100	N or ↑	↑	N or ↑	N	N or ↑	↑	N or ↑
Platelet count	N	N	N or ↓	N	N	N	N or ↓
Factor VIII activity	N or ↓	N or ↓	N or ↓	↓ (discrepantly low compared to VWF antigen)	N or ↓	Markedly ↓	N or ↓
VWF Antigen (VWF:Ag)$	↓	↓	N or ↓	N	↓	Markedly ↓	N or ↓
Ristocetin cofactor activity (VWF R:Co)$	↓	↓	N or ↓	N	↓ (discrepantly low compared to VWF antigen)	Markedly ↓	N or ↓
Low dose ristocetin induced platelet aggregation (LDRIPA)	Absent	Absent	Present	Absent	Absent	Absent	Present
VWF multimer analysis	N	Absence of HMWM	Absence of HMWM	N	N or ↑ HMWM	Absent	Absence of HMWM

Abbreviations: ↑, indicates prolonged; ↓, indicates decreased; AD, autosomal dominant; AR, autosomal recessive; DDAVP, desmopressin acetate; HMWM, high molecular weight multimers; N, normal; PFA, platelet function analyzer.

$Laboratory interpretation of von Willebrand factor levels should be interpreted in the context of the patient's blood group.

Reproduced with permission from Nelson Textbook of Pediatrics, 17th edn, Chapter 469, Figure 469-I (Saunders/Elsevier).

E. Diagnosis of VWD

- Important components of the diagnosis of VWD include: personal history of bleeding, family history of bleeding and abnormal laboratory testing for VWD.
- Screening coagulation tests: PT and APTT are usually normal; the APTT may be prolonged due to low FVIII levels. Bleeding times and whole blood platelet function analyzers (PFA-100) are neither sensitive nor specific enough to rely on for screening for VWD therefore specific assays for VWF must be performed.
- VWF laboratory assays:
  - **VWF antigen (VWF:Ag) assay:** This quantitative immunoassay measures the actual concentration of VWF protein in blood plasma.
  - VWF function analysis:
    - **The ristocetin cofactor assay (VWF:RCo)** is a pharmacologic assay that measures the ability of VWF to bind platelet GPIb in the presence of ristocetin. Ristocetin, a positively charged antibiotic, induces structural change in VWF and exposes the domain for binding to platelet GPIb/IX/V complex. This assay is based on the ability of patient plasma to induce agglutination of formalin-fixed platelets in the presence of a fixed concentration of ristocetin. The level of VWF functional activity in a blood sample is assessed by comparing its ability to induce platelet agglutination with that of various dilutions of known normal pooled human plasma.
    - The adhesive function of VWF can also be measured by the *collagen binding assay* (VWF:CBA), in which microtitre wells are coated with collagen which preferentially binds large VWF multimers.
  - **Factor VIII activity:** Measured using a standard clotting factor assay based on the APTT.
  - **VWF multimer analysis:** These tests are available in specialized coagulation laboratories. The full range of VWF multimers within plasma are best demonstrated after fractionation on a low concentration agarose gel. The VWF multimers are then visualized with radiolabeled anti-VWF antibody (Figure 11.1).
  - **Specialized assays:**
    - Following a diagnosis of VWD, additional functional assays may be used to determine the affinity of VWF for FVIII or platelets. These assays may assist in determining certain qualitative subtypes of VWD
    - **Ristocetin-induced platelet aggregation (RIPA):** This assay is similar in principle to the test performed for VWF:RCo activity, except that the patient's own platelets are used to evaluate the sensitivity of the patient's VWF-platelet aggregation in response to ristocetin.
- **Interpretation of VWF diagnostic assays:** VWF antigen and functional assays should be interpreted in the context of VWF multimer assays. In general, a proportionate decrease in VWF antigen, VWF functional activity and FVIII activity accompanied by a normal distribution of multimers of

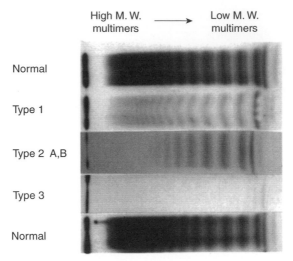

High M. W. → Low M. W.
multimers   multimers

Normal

Type 1

Type 2 A,B

Type 3

Normal

Figure 11.1 Von Willebrand multimer analysis. (Reproduced with permission from Pruthi RK. A practical approach to genetic testing for von Willebrand Disease. Mayo Clinic Proceedings 2006;81(5):679–91.)

VWF (from low to high molecular weight) indicates a quantitative defect. Lack of concordance of the functional and antigen assays or an abnormal distribution of VWF multimers indicates a qualitative defect. Additional specialized assays may be used to identify the specific qualitative defect.

F. Clinical subtypes of VWD

- **VWD subtypes:** VWD is classified into three major subtypes: type 1, type 2 and type 3 (Table 11.2). It is best understood as either quantitative deficiency (type 1 or type 3) or a qualitative deficiency (type 2A, 2B, 2N, 2M).
- **Prevalence of VWD subtypes:** Most cases, ~85%, appear to have a partial quantitative deficiency of VWF (type 1 VWD) with variable bleeding tendency. About 20–30% patients have qualitative variants (type 2 VWD), due to a dysfunctional VWF. These patients are clinically more homogeneous and exhibit moderate bleeding tendency. Type 3 VWD is rare, ~5%, and the patients have a moderate to severe bleeding diathesis because of the virtual absence of VWF and concurrent deficiency of FVIII.
- **Mode of inheritance:** Type 1, 2A, 2B, 2M are inherited in an autosomal dominant fashion while type 2N and type 3 are inherited in an autosomal recessive fashion.
- **Pathophysiology and its implications on management:**
  - **Type 1 VWD:** This subtype may be caused by mutations that results in decreased synthesis or promote increased clearance of VWF from circulation. Proportionate reductions in VWF:Ag, VWF:RCo, and FVIII activity and a normal distribution of VWF multimers is consistent with type I

VWD. These patients respond to pharmacological agents such as DDAVP which act to raise endogenous levels of VWF through release from endothelial storage granules.

- **Type 2A VWD:** Is typically caused by mutations that interfered with the assembly or secretion of HMW multimers of VWF or that increase the susceptibility of VWF to proteolysis. This results in a disproportionate reduction in VWF:RCo compared to VWF:Ag and deficit of HMW multimers. Although these patients may respond to DDAVP, VWF concentrates are often required for the treatment of moderate to severe bleeding.

- **Type 2B VWD:** This subtype is caused by "gain of function" mutation in the A1 region of VWF leading to spontaneous binding of VWF to platelets which leads to proteolytic degradation and depletion of the HMW multimers and platelets. These patients typically present with thrombocytopenia, reduced VWF levels and absence of HMW multimers. The laboratory diagnosis relies on the demonstration that the "hyperreactive" VWF binds to platelets resulting in agglutination in the RIPA at low concentration of ristocetin. Since DDAVP can release these "hyperreactive" VWF multimers, this can worsen the thrombocytopenia, and should be used with caution in this subtype of VWD. These patients are usually treated with VWF concentrates. Type 2B VWD must be distinguished from platelet-type VWD or pseudo-VWD where mutations within the GP1b/IX/V platelet receptor results in increased binding of platelets to VWF. Since the defect is in the platelets, standard treatment options for VWD are not effective. Such patients may require treatment with normal platelets to control the bleeding.

- **Type 2M:** This describes VWF variants that exhibit decreased VWF-dependent platelet adhesion despite the presence of HMW multimers. This results in laboratory results where the VWF:RCo assay is disproportionately decreased compared to VWF:Ag. The distinction from type 2A VWD depends on VWF multimer analysis. Pharmacological treatment with DDAVP is generally effective for the treatment of bleeding manifestations.

- **Type 2N:** This type is caused by genetic mutations in the FVIII binding domain of VWF. This results in rapid clearance of FVIII from plasma and results in low residual FVIII plasma levels. This subtype of VWD has been referred to as "autosomal hemophilia" or the "Normandy" variant. Patients will have normal VWF:Ag and VWF:RCo levels but decreased FVIII activity (<10%). The laboratory diagnosis relies on a specific binding assay that confirms the decreased binding affinity of VWF for FVIII. The majority of patients will still respond to DDAVP treatment as FVIII is released from storage granules along with VWF, though the half-life of the endogenous FVIII will remain very short. If FVIII levels are <5%, then treatment with VWF-containing FVIII concentrates should be considered to treat major bleeding events.

▪ **Type 3 VWD:** This subtype is characterized by undetectable levels of VWF:Ag and VWF:RCo and complete absence of VWF on multimer analysis. FVIII levels are usually very low (1–9%). Such VWD patients have the most severe bleeding manifestations and may exhibit a clinical phenotype similar to moderate hemophilia A. These patients do not respond to DDAVP and require VWF concentrates for the treatment of bleeding.

G. Treatment of VWD

- The principles of treatment of bleeding in patients with VWD include: (1) increasing functional VWF levels and (2) enhancing clot stability.
- Specific treatment options to raise VWF levels include DDAVP and VWF concentrates. Adjuvant therapies such as antifibrinolytics and local hemostatic agents are used to enhance clot stability. Hormone suppression therapy can be used to control menorrhagia; estrogens are also shown to increase VWF levels.
- **DDAVP:** DDAVP is generally used as a first line of therapy in patients with type 1, 2A, 2M, and 2N VWD with or without adjuvant therapies.
- **VWF concentrates:** Plasma-derived VWF concentrates contain HMW multimers of VWF as well as FVIII. These are usually recommended for the treatment of severe bleeding in patients with VWD or for any other bleeding episodes which are unresponsive to therapy. Similar to hemophilia, for major bleeding episodes, the levels of VWF should be raised to 80–100% and for minor bleeding events the level should be raised up to 30–50%. The dosing of VWF concentrates is calculated based on the Ristocetin cofactor units. One unit per kg of ristocetin cofactor activity raises the plasma VWF:RCo activity by ~1%. The half-life of VWF:RCo activity after infusion is ~10–12 hours. Further maintenance treatment with VWF concentrates depends upon the severity of bleeding and the initial response to factor concentrate treatment.

H. Acquired abnormalities of VWF

Alterations in amount and function of VWF has been reported in following pathologic states:

- Acquired VWD secondary to autoantibody formation is described in autoimmune disorders (SLE or scleroderma), lymphoma, leukemia, multiple myeloma and monoclonal gammopathies. These antibodies do not inhibit the function of VWF but reduce the half-life of VWF by enhancing its clearance.
- Wilms' tumor due to adsoption of VWF on tumor cells.
- Hypothyroidism due to decreased synthesis of VWF.
- Congenital heart disease such as ventriculoseptal defect, aortic stenosis and pulmonary hypertension may cause loss of the HMW multimers of VWF and may mimic type 2A.

- Vascular malformations (angiodysplasia, giant hemangiomas and telangiectasia) have been associated with abnormal synthesis and clearance of VWF multimers.

IV. Rare bleeding disorders

A. Overview
Qualitative and quantitative deficiencies of coagulation factors such as fibrinogen, prothrombin, factor V, combined deficiency of factors V and VIII, factor VII, factor X, factor XI, factor XIII, and multiple deficiencies of vitamin K-dependent coagulation factors are collectively known as rare bleeding disorders (RBD).

B. Epidemiology
- These disorders are usually transmitted in an autosomal recessive manner. Therefore they can affect both males and females equally.
- The prevalence of RBD is low ranging from 1:500,000 for FVII deficiency to 1:2,000,000 for prothrombin and factor XIII deficiency.
- Ethnic/racial predisposition: The prevalence of RBDs is significantly increased by a high rate of consanguinity in the population, such as Middle Eastern communities. FXI deficiency is more commonly seen in Ashkenazi Jews.

C. Bleeding manifestations
- In general, the bleeding patterns among patients with RBDs are quite variable and, unlike hemophilia, the coagulation factor levels do not necessarily correlate with the severity of the bleeding.
- Patients with severe deficiencies (factor levels <10%) tend to have relatively severe symptoms.
- Overview of bleeding symptoms: The majority of these patients can be asymptomatic and present with hemorrhages after hemostatic challenge such as menstruation, and surgical procedures. Rarely patients with severe deficiency can present with symptoms of mucocutaneous bleeding, hemarthosis, and deep muscle hematoma. Life-threatening bleeding events, such as CNS appear to be less frequent than that in hemophilia, except in patients with factor XIII deficiency. About 24% patients with severe factor XIII deficiency (FXIII <1%) present with spontaneous ICH in the newborn period. It is also the major cause of death in midlife in patients with factor XIII deficiency. Besides bleeding symptoms, patients with dysfibrinogenemia and afibrinogenemia can present with strokes or thromboembolic events. Women with dysfibrinogenemia or afibrinogenemia can present with miscarriages.

D. Diagnosis of RBDs
- Detailed clinical history and a high index of suspicion is the key to diagnose RBDs. The majority of these patients are diagnosed either due to the

positive family history or history of unexpected bleeding when exposed to hemostatic challenge such as menstruation, labor and delivery and surgical procedures.

- Screening coagulation tests such as PT and APTT are usually sensitive enough to detect each of the coagulation factors except for factor XIII (see Chapter 10).
- Thrombin time (TT) is prolonged with fibrinogen deficiency.
- In patients with suspected functional abnormalities of the proteins such as dysfibrinogenemia and dysprothrombinemia, immunogenic assays are required to quantitate the antigen level in addition to measurement of functional levels.
- Factor XIII deficiency: Since all the screening tests are normal in patients with factor XIII deficiency, a specific assay, the 5 M urea clot solubility assay, is required to diagnose factor XIII deficiency. Since factor XIII is required for the cross-linking of fibrin monomers, this diagnostic test is based upon the observation that there is an increased solubility of the clot because of the failure to cross-link the fibrin monomers. The normal clot remains insoluble in the presence of 5 M urea, whereas the clot formed from a patient with factor XIII deficiency dissolves rapidly within hours. It is important to note that this method detects only severe factor XIII deficiency (with activity typically below 0.5 to 3%). More specific immunologic assays for factor XIII quantitation are also available in specialized laboratories and measure less severe forms of factor XIII deficiency.
- Scope of genetic testing for the diagnosis of RBDs: Unlike hemophilia, the molecular pathology of RBDs is not well-described. Therefore genetic testing for the diagnosis of RBDs is not available for clinical use.

E. Management of RBDs
- Similar to hemophilia, the management of RBDs focuses on treatment of acute bleeding events through factor replacement therapy.
- Specific concentrates for fibrinogen, factor VII, and factor XIII are available (Table 11.3). Prothrombin complex concentrates contain factors II, VII, IX and X and may be suitable for deficiencies of prothrombin or factor X. For the other RBDs, fresh frozen plasma remains an option for the treatment or prevention of major bleeding events. Conventionally, 10–20 mL/kg of FFP will often increase the factor levels by 10–20%. Volume overload and the potential for transmission of blood-borne pathogens discourage their routine use.

V. Miscellaneous bleeding disorders: deficiencies of inhibitors of fibrinolytic pathway

- **Deficiency** of either of the two inhibitors of plasmin, α-2 antiplasmin and plasminogen activator inhibitor-1 (PAI-1), results in increased plasmin generation and premature lysis of fibrin clots leading to a bleeding tendency.

Table 11.3 Characteristics and management of rare coagulation factor deficiencies and miscellaneous bleeding disorders

Coagulation disorder	Mode of inheritance	Diagnostic test	Specific treatment
FII deficiency Dysprothrombinemia	AR	Prolongation of PT and PTT Mixing studies: correction FII activity	FFP, PCC
FV deficiency	AR	Prolongation of PT and PTT Mixing study: correction FV activity	FFP, platelet transfusion
FX deficiency	AR	Prolongation of PT and APTT Mixing study: correction FX activity	FFP, PCC
Afibrinogenemia Hypofibrinogenemia Dysfibrinogenemia	AR/AD	Prolongation of PT, APTT and TT Mixing study: Correction Fibrinogen activity Fibrinogen antigen	Cryoprecipitate Fibrinogen concentrates FFP
Severe FXIII deficiency	AR	PT, APTT, TT: Normal Urea clot solubility test: early clot lysis F XIII quantitation	FXIII concentrates (FibroGammin-P) FFP
Miscellaneous bleeding disorders			
Disorders of fibrinolytic pathway: PAI-1 deficiency α_2-antiplasmin deficiency	AR	Clot lysis time <60 minutes PAI-1 activity and antigen levels α_2-antiplasmin activity and antigen levels	Antifibrinolytic agents: EACA, Tranexamic acid FFP

Abbreviations: AD, autosomal dominant; AR, autosomal recessive; CNS, central nervous system; EACA, epsilon amino caproic acid; F, factor; FEIBA, factor eight inhibitor bypassing activity; FFP, fresh frozen plasma; PAI-1, plasminogen activator inhibitor-1; PCC, prothrombin complex concentrates; PT, prothrombin time; PTT, partial thromboplastin time; TT, thrombin time; XR, X-linked recessive.
Mucocutaneous bleeding involves bruising, epistaxis, subcutaneous hematoma formation, epistaxis, menorrhagia.

- **Clinical symptoms:** These patients can experience mucocutaneous bleeding but rarely have joint hemorrhages.
- **Diagnosis:** The commonly used screening coagulation tests are normal in patients with these RBDs. Specific tests such as the euglobulin clot lysis time that measures fibrinolytic activity is shortened in the presence of these deficiencies. Specific assays for alpha-2-antiplasmin and PAI-1 quantitation are available at specialized laboratories.
- **Treatment of bleeding:** Antifibrinolytic drugs such as epsilon aminocaproic acid and tranexamic acid are the cornerstones of management of bleeding in these patients (Table 11.3). Rarely FFP is used as a source of these proteins to control severe bleeding.

Further reading

Dimichele D, Rivard G, Hay C, Antunes S. Inhibitors in haemophilia: clinical aspects. Haemophilia 2004;10(Suppl 4):140–5.

Mann KG. Biochemistry and physiology of blood coagulation. Thromb Haem 1999;82:165–74.

Mannucci PM, Tuddenham EG. The hemophilias—from royal genes to gene therapy. N Engl J Med 2001;344(23):1773–9.

Mannucci PM. Hemostatic drugs. New Engl J Med 1998;339(4):245–53.

Mannucci PM. Treatment of von Willebrand's disease. New Engl J Med 2004;351:83–94.

Peyvandi F, Palla R, Menegatti M, Mannucci PM. Introduction. Rare bleeding disorders: general aspects of clinical features, diagnosis and management. Semin Thromb Hemost 2009;35(4):349–55.

Pipe SW, High KA, Ohashi K, Ural AU, Lillicrap D. Progress in the molecular biology of inherited bleeding disorders. Haemophilia 2008;14(Suppl 3):130–7.

Pipe SW. Recombinant clotting factors. Thromb Haem 2008; 99(5):840–50.

12 | Acquired Bleeding Disorders

Howard A. Liebman

University of Southern California—Keck School of Medicine, Los Angeles, CA, USA

I. Introduction

Physiologic hemostasis results from the coordinated interaction of two systems; platelet activation with the subsequent formation of a platelet plug and the coagulation factor cascade leading to the generation of thrombin and fibrin plug formation. Congenital or acquired defects or deficiencies in either system can result in a bleeding disorder. The diagnosis of any bleeding disorder requires the taking of a careful history, physical examination and the use of specific clinical laboratory coagulation assays. The primary objective of this chapter is to provide an outline to the systematic approach to the diagnosis of acquired bleeding disorders. A listing of the common acquired bleeding disorders and their relationship to either defects in platelet plug formation, fibrin clot formation or both systems are listed in Table 12.1. Acquired defects in hemostasis are the most frequent cause of unexpected bleeding and a systematic approach to diagnosis is essential to providing appropriate therapy.

II. Diagnosis

A. Medical and bleeding history

A careful medical history is an essential first step in the diagnosis of an acquired bleeding history. While most inherited or congenital bleeding disorders have their onset during childhood, patients with mild hemophilia (factors VIII or IX >10% of normal levels), factor XI deficiency or type I von Willebrand disease may not present with major bleeding until adulthood after a hemostatic challenge. Therefore, the history should include questions regarding previous hemostatic challenges including surgery, dental procedures, trauma, contact sports, menstrual history, pregnancy and delivery.

Concise Guide to Hematology, First Edition. Edited by Alvin H. Schmaier, Hillard M. Lazarus.
© 2012 Blackwell Publishing Ltd. Published 2012 by Blackwell Publishing Ltd.

Table 12.1 Common acquired bleeding disorders grouped by defects in either platelet plug formation, coagulation cascade defects or both

Platelet plug formation defects	Coagulation cascade defects	Defects in both platelet plug formation and coagulation cascade
Immune thrombocytopenia	Anticoagulants: warfarin,	Advanced liver disease
Drug induced	heparins, direct thrombin	Disseminated
thrombocytopenia	inhibitors	intravascular
Antiplatelet medications:	Fibrinolytic drugs	coagulation
aspirin, thienopyridines,	Coagulation factor inhibitors	
GPIIb/IIIa inhibitors	Vitamin K deficiency	
Monoclonal immunoglobulins	Super warfarin ingestion	
	Massive transfusion	

The medical history should include a history of other medical disorders and co-morbidities such as liver or renal disease which are associated with acquired defects in hemostasis. Patients with a history of autoimmune disorders such as lupus erythematosis, rheumatoid arthritis or immune thyroid disease develop auto-antibodies directed against platelets resulting in immune thrombocytopenia or inhibitory antibodies directed against coagulation factors. The history should include all medication and supplements taken by the patient. Certain drugs can affect platelet function or induce drug-associated immune thrombocytopenia. Finally a careful family history determines if the patient may have a mild inherited bleeding disorder.

B. Physical examination

Physical examination assists in determining whether bleeding is the result of an acquired hemostatic defect in platelet plug formation or fibrin clot formation. Epistaxis, gum bleeding, ecchymosis and petechae suggest a defect in platelet plug formation as occurs with thrombocytopenia or platelet dysfunction. However, extensive ecchymosis are also seen with such disorders as spontaneous coagulation factor VIII inhibitors. An enlarged liver and spleen, abdominal ascites and jaundice suggest advanced liver disease with decreased production of clotting factors and trapping of platelets in an enlarged spleen (hypersplenism). Fever and hypotension are associated with sepsis and the development of acute thrombocytopenia and disseminated intravascular coagulation.

Rarer associations with physical findings even include the presence of gastrointestinal bleeding with the finding of a loud systolic heart murmur on cardiac auscultation consistent with severe aortic stenosis. Severe aortic stenosis has been associated with acquired type IIa von Willebrand disease and episodic gastrointestinal bleeding (Heyde's syndrome). In Heyde's syndrome bleed occurs secondary to a combination of gastrointestinal angiodysplasia and acquired von Willebrand disease secondary to accelerated von Willebrand factor cleavage induced by the high sheer forces occurring with the blood flow through the narrowed aortic valve.

By integrating patient history and physical examination findings a preliminary differential diagnosis frequently is formulated that assists in selecting diagnostic laboratory tests.

C. Laboratory diagnostic tests

There are four readily available laboratory screening tests that can be used to evaluate general hemostasis in patients with active bleeding. These include the complete blood count including the platelet count, prothrombin (Quick) time (PT), activated partial thromboplastin time (APTT), and quantitative fibrinogen (see Chapter 10). Thrombocytopenia is the most frequent acquired platelet disorder with spontaneous major bleeding rarely seen in platelet counts greater than 10,000/µL. Acquired functional platelet defects are evaluated in the clinical laboratory with instruments such as the platelet function analyzer or template bleeding time test. Nearly all acquired defects in platelet function are associated with the use of antiplatelet drugs such as aspirin, $P2Y_{12}$ ADP receptor antagonists (clopidogrel, ticlopidine, prasugel), platelet integrin antagonists ($\alpha_{2b}\beta_3$ or glycoprotein IIb/IIIa antagonists- abciximab, tirofiban, and eptifabatide) (see Table 12.1). Primary platelet function defects are quite uncommon.

Prolongation of the PT and/or APTT tests are characterized to determine whether the laboratory defect is due to either a deficiency of a coagulation factor or an acquired coagulation factor inhibitor by performing a mixing study. Mixing patient plasma with normal pooled plasma in equal amounts (50/50 mix) will provide sufficient amounts of a missing coagulation factor in a patient with a deficiency to correct an abnormal coagulation test into the normal range. If there is a coagulation factor inhibitor present in the patient plasma, the mixing test will not correct into the normal range. Most acquired inhibitors associated with bleeding are antibodies directed against a specific coagulation factor such as factor VIII or factor X (see Table 12.1). However, occasional bleeding results from an overdose of unfractionated heparin (UFH), or any anticoagulant, which would result in a prolonged APTT that would not correct in the mixing study. Any anticoagulant appears as an "inhibitor" on a mixing study.

III. Acquired bleeding associated with defective platelet plug formation alone

Patients with normal screening tests for fibrin plug formation, PT, APTT and fibrinogen are most frequently found to have quantitative or qualitative defects in platelets. Thrombocytopenia is the most frequent platelet abnormality associated with an acquired bleeding disorder. The differential diagnosis of congenital or acquired thrombocytopenias is discussed in the chapters on platelet disorders (Chapters 13 and 14). It should be emphasized that in the evaluation of acquired bleeding disorders due to thrombocytopenia, a careful review of the blood smear is necessary in formulating a differential diagnosis.

Medications used to inhibit platelet function are important agents in the management of arterial thrombotic disease and are utilized for either primary or secondary prevention of stroke or myocardial infarction. All antiplatelet agents can be associated with an increased risk of bleeding. Aspirin effectively inhibits the synthesis of thromboxane, an important amplifying agonist for platelet aggregation by its irreversible inactivation of platelet cyclooxygenase. The thienopyridine drugs, ticlopidine, clopidogrel and prasugrel, are inhibitors of the $P2Y_{12}$ platelet ADP receptor. They are used in patients with coronary artery vascular disease and patients who have had coronary stents placed. They are frequently used in combination with aspirin and result in potent inhibition of platelet aggregation. An increased risk of bleeding also has been noted in patients taking sensitive serotonin release inhibitors (SSRI) antidepressants, particularly when combined with other antiplatelet agents such as aspirin. SSRI produce an acquired storage pool disorder of platelets (see Chapter 13). Glycoprotein IIb/IIIa inhibitors, abciximab, tirofiban, and eptifabatide, are agents that block the ability of this important platelet receptor necessary for platelet aggregation. They are used primarily in the immediate period after pericutaneous coronary intervention to prevent reocclusion of a vessel after angioplasty. They are potent inhibitors of platelet function, but can also be associated with the rare development of acute thrombocytopenia. In most cases of bleeding due to medication induced-platelet dysfunction, transfusion of normal platelet concentrates can correct the bleeding diathesis.

Additional acquired platelet defects are seen following cardiopulmonary bypass surgery with partial release of alpha granules from platelets that have traveled through the membrane oxygenator heart lung machine. Renal failure also is associated with an acquired platelet defect, particularly in patients with anemia due to the deficiency of erythropoietin. The use of supplemental erythropoietin in patients with renal failure to maintain a near normal hemoglobin when combined with renal dialysis rapidly can correct platelet dysfunction. Patients with high concentrations of monoclonal immunoglobulins, as occurs with multiple myeloma and Waldenström's macroglobulinemia, can have a significant defect in platelet function due to the immunoglobulin non-specifically binding to and inhibiting platelet receptor function. Patients with multiple myeloma and Waldenström's macroglobulinemia also have defects in their coagulation factor assays, but bleeding episodes appear to be primarily due to platelet dysfunction. Treatment of the underlying plasma cell disorders to reduce the monoclonal immunoglobulin, either alone or combined with plasmapheresis, often corrects the platelet disorder.

IV. Acquired bleeding due to defects coagulation cascade alone

A. Anticoagulants and bleeding

The most common cause of acquired bleeding associated with defects in coagulation factor cascade function are in patients receiving oral or parenteral anticoagulants. The three commonly used families of anticoagulants are the oral vitamin K antagonists (warfarin); heparin type anticoagulants (unfractionated heparin [UFH], low molecular weight [LMW] heparins and fondaparinux); and the direct thrombin inhibitors (lepirudin, argatroban, bivalirudin, dabigatran). Also fibrinolytic agents (tissue plasminogen activator, single-chain urokinase plasminogen activator, plasmin) used to dissolve formed clots can result in major bleeding.

The oral vitamin K antagonists (VKA) (warfarin) inhibit the intracellular recycling of vitamin K resulting in a decrease in the functional vitamin K-dependent coagulation factors, factors II, VII, IX and X, as well as protein C and S in blood. Vitamin K antagonists are predominately agents used for primary or secondary (after a thrombotic event) prophylaxis. The safety of VKA therapy is achieved by monitoring the anticoagulant effect using the prothrombin time assay and converting the results to an international normalized ratio (INR). Studies have shown that a target INR of 2.5 (2.0 to 3.0) is generally safe in regards to bleeding and effective in preventing thrombosis. When a patient has an INR between 2 and 3, there are 5–15% functional vitamin K-dependent factors to maintain hemostasis. With careful monitoring the risk of major bleeding is 0.3 to 0.5%/year. However, the bleeding risk doubles with an INR greater than 3.0. The most feared complication is intracerebral bleeding which in nearly all cases is fatal. Important additional risk factors associated with an increased risk of bleeding on VKA include renal failure, age greater than 70 years, anemia and concomitant antiplatelet therapy. Treatment of bleeding on VKA is to give vitamin K and with major bleeding replace the missing coagulation factors with fresh frozen plasma, prothrombin complex concentrates, or recombinant FVIIa. Intracerebral hemorrhage on warfarin treatment is treated with prothrombin concentrate complex for rFVIIa infusion.

Heparin type anticoagulants mediate their inhibitory effect by activating the coagulation factor serine protease inhibitor antithrombin. The negatively charged heparins upon binding to lysine residues on antithrombin convert the protein from a slow acting inhibitor to a rapid acting inhibitor of thrombin, factor Xa and factor IXa. The size of the heparin molecule determines the specificity of the antithrombin activated coagulation inhibition. Smaller heparin molecules (i.e., <10 disaccharide units) (e.g., LMW heparin) preferentially inhibit factor Xa with less thrombin inhibition. The smallest heparin-like molecule, fondaparinux, is a synthetic pentasaccharide which upon binding antithrombin results in factor Xa inhibition alone. The heparin anticoagulants are broadly used for treatment of acute thromboembolism, medical and surgical prophylaxis, prevention of ischemic coronary events, and with various pericutaneous interventions. Due to their broad use, bleeding events are related to the indication (treatment or prophylaxis), patient situation (surgery or medical indication), dose of the heparin agent and additional cofactors that may increase the bleeding risk (age, renal insufficiency, antiplatelet therapy, post-surgical prophylaxis).

Bleeding risk appears to be the greatest with the use of UFH with major bleeding as high as 3% some trials. Despite monitoring by the APTT ratio, UFH can be associated with a bleeding risk of up to 2%. LMW heparin and fondaparinux are renally cleared from blood and their use in patients with renal insufficiency may be associated with a greater bleeding risk. Bleeding in patients receiving heparin anticoagulants is treated with supportive transfusions until the drug is cleared. Drug metabolism is usually 4–10 hours, depending upon the heparin preparation or fondaparinux. UFH can be reversed with infusions of protamine. A rare complication of heparin use is the development of heparin-induced thrombocytopenia and thrombosis syndrome (1–2% of patients who receive the medication [see Chapter 14]. This situation is rarely associated with bleeding, but is frequently associated the development of venous and arterial thrombosis due to heparin activating platelets leading to thrombosis.

The direct thrombin inhibitors inhibit thrombin by interacting with its active site, exosites, or both and their bleeding risk is proportional to their affinity towards thrombin, dose, half-lives, and clearance mechanisms. Argatroban is metabolized by the liver and thus its removal is altered in liver disease. Lepirudin, bivalirudin, and dabigatran are renally cleared and thus toxicity is more likely in patients with renal disease. These agents are primarily used to treat patients with heparin-induced thrombocytopenia, but have some indications for medical (alterative agents for cardiac catheterization, e.g., bivalirudin) and surgical prophylaxis. Dabigatran is used to prevent clots in atrial fibrillation. Their anticoagulant effects are not reversible and bleeding events are treated with supportive transfusions until the direct thrombin inhibitor is cleared from the blood.

B. Coagulation factor inhibitors

Coagulation factor inhibitors are rare acquired causes of major bleeding with abnormal coagulation assays. The most common are factor VIII and factor V inhibitor and acquired von Willebrand disease. Factor VIII inhibitors are antibodies that neutralize factor VIII activity resulting in acquired hemophilia. They develop most often in the elderly, younger women postpartum, patients with autoimmune disorders and patients with lymphoproliferative malignancies. Patients with factor VIII inhibitors have a prolonged APTT assay that does not correct with a mixing study. Patients with high inhibitory titers can have spontaneous soft tissue and intramuscular bleeding. Less commonly seen are acquired factor V inhibitors that result in both a prolonged

PT and APTT assay that does not correct with a mixing study. The development of factor V inhibitors occurs in a similar population to that of factor VIII inhibitors with the addition of individuals exposed to bovine thrombin preparation used for surgical hemostasis.

Bleeding in patients with factor VIII inhibitors can be treated with activated prothrombin complex products or recombinant factor VIIa to bypass the block in the coagulation cascade due to the loss of factor VIII co-factor activity. Patients are also given immunosuppressive drugs to suppress the production of the inhibitory antibody. Patients with Factor V inhibitors are frequently treated with a similar therapeutic approach. In some patients with high titer inhibitors against factor V, plasmapheresis may also be employed.

Acquired von Willebrand disease is associated with a prolongation of the APTT and platelet function studies. The disorder is different from factor VIII or V inhibitors in that the acquired antibody against von Willebrand factor does not inhibit the activity of the factor, but clears it with its associated factor VIII from the blood. The disease frequently develops in patients with monoclonal immunoglobulin disorders such as benign monoclonal gammopathy, multiple myeloma or Waldenström macroglobulinemia. Bleeding events in patients with acquired von Willebrand disease respond to treatment with infusions of von Willebrand factor concentrates, desmopressin (DDAVP) and intravenous immunoglobulin. Immunosuppressive agents are less effective in removing the antibodies in this disorder.

C. Other disorders

Vitamin K deficiency is a less common cause of prolongation of coagulation assays. It is rarely observed, but can occur in patients who are not eating and on long-term antibiotics. It is seen most commonly in patients receiving intravenous feedings due to serious illness. A disorder in newborn infants due to vitamin K deficiency has generally disappeared from western societies since newborn infants are now given an injection of vitamin K at birth. Occasionally a patient who has attempted suicide with the long activating superwarfarin rodenticide, brodifacoum, will present with major bleeding. These patients will be treated similar to warfarin associated bleeding, but will require long-term vitamin K supportive care until the drug is cleared from the liver which can take months.

Massive transfusion has been defined as the replacement of more than 1.5 blood volume in 24 hours. For example, in the 70 kg man, 7% of body weight, or 4.9 kg or L, is the blood volume ($\approx$16–19 units, assuming that a unit of blood is 250–300 mL). Hemostatic failure can result from dilution of clotting factors, DIC, or acquired platelet dysfunction. Dilutional coagulopathy results from replacement with packed red blood cells and normal saline and lack of clotting factors or platelets. Additionally, each unit of infused blood product contains approximately 1/6th volume of anticoagulant usually consisting of acid citrate dextrose. This anticoagulant chelates free calcium, making it less available for blood coagulation reactions. Thus patients become functionally calcium depleted. Tests of hemostasis typically show prolongation of PT and APTT, reduced fibrinogen, and thrombocytopenia. This condition is seen after major hemorrhage associated with surgery or in battlefield management of acute wounds. Current management trends treat massive wounds with 1 unit of fresh frozen plasma for every unit of red blood cells infused. Calcium replacement is also needed to overcome the anticoagulant chelation of ionized calcium.

V. Acquired bleeding due to defects in both platelet plug formation and coagulation cascade

Liver disease is the most common disorder associated with acquired abnormalities in platelets and coagulation factors. The liver is the primary site for the synthesis of all coagulation factors except von Willebrand factor and factor VIII. Severe hepatocellular disease can result deficiencies leading to prolongations in both the PT and APTT assays. With hepatic cirrhosis, there is increased portal venous hypertension resulting in splenic enlargement, sequestration of platelets and ultimately thrombocytopenia. The latter can be particularly significant in patient with hepatitis C cirrhosis since this virus is associated with an additional immune platelet destruction. In addition, there is some evidence that patients with advanced liver disease have excessive fibrinolytic activity. Major bleeding in patients with advanced liver disease with hepatic cirrhosis is treated with coagulation factor replacement via fresh frozen plasma and platelet concentrates. Patients with increased fibrinolytic activity may benefit from the addition of a fibrinolytic inhibitor such as epsilon aminocaproic acid (AMICAR).

Systemic activation of coagulation leads to a syndrome of coagulation factor and platelet consumption. Disseminated intravascular coagulation (DIC) is a syndrome associated with a number of systemic disorders (see Chapter 14). It can occur with severe bacterial and viral infections, large volume tissue trauma, heparin-induced thrombocytopenia, hypotension due to blood loss or metastatic cancer and several obstetrical castrophes such as placenta previa, abruption placenta, and retained dead fetus. These disorders result in generalized thrombin generation with coagulation factor consumption, platelet activation and induction of secondary fibrinolysis. There are two forms of DIC, an acute variety mostly associated with a hyperfibrinolytic state and a bleeding disorder. This form of DIC is most commonly recognized. Patients with acute DIC have prolongations of both the PT and APTT assays, may have low plasma fibrinogen levels, thrombocytopenia and elevations of markers of thrombin generation such as the D-dimer test. The D-dimer assay, that best characterizes this condition, measures thrombin-cleaved, insoluble cross-linked fibrin that has been liberated by generated plasmin (Chapter 9). Finding evidence for simultaneous thrombin and plasmin formation is the biochemical characterization of DIC. Treatment is supportive with transfusion of coagulation factors and platelets, but success and patient survival is dependent on reversal of the initiating cause. The second form of DIC is the so-called chronic variety, associated with malignancy, connective tissue disorders and antiphospholipid antibody syndrome. This form of the disorder is clinically associated with vasculitis and thrombosis. In the laboratory, one may find a positive d-dimer, normal PT and APTT and the fibrinogen may be normal or elevated. Treatment for this condition is directed towards the underlying disease.

Further reading

Feinstein DI. Immune coagulation disorders. Chapter 60. In: Colman R, Hirsh J, Marder VJ, Clowes AW, George JN, eds. Hemostasis and Thrombosis: Basic Principles and Clinical Practice, 4th edn. Philadelphia, PA: Lippincott Williams & Wilkins, 2001:1003–1020.

Liebman HA, Weitz IC: Disseminated intravascular coagulation. Chapter 132. In: Hoffman R, Benz EJ, Shattil SJ, Furie B, Cohen HJ, Silbertein L, McGlave P, eds. Hematology: Basic Principles and Practice, 5th edn. New York, NY: McGraw-Hill, 2008:2231–6.

Patrono C, Balgent C, Hirsh J, Roth G. Antiplatelet drugs. American College of Chest Physicians Evidence Based Clinical Practice Guidelines, 8th edn. Chest 2008;133 (Supplement):199S–233S.

Schulman S, Beyth RJ, Kearon C, Levine MN. Hemorrhagic complications of anticoagulant and thrombolytic treatment. American College of Chest Physicians Evidence Based Clinical Practice Guidelines, 8th edn. Chest 2008;133(Supplement):257S–298S.

13 Platelet Function in Hemostasis and Inherited Disorders of Platelet Number and Function

A. Koneti Rao and David W. Essex

Sol Sherry Thrombosis Research Center, Temple University School of Medicine, Philadelphia, PA, USA

I. Platelet structure

Blood platelets are anucleate fragments derived from bone marrow megakaryocytes. They are 1.5–3.0 μm in diameter with a volume of ~7 fL. Electron microscopy reveals a fuzzy coat (glycocalix) on the platelet surface composed of membrane glycoproteins (GP), glycolipids, mucopolysaccharides and plasma proteins. The plasma membrane is a bilayer of phospholipids in which cholesterol, glycolipids and glycoproteins are embedded. Platelets have an elaborate channel system, the open canalicular system, which is composed of invaginations of the plasma membrane. In addition, they have a dense tubular system, a closed-channel network derived from the smooth endoplasmic reticulum; it is the major site of platelet thromboxane synthesis. The discoid shape of resting platelets is maintained by a cytoskeleton consisting of a spectrin membrane skeleton, a microtubule coil, and an actin scaffold.

Platelets contain several organelles: mitochondria and glycogen stores, lysosomes, dense granules and alpha granules. The dense (δ) granules contain calcium, ATP, ADP, magnesium and serotonin. The alpha (α) granules contain numerous proteins, including β-thromboglobulin (βTG) and platelet factor 4 (PF4), which are considered platelet-specific, several higher molecular mass coagulation factors, (e.g., fibrinogen, factor V, high molecular weight kininogen, factor XIII), von Willebrand factor (vWF), growth factors (e.g., platelet-derived growth factor, vascular endothelial growth factor), protease inhibitors (e.g., plasminogen activator inhibitor-1, C1 inhibitor, amyloid-β-protein precursor), thrombospondin, P-selectin. albumin and IgG. The lysosomes contain acid hydrolases and other enzymes.

Concise Guide to Hematology, First Edition. Edited by Alvin H. Schmaier, Hillard M. Lazarus.
© 2012 Blackwell Publishing Ltd. Published 2012 by Blackwell Publishing Ltd.

II. Platelet function in hemostasis

A. Adhesion

Following injury to the blood vessel, platelets adhere to exposed subendothe-lial collagen (adhesion), which involves among other events the interaction of a plasma protein, von Willebrand factor (vWF), and a specific glycoprotein complex on the platelet surface, glycoprotein (GP) Ib–IX–V (Figure 13.1). This interaction is particularly important for platelet adhesion under conditions of high shear stress (i.e., high blood flow). Glycoprotein VI also contributes to platelet adhesion to collagen under conditions of flow.

B. Aggregation

Adhesion is followed by recruitment of additional platelets which form clumps, a process called aggregation. This process involves binding of fibrino-gen to specific platelet surface receptors—a complex comprised of glycopro-teins IIb and IIIa (GPIIb–IIIa, integrin $\alpha IIb\beta_3$) (Figure 13.1). Binding of fibrinogen to platelets is a prerequisite for aggregation. On platelet activation, the GPIIb–IIIa complex undergoes a conformational change and acquires the ability to bind fibrinogen.

C. Secretion (release reaction)

Activated platelets release contents of their granules including from dense granule, alpha granules and the lysosomal vesicles. ADP and serotonin released from the dense granules further enhance the platelet activation proc-esses. For example, ADP released from the granules interacts with receptors on platelets to enhance the activation process.

D. Platelet procoagulant activities

Several key enzymatic reactions of blood coagulation occur on the platelet membrane lipoprotein surface. During platelet activation negatively charged phospholipids, especially phosphatidylserine, translocate from the inner aspect of the plasma membrane to the platelet surface (Figure 13.1). This translocation is an essential step in accelerating specific coagulation reactions that occur on the platelet surface and leading to thrombin generation.

III. Platelet activation mechanisms

A number of physiological agonists interact with receptors on the platelet surface to induce responses, including a change in platelet shape from discoid to spherical, aggregation, secretion, and thromboxane A_2 (TxA_2) production. Selected aspects of platelet activation are shown in Figure 13.1. Activation of platelet surface receptors initiates the production of several intracellular mes-senger molecules, including products of hydrolysis of phosphoinositide by phospholipase C (diacylglycerol and inositol 1,4,5-triphosphate), TxA_2 and cyclic nucleotides (cAMP) (Figure 13.1). These induce or modulate the various

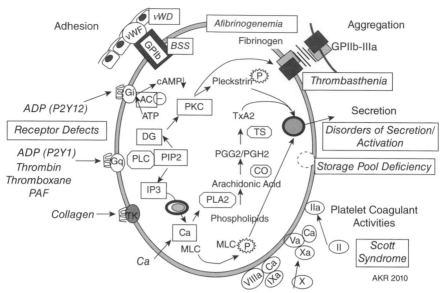

Figure 13.1 Schematic representation of selected aspects of platelet responses to activation and inherited disorders of platelet function. Following vessel wall injury, platelets adhere to subendothelium and this is mediated by binding of vWF to platelet GPIb (left upper section of figure). Platelet aggregation is mediated by the interaction of fibrinogen with the GPIIb–IIIa complex on platelet surface (right upper corner). Platelets possess receptors for several agonists, such as ADP, thrombin, thromboxane A_2 and collagen. Receptor activation results in the formation of intracellular mediators that regulate the end-responses, such as aggregation and secretion. Activation of intracellular enzymes on receptor activation is mediated by GTP-binding proteins (G). Responses to collagen are mediated by tyrosine kinase (TK)-dependent mechanisms. Receptor activation leads to hydrolysis of phosphatidylinositol bisphosphate (PIP_2) to form diacylglycerol (DAG), which activates protein kinase C (PKC), and inositoltrisphosphate (IP_3), which mediates the rise in cytoplasmic Ca^{2+} levels. This increase in Ca^{2+} levels leads to other responses, such as activation of myosin light chain kinase (MYLK) to phosphorylate myosin light chain (MLC) and activation of phospholipase A_2 (PLA_2), which mediates the release of free arachidonic acid from phospholipids. Arachidonic acid is converted by cyclooxygenase (CO) and thromboxane synthase (TS) to thromboxane A_2. As a result of several of these mechanisms, platelets release granule contents (secretion). Moreover, platelets play a major role in blood coagulation mechanisms by providing the membrane surface on which several of the key reactions occur (platelet coagulant activities). The coagulation factors are shown by Roman numerals in circles. The figure also shows some of the inherited disorders of platelet function. *Disorders of adhesion* arise due to defects/ deficiency in GPIb complex (Bernard–Soulier syndrome, BSS) or in plasma vWF (von Willebrand disease, vWD). *Disorders of aggregation* arise due to defects in GPIIb-IIIa on platelets or the absence of plasma fibrinogen (right upper corner). *Defects in platelet activation mechanisms and secretion* may occur secondary to deficiencies of platelet surface receptors (receptor defects) and defects at the level of G-proteins and in other signal transduction events (described in the text). In *storage pool deficiency*, secretion is impaired because the granules or their contents are decreased. Several patients have been described with *defects in thromboxane A_2 synthesis* due to deficiencies of phospholipase A_2, cyclooxygenase or thromboxane synthase. In the Scott syndrome the contribution of platelets to the coagulation system is impaired. (Modified with permission from Rao AK. Am J Med Sci 1998;316:69–77.)

platelet responses such as the rise in cytoplasmic Ca^{2+} concentration, protein phosphorylation, aggregation, secretion, and TxA_2 production. The interaction between the platelet surface receptors and the key intracellular enzymes (e.g., phospholipases A_2 and C, adenylyl cyclase) is mediated by a group of GTP-binding proteins that function as molecular switches. Platelet activation results in a rise in cytoplasmic ionized calcium concentration. $InsP_3$ functions as a messenger to mobilize Ca^{2+} from intracellular stores. Diacylglycerol activates protein kinase C (PKC) resulting in the phosphorylation of several proteins. PKC activation plays a major role in platelet secretion and in the activation of GPIIb-IIIa. GTP-binding protein Gαq mediates the activation of phospholipase C-β2 on activation of platelet $P2Y_1$-ADP, thrombin, thromboxane and other receptors. Gαi mediates the inhibition of adenylyl cyclase on platelet activation with $P2Y_{12}$-ADP receptor and other receptors. Lastly, Gαs stimulates adenylyl cyclase to increase cAMP levels in platelets. Numerous other mechanisms, such as activation of tyrosine kinases and phosphatases, are also triggered by platelet activation.

IV. Regulation of platelet number

Platelets are produced from bone marrow megakaryocytes; approximately 1×10^{11} platelets are produced daily. The normal platelet count is 150,000–400,000/μL (Atlas Figure 8). Platelets have a life-span in blood of 7–10 days. The number of circulating platelets is regulated by thrombopoietin (TPO), which is synthesized in the liver and binds to megakaryocytes and hematopoietic stem cells via the TPO receptor, c-Mpl. Because of this binding, there is an inverse relationship between platelet mass and circulating TPO levels.

V. Inherited disorders of platelets

Two categories of inherited platelets disorders are recognized: disorders associated with thrombocytopenia and those characterized by impaired platelet function. Some patients may have a combination of inherited thrombocytopenia and platelet dysfunction.

VI. Inherited thrombocytopenias

The clinical spectrum of inherited thrombocytopenias ranges from severe bleeding early in life to being asymptomatic into adulthood. It is important to distinguish between immune thrombocytopenias and the hereditary thrombocytopenias in order to avoid unnecessary potentially harmful treatment. Inherited thrombocytopenias can be classified by the inheritance pattern, clinical features (age of presentation or presence of associated non-platelet abnormalities) or platelet size. Platelet size on the peripheral blood smear provides diagnostic clues. These disorders are described here based on the inheritance pattern. Table 13.1 shows them classified by platelet size.

Table 13.1 Inherited thrombocytopenias classified by platelet size		
Large/giant platelets (MPV >11 fL)	Normal platelets (MPV 7–11 fL)	Small platelets (MPV <7 fL)
MYH9 thrombocytopenias* (e.g., May–Hegglin anomaly) Mediterranean thrombocytopenia* Paris–Trousseau thrombocytopenia* Gray platelet syndrome* Velocardiofacial/DiGeorge syndrome* Bernard–Soulier syndrome† GATA1 mutations**	RUNX1 abnormalities* Congenital amegakaryocytic thrombocytopenia† Thrombocytopenia with absent radii†	Wiskott–Aldrich syndrome** X-linked thrombocytopenia**
MPV = mean platelet volume. *Autosomal dominant inheritance. †Autosomal recessive inheritance. **X-linked disorder.		

A. Autosomal dominant thrombocytopenias

1. MYH9-related thrombocytopenia syndromes

These syndromes are caused by mutations in the *MYH9* gene that encodes non-muscle myosin-heavy chain IIa and includes the May–Hegglin anomaly and other entities with associated clinical features such as nephritis, deafness and cataracts. The thrombocytopenia is mild to moderate with large or giant platelets and mild bleeding. Neutrophils have large blue cytoplasmic inclusions called Döhle-like bodies (Atlas Figure 30) which is non-muscle myosin heavy-chain IIA in the May–Hegglin variant (Figure 13.2).

2. Mediterranean macrothrombocytopenia

This disorder is a relatively common mild form of macrothrombocytopenia in southern Europe and is without significant bleeding. The thrombocytopenia is identified incidentally during routine blood testing. This disorder is due to a mutation in GpIbα with impaired expression.

3. RUNX1-related mutations

These patients have mild bleeding but have a marked predisposition for acute leukemia and familial platelet dysfunction. They have mutations or deletions in hematopoietic transcription factor RUNX1.

4. Paris–Trousseau thrombocytopenia

Platelets are larger than normal in this disorder and are characterized by giant α-granules. It is associated with mutations involving transcription factor FLI-1 and the bone marrow has increased immature megakaryocytes. Mental retardation, facial and cardiac abnormalities are associated features.

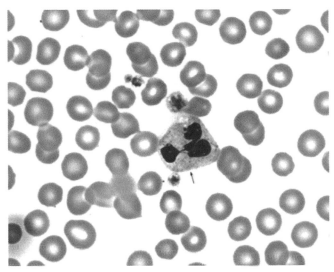

Figure 13.2 Peripheral smear showing a giant platelet and a granulocyte inclusion called Dohle bodies in a patient with May Hegglin syndrome. (Reprinted with permission from Lazarchick J et al. ASH Image Bank 2008;8-00023.)

5. Gray platelet syndrome
This entity is characterized by reduced or absent α-granules in platelets that appear gray color on Wright–Giemsa stain. The defects are in granule formation and targeting of proteins to the granules. Some of these patients have macrothrombocytopenia.

6. Velocardiofacial/DiGeorge syndrome
These syndromes are caused by deletions in chromosome 22 and have only mild thrombocytopenia without significant bleeding. They are characterized by cardiac abnormalities, parathyroid and thymus insufficiencies, cognitive impairment, and, in some, facial abnormalities.

B. Autosomal recessive thrombocytopenias
1. Congenital amegakaryocytic thrombocytopenia
This entity is a severe thrombocytopenia (<10,000 platelet/μL) that presents in the newborn with absence of megakaryocytes in the bone marrow. Affected infants are identified within days to weeks of birth because of bleeding. Leukocyte and erythrocyte production is decreased leading to pancytopenia by the second decade. This disorder is caused by mutations in the thrombopoietin receptor *c-Mpl*.

2. Thrombocytopenia with absent radii (TAR)
Affected individuals have shortened or absent forearms bilaterally due to defects in radius development with severe thrombocytopenia at birth

requiring platelet transfusion. Thrombocytopenia becomes less severe during the first year of life.

3. Bernard–Soulier syndrome
This macrothrombocytopenia has marked platelet dysfunction with severe bleeding (see below). The mutation is in the GpIb, which forms the binding site on platelets for vWF.

C. X-linked disorders
1. Wiskott–Aldrich syndrome (WAS)
This syndrome affects males with moderate to severe microthrombocytopenia, immunodeficiency and eczema. WAS usually presents within the first year of life with bruising and bleeding and recurrent infections with eczema developing after the first year. The underlying defect is a mutation in the WAS protein (WASP) that links the cellular cytoskeleton with signal transduction pathways. The thrombocytopenia often improves after splenectomy. Stem cell transplantation is curative. A large proportion of patients with mutations in WASP exhibit a milder form of X-linked thrombocytopenia. These patients have residual WASP and do not have significant eczema or immunodeficiency.

2. GATA-1 mutation X-linked macrothrombocytopenia with dyserythropoiesis
This disorder has marked thrombocytopenia (10,000–40,000/μL) with bruising and severe bleeding, and a variable degree of anemia. It is caused by mutations in the hematopoietic transcription factor GATA-1. The bone marrow is hypercellular with dysplastic features in the megakaryocytic and erythroid lineages.

VII. Inherited disorders of platelet function

A. General features
Patients with inherited disorders of platelet function are characterized by mucosal bleeding (epistaxis, menorrhagia, gastrointestinal bleeding) and cutaneous bleeding. There is a wide variability in bleeding manifestations.

B. Evaluation of platelet function
1. Platelet count and size and peripheral blood smear
The evaluation of patients with inherited platelet defects starts with a platelet count and examination of the peripheral smear to detect alterations in platelet morphology. If the platelet count is normal, approximately 8–15 platelets are visible in each oil-immersion (×1000) field; one platelet is observed for every 20 erythrocytes.

2. Bleeding time
The bleeding time test involves making an incision on the volar surface of the forearm under standardized conditions (i.e., with a blood pressure cuff inflated to 40 mmHg) and monitoring the time it takes for the bleeding to stop (normal range is 2–8 min). It is prolonged in many patients with von Willebrand's

disease, disorders of platelet function and when platelet counts are less than 70,000/ul, and in certain connective tissue disorders like pseudoxanthoma elastica and scurvy. It is not used frequently any more due to its variability.

3. Platelet aggregation studies

These are performed using platelet-rich plasma (PRP) prepared from blood. Light transmission through a glass cuvette containing PRP is monitored in an instrument called the aggregometer. Following addition of an agonist (e.g., ADP, collagen, epinephrine, arachidonic acid, and ristocetin) platelets in a stirred cuvette form clumps thereby increasing the light transmission, which is recorded. On addition of an agonist (e.g., ADP, epinephrine) to normal platelets there is an initial wave of aggregation (primary wave), which is followed by release of granule contents and thromboxane production leading to a secondary wave and irreversible aggregation. With agonists such as, thrombin, collagen and arachidonic acid only one large wave of is generally discerned without a distinct second wave. Platelet dense granule secretion is measured, by monitoring the release of ATP or using radioactive 5-hydroxytryptamine (serotonin), which is incorporated by platelets into the dense granules.

4. Platelet function analyzer (PFA-100)

The platelet function analyzer (PFA)-100 measures platelet adherence under shear by passing whole blood through an aperture in a membrane coated with collagen in combination with ADP or epinephrine. The time to closure of the aperture is measured. In many disorders of platelet function the closure time is prolonged.

C. Classification of inherited disorders of platelet function

Box 13.1 provides a classification of inherited disorders of platelet function based on the platelet function or responses that are abnormal (Figure 13.1). Not all of the disorders are due to a defect in the platelets *per se*. Some, such as the von Willebrand disease (vWD) and afibrinogenemia, result from deficiencies of plasma proteins essential for platelet-endothelial and platelet-platelet interactions. In many patients with inherited platelet dysfunction, the underlying molecular mechanisms remain unknown.

D. Disorders of platelet adhesion

In patients with defects in platelet-vessel wall interactions, adhesion of platelets to subendothelium is abnormal. The two disorders in this group are von Willebrand disease (vWD) (see Chapter 11) due to a deficiency or abnormality in plasma vWF, and the Bernard–Soulier syndrome (BSS) in which platelets are deficient in GP Ib (and GP V and GP IX). In both disorders, platelet-vWF interaction is compromised.

1. Bernard–Soulier syndrome (BSS)

BSS is a rare autosomal recessive platelet function disorder resulting from an abnormality in platelet GP Ib–IX–V complex, which mediates the binding of vWF to platelets. GP Ib exists in platelets as a complex consisting of

---

Box 13.1 Inherited disorders of platelet function

1. **Defects in platelet-vessel wall interaction (disorders of adhesion)**
   (a) von Willebrand disease (deficiency or defect in plasma vWF)
   (b) Bernard–Soulier syndrome (deficiency or defect in GPIb)
2. **Defects in platelet-platelet interaction (disorders of aggregation)**
   (a) Congenital afibrinogenemia (deficiency of plasma fibrinogen)
   (b) Glanzmann's thrombasthenia (deficiency or defect in GPIIb–IIIa)
3. **Disorders of platelet granules, secretion and activation**
   (a) Disorders of granules
      (i) Storage pool deficiency (δ, α, $\alpha\delta$)
      (ii) Quebec platelet disorder
   (b) Disorders of platelet activation and signal transduction mechanisms
      (i) Defects in platelet agonist receptors (thromboxane A_2, ADP receptors ($P2Y_{12}$), epinephrine, platelet activating factor)
      (ii) GTP-binding protein defects (Gαq deficiency, Gαi1 deficiency, Gαs hyperfunction,
      (iii) Phospholipase C-β_2 deficiency and defects in phospholipase C activation, calcium mobilization, and protein phosphorylation (PKC-θ deficiency)
   (c) Defects in thromboxane A_2 synthesis (deficiency of phospholipase A_2, cyclooxygenase, or thromboxane synthase)
4. **Disorders of platelet coagulant–protein interaction (Scott syndrome)**
5. **Other disorders**
   (a) Defects related to cytoskeletal/structural proteins
      (i) Wiskott–Aldrich syndrome
   (b) Abnormalities of transcription factors leading to functional defects
      (i) RUNX1 mutations (familial platelet dysfunction with predisposition to acute myelogenous leukemia)
      (ii) GATA-1 mutations

---

glycoproteins Ib, IX and V, and it is reduced in the BSS due to mutations in GPIb. The bleeding time is markedly prolonged, platelet counts are moderately decreased and platelets are markedly increased in size. In platelet aggregation studies, the responses to ADP, epinephrine and collagen are normal. Characteristically, the aggregation in platelet-rich plasma in response to the antibiotic ristocetin is decreased or absent, a feature shared with patients with vWD. However, unlike in vWD, plasma vWF and factor VIII are normal in BSS. The diagnosis of BSS is established by demonstrating decreased platelet surface GPIb, most commonly by flow cytometry.

E. Disorders of platelet aggregation

Binding of fibrinogen to the GPIIb–IIIa (integrin αIIbβ_3) complex is a prerequisite for platelet aggregation. Disorders characterized by abnormal platelet-platelet interactions (aggregation disorders) arise because of a quantitative or qualitative abnormality of the platelet membrane GP IIb–IIIa complex, which binds fibrinogen (Glanzmann thrombasthenia). In the absence of plasma fibrinogen (inherited afibrinogenemia) also platelet aggregation is absent. In general, as little as 50 µg/mL fibrinogen is adequate for normal platelet aggregation.

1. Glanzmann thrombasthenia

Glanzmann thrombasthenia is a rare autosomal recessive disorder character- ized by markedly impaired platelet aggregation, a prolonged bleeding time, and severe mucocutaneous bleeding manifestations. In thrombasthenia there is a quantitative or qualitative defect in this complex arising due to a mutation in either GP IIb or GP IIIa gene. Because of this, fibrinogen binding to platelets and aggregation are impaired. Clot retraction, a function of the interaction of GP IIb–IIIa (αIIbβ_3 integrin) with the platelet cytoskeleton, is also impaired. The diagnostic hallmark of thrombasthenia is absence or marked decrease of platelet aggregation in response virtually to all agonists (except ristocetin), with absence of both the primary and the secondary wave of aggregation (Figure 13.3). Platelet dense granule secretion may be decreased with weak

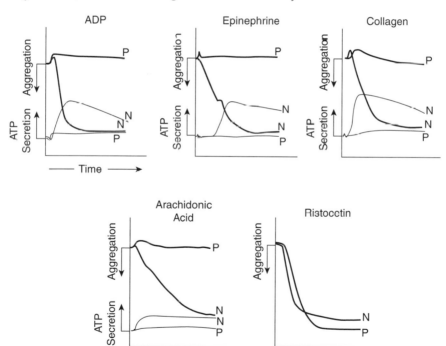

Figure 13.3 Aggregation and ATP secretion studies in Glanzmann thrombasthenia performed using a lumi-aggregometer and platelet-rich plasma (PRP). Shown are aggregation (upper tracings in each panel) and ATP secretion (lower tracings) in the patient (P) and a healthy subject (N) in response to ADP (7.5 µM), epinephrine (7.5 µM), collagen (1 µg/mL), ristocetin (1.5 mg/mL) and arachidonic acid (1 mM). With all agonists except ristocetin neither the primary wave nor the secondary wave of aggregation are noted in the patient, and secretion is decreased.

agonists (e.g., ADP, epinephrine) but normal on activation with thrombin. Heterozygotes have ~50% of platelet GP IIb–IIIa complexes, have no bleeding symptoms and the platelet aggregation responses are normal. The diagnosis of thrombasthenia is established by demonstrating a defect or deficiency of the integrin receptor, generally by flow-cytometry.

2. Inherited afibrinogenemia
Although inherited afibrinogenemia is also characterized by an absence of platelet aggregation responses, the PT, APTT, and thrombin time are markedly prolonged, whereas they are normal in thrombasthenia.

F. Disorders of platelet granules, secretion and activation
Patients lumped in this heterogeneous group are generally characterized by impaired dense granule secretion and absence of the second wave of aggregation upon stimulation of platelet-rich plasma with ADP or epinephrine; responses to collagen, thromboxane analog (U46619), or arachidonic acid may also be decreased. Platelet function is abnormal in these patients either when the granule contents are diminished as in storage pool deficiency (SPD) leading to decreased secretion or when signaling mechanisms are impaired leading to decreased aggregation and secretion (Box 13.1).

1. Deficiency of granule stores (storage pool deficiency)
The term storage pool deficiency refers to patients with deficiencies in platelet content of dense granules (δ-SPD), alpha-granules (α-SPD, gray platelet syndrome) or both types of granules (αδ-SPD).

Patients with *δ-storage pool deficiency* (δ-SPD) have a mild to moderate bleeding diathesis associated with a prolonged bleeding time. In the platelet studies, the second wave of aggregation in response to ADP and epinephrine is usually absent or blunted and the collagen response is markedly impaired (Figure 13.4). Normal platelets possess 3–8 dense granules (each 200–300 nm in diameter). Under the electron microscope, dense granules are decreased in SPD platelets. By direct biochemical measurements, the platelet ATP and ADP contents are decreased along with other dense granule constituents. δ-SPD has been reported in association with other inherited disorders such as the Hermansky–Pudlak syndrome (HPS) (characterized by oculocutaneous albinism and increased reticuloendothelial ceroid, and associated with mutations in the *HPS* and other genes), the Chediak–Higashi syndrome (defect in *LYST* or *CHS1* gene, see Chapter 16), the Wiskott–Aldrich syndrome (*WASP* gene defect), and the thrombocytopenia-absent-radii (TAR) syndrome. There is a large group of HPS patients in northwest Puerto Rico.

Chediak–Higaski syndrome is a rare autosomal recessive disorder characterized by SPD, oculocutaneous albinism, immune deficiency, neurological symptoms and presence of giant cytoplasmic inclusions in different cells.

Patients with the *"gray-platelet syndrome"* (GPS) have an isolated deficiency of platelet α-granule contents. The platelets have a gray appearance with

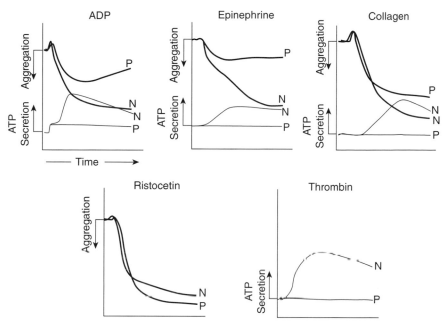

Figure 13.4 Aggregation and ATP secretion studies in δ-storage pool deficiency. Shown are responses the patient (P) and a healthy subject (N) to ADP (7.5 µM), epinephrine (7.5 µM), collagen (1 µg/mL), ristocetin (1.5 mg/mL) and thrombin (2 U/mL). In the patient only the primary wave of aggregation is noted with ADP and epinephrine; aggregation is blunted with collagen. Secretion is decreased with all agonists except ristocetin. With thrombin only secretion is shown because addition of thrombin induces clotting of fibrinogen and does not permit recording of aggregation.

paucity of granules on the peripheral blood smears. These patients have a bleeding diathesis, mild thrombocytopenia and a prolonged bleeding time. The platelets are deficient in α-granule proteins including platelet factor-4, β-thromboglobulin, and vWF. Platelet aggregation responses to ADP and epinephrine are normal in most patients; in some patients aggregation responses to thrombin, collagen, and ADP are impaired.

The *Quebec platelet disorder (QPD)*, another disorder affecting the platelet granules, is an autosomal dominant disorder associated with delayed bleeding and abnormal proteolytic degradation of α-granule proteins (including fibrinogen, factor V, vWF, thrombospondin, multimerin and P-selectin) due to increased amounts of platelet urokinase type plasminogen activator (uPA). This results from duplication of a 78 kb segment that includes *PLAU*, the gene for uPA.

G. Defects in platelet activation mechanisms

Signal transduction mechanisms encompass processes that are initiated by the interaction of agonists with specific platelet receptors and include responses such as G-protein activation and activation of phospholipase C and phospholipase A_2 (Figure 13.1).

Patients with receptor defects have impaired responses because of an abnormality in the platelet surface receptor for a specific agonist. Such defects have been documented for receptors for ADP ($P2Y_{12}$), thromboxane A_2, collagen (GP VI or GPIa/IIa; $\alpha_2\beta_1$), and epinephrine (Figure 13.1). Patients with the ADP receptor abnormalities have had a defect in the $P2Y_{12}$ ADP receptor, which is coupled to inhibition of adenylyl cyclase mediated by the G-protein $G\alpha i$ (Fig 13.1).

G-proteins link surface receptors and intracellular effector enzymes and *defects in G-protein activation* have impaired signal transduction. Patients with platelet defects in G-proteins $G\alpha q$, $G\alpha i1$ and $G\alpha s$ have been described.

Patients have been described with impaired signal transduction due to *defects in phospholipase C activation, calcium mobilization and pleckstrin phosphorylation* (Figure 13.1). Defects in phospholipase C-$\beta 2$ and protein kinase C-θ have been documented.

A major platelet response to activation is liberation of arachidonic acid from phospholipids and its subsequent oxygenation to thromboxane A_2. Patients have been described with impaired thromboxane synthesis due to *inherited deficiencies of cyclooxygenase and thromboxane synthase* and *phospholipase A_2*.

H. Disorders of platelet procoagulant activities
Platelets provide the surface on which several specific key enzymatic reactions occur (Figure 13.1). Platelet activation results in a redistribution of phospholipids with expression of phosphatidylserine on the outer surface. This phospholipid translocation is essential to the expression of platelet procoagulant activities. A few patients have been described in whom the platelet contribution to blood coagulation is impaired and this is referred to as the *Scott syndrome*. In these patients the bleeding time and platelet aggregation responses have been normal.

I. Other abnormalities
Platelet function abnormalities have been described in the *Wiskott–Aldrich syndrome* (WAS), and in patients with mutations in transcription factors, RUNX1, and GATA-1; all three are also associated with thrombocytopenia.

J. Therapy of inherited platelet function defects
Because of the wide variation in bleeding manifestations, management of these patients needs to be individualized. Platelet transfusions are indicated in the management of clinically relevant bleeding and in preparation for surgical procedures. Transfusion therapy has potential risks including alloimmunization in patients lacking specific platelet glycoproteins. For example, patients with thrombasthenia and BSS may develop antibodies against GP IIb–IIIa and GPIb, respectively, that compromise the efficacy of subsequent platelet transfusions. An alternative to platelet transfusions is intravenous administration of DDAVP, which induces the release of vWF from endothelial cells and shortens the bleeding time in some patients with platelet function

defects. Infusion of recombinant factor VIIa has been used in the management of bleeding events in thrombasthenia and other inherited defects. It induces increased thrombin generation *in vivo*. DDAVP and recombinant FVIIa are not currently FDA approved for management of patients with inherited platelet defects.

Further reading

Coller BS, French DL, Rao AK. Hereditary qualitative platelet disorders. In: Kaushansky K, Lichtman M, Beutler E, Kipps T, Seligsohn U, Prchal J, eds. Williams Hematology, 8th edn. New York: McGraw-Hill, 2010:1933–70.

Drachman JG. Inherited thrombocytopenia: when a low platelet count does not mean ITP. Blood 2004;103:390–8.

Nurden P, Nurden AT. Congenital disorders associated with platelet dysfunctions. Thromb Haemost 2008;99:253–63.

Rao AK. Hereditary disorders of platelet secretion and signal transduction. In: Colman RW, Marder VJ, Clowes AW, George JN, Goldhaber SZ, eds. Hemostasis and Thrombosis: Basic Principles and Clinical Practice, 5th edn. Philadelphia: Lippincott Williams & Wilkins, 2006:961–74

CHAPTER 14

14 Acquired Thrombocytopenia

Theodore E. Warkentin[1] and Andrew E. Warkentin[2]

[1]Michael G. DeGroote School of Medicine, McMaster University, Hamilton, ON, Canada
[2]University of Toronto, Toronto, ON, Canada

I. Introduction

Thrombocytopenia (combination of medical terms, "thrombocyte" [*platelet*] and "penia" [*deficiency*], based upon Greek "thrombos" [*clot*]; "kytos" [*container*, with modern meaning of *cell*]; and "penia" [*poverty*]) indicates reduced platelet count numbers. Depending on its cause, thrombocytopenia can indicate increased risk of bleeding, thrombosis, and/or mortality. Thus, when faced with a thrombocytopenic patient, the clinician's key question is: *what is the probable cause of the patient's thrombocytopenia?* The answer will point to the appropriate prognostic and therapeutic considerations.

II. Definition

The normal platelet count range is approximately 150,000 to 400,000/μL (150 to 400×10^9/L); thus, "thrombocytopenia" usually indicates a platelet count <150,000/μL. Conceptually, thrombocytopenia infers any pathological reduction in platelet numbers, and thus a large decrease in the platelet count that does not necessarily fall below 150,000/μL can also indicate thrombocytopenia, e.g., a >50% platelet count fall from 400,000 to 175,000/μL during the second postoperative week as a sign of heparin-induced thrombocytopenia (HIT). Thrombocytopenia can be classified as mild (100,000–150,000/μL), moderate (50,000–100,000/μL), severe (<50,000/μL) or very severe (<20,000/μL).

III. Clinical features of thrombocytopenia

A. **Hemorrhage** is a potential complication of thrombocytopenia (Table 14.1).
B. **Sites of bleeding**
    1. **Cutaneous** (various types of purpura, e.g., petechiae [pin-point hemorrhages located in regions of increased hydrostatic pressure, e.g., dorsa

Concise Guide to Hematology, First Edition. Edited by Alvin H. Schmaier, Hillard M. Lazarus.
© 2012 Blackwell Publishing Ltd. Published 2012 by Blackwell Publishing Ltd.

Table 14.1 Clinical manifestations of thrombocytopenia	
Clinical context	*Clinical manifestations*
Bleeding (increased risk seen with many causes of thrombocytopenia)	
Platelet count, <75,000 to 100,000/µL	Increased bleeding with surgery and trauma
Platelet count, <20,000/µL	Increased risk of spontaneous mucocutaneous hemorrhage
Platelet count, <10,000/µL	Increased risk of spontaneous intracranial hemorrhage
Thrombosis (increased risk depends on particular cause of thrombocytopenia)	
Heparin-induced thrombocytopenia	Thrombosis, especially large veins and arteries
Disseminated intravascular coagulation	Thrombosis, especially microvascular
Thrombotic microangiopathy (TTP, HUS)	Thrombosis, especially small arteries/ arterioles (CNS, renal)

of feet in ambulatory patients, lower back in bedridden patients, upper chest/face in ventilated patients], or ecchymoses [purpura >2 mm in diameter], often associated with trauma, e.g., venipuncture sites).

2. **Mucosal** (epistaxis, menometrorrhagia [heavy, irregular menstrual periods], hemorrhagic bullae in mouth [blood blisters], gastrointestinal [GI] or genitourinary [GU] bleeding.

3. **Central nervous system (CNS).**

C. **Thrombosis** is a feature of certain thrombocytopenic disorders (Table 14.1).

1. **Large vein and/or artery thrombosis** is typical of HIT and cancer-associated disseminated intravascular coagulation (DIC).

2. **Microvascular thrombosis** can complicate thrombocytopenia associated with DIC; sometimes, acral (distal extremity) ischemic necrosis occurs despite palpable limb pulses.

3. **Small artery/arteriolar thrombosis** is characteristic of thrombotic thrombocytopenic purpura (TTP) and hemolytic-uremic syndrome (HUS).

D. **Increased mortality** is associated with thrombocytopenia in critically-ill patients with multi-organ failure.

IV. Classification of thrombocytopenia

There are five general mechanisms of thrombocytopenia (Table 14.2), plus pseudothrombocytopenia:

A. **Decreased platelet production** (marrow disorders).

B. **Hemodilution** (e.g., postoperative).

C. **Sequestration** (hypersplenism).

D. **Increased platelet consumption** (thrombin- and von Willebrand factor [VWF]-mediated).

Table 14.2 Classification of thrombocytopenia

Classification	Picture	Mechanisms
Decreased platelet production	Pancytopenia or isolated thrombocytopenia*	Injured or abnormal stem cells result in reduction in all three cell lines
Hemodilution	Bicytopenia or pancytopenia	Administration of fluids, especially during surgery, associated with abrupt decrease in concentration of platelets and red cells; white cell count may remain normal or increase due to acute inflammation
Sequestration	Pancytopenia	Hypersplenism (trapping of all three cell lines in enlarged spleen)
Increased platelet consumption	Isolated thrombocytopenia (DIC) or thrombotic microangiopathy (TTP, HUS)	Increased thrombin generation explains thrombocytopenia in DIC; increased VWF-platelet-subendothelial interactions are associated with thrombotic microangiopathy in TTP and HUS
Increased platelet destruction	Isolated thrombocytopenia	Antibody-mediated platelet clearance by mononuclear-phagocytic (reticuloendothelial) system (auto-, allo-, and drug-dependent antibodies); exception: platelet-activating antibodies characterize HIT
Pseudothrombo-cytopenia	Platelet clumps or platelet rosetting on neutrophils	Spurious thrombocytopenia that results when electronic particle counter fails to identify platelets

*Certain disorders of decreased platelet production result in isolated thrombocytopenia, rather than pancytopenia: e.g., MYH9-associated macrothrombocytopenia, alcohol-induced thrombocytopenia, acquired amegakaryocytic thrombocytopenia, and some patients with myelodysplasia.

E. **Increased platelet destruction** (immune-mediated).

F. **Pseudothrombocytopenia** (spurious thrombocytopenia).

V. Decreased platelet production

A. Pancytopenia

Many bone marrow disorders feature reduction in circulating red cells, white cells, and platelets ("pancytopenia") (Table 14.3). Bone marrow megakaryocytes are usually decreased in number, either in the setting of marrow aplasia/hypoplasia, or because of replacement by fibrosis, tumor, or hypercellular (megaloblastic) marrow.

1. **Primary bone marrow disorders (congenital/hereditary)** (see Chapters 13 and 18).
   (a) Fanconi anemia.
   (b) Miscellaneous hereditary aplastic anemia.
   (c) Congenital (intrauterine) infections

Table 14.3 Thrombocytopenia caused by decreased platelet production	
Congenital/hereditary	*Acquired*
Pancytopenia	
Primary bone marrow disorders	Primary bone marrow disorders:
Fanconi anemia	acquired aplastic anemia,
Miscellaneous aplastic anemias	leukemia, myelodysplasia
Dykeratosis congenita	Bone marrow infiltration:
Schwachmann–Diamond syndrome	Metastatic cancer
Congenital intrauterine infection	Myelofibrosis
Rubella	Infectious diseases (e.g.,
Cytomegalovirus	tuberculosis)
Herpes virus	Bone marrow injury:
Echovirus	Drugs (e.g., chemotherapy,
Toxoplasmosis	chloramphenicol)
Syphilis	Chemicals (e.g., benzene)
	Radiation
	Megaloblastic anemia (B_{12} or folate
	deficiency)
	Copper deficiency
Isolated thrombocytopenia	
Thrombocytopenia-absent radius (TAR) syndrome	Alcohol-induced thrombocytopenia
Miscellaneous syndromic hypomegakaryocytic	Iron depletion or repletion
thrombocytopenia	Acquired amegakaryocytic
Congenital amegakaryocytic thrombocytopenia	thrombocytopenia
Wiskott–Aldrich syndrome (WAS) and variant WAS	
MYH9-associated thrombocytopenia*	

*Hereditary thrombocytopenia may not be recognized until adulthood, and thus mimic an "acquired" thrombocytopenia, if previous platelet count values from childhood and infancy are not available.

2. **Primary bone marrow disorders (acquired)** (see Chapters 18 and 19):
   (a) Acquired aplastic anemia.
   (b) Leukemia.
   (c) Myelodysplasia.
3. **Bone marrow infiltration:**
   (a) Metastatic cancer to the bone marrow, most often breast and prostate cancer, causes "myelophthisis", manifesting as leukoerythroblastosis (left shift in circulating granulocytes—metamyelocytes, myelocytes, promyelocytes, and rarely myeloblasts—and nucleated red blood cells) and "tear drop" red cells (dacrocytes).
   (b) Myelofibrosis with myeloid metaplasia also produces myelophthisis due to fibrotic infiltration (see Chapter 18).
   (c) Infectious diseases sometimes cause marrow infiltration by microbes, e.g., disseminated tuberculosis or histoplasmosis in AIDS.
4. **Bone marrow injury.** Rapidly dividing marrow progenitor cells are susceptible to a variety of injuries:

(a) Drugs. Antineoplastic agents produce predictable, transient pancyto-penia; a few drugs (e.g., chloramphenicol, penicillamine, gold, car-bamazepine) rarely cause idiosyncratic (immune-mediated) aplastic anemia.

(b) Chemicals such as benzene can cause bone marrow injury.

(c) Radiation causes predictable pancytopenia, and in large amounts pro-duces fatal marrow failure.

5. **Nutritional disorders:**

(a) Megaloblastic anemia due to vitamin B_{12} or folate deficiency can produce pancytopenia; marked red cell macrocytosis is a clue.

(b) Copper deficiency complicating total parenteral nutrition or after bowel surgery is a rare cause of pancytopenia.

B. Isolated thrombocytopenia

Certain megakaryocytic disorders produce isolated thrombocytopenia (Table 14.3). Bone marrow aspirate/biopsy can reveal a "hypomegakaryocytic" picture (reduced/absent megakaryocytes) whereas normal megakaryocyte numbers suggest ineffective thrombopoiesis.

1. **Hypomegakaryocytic:**

(a) Thrombocytopenia-absent radius (TAR) syndrome features bilateral absent radii and hypomegakaryocytic thrombocytopenia (also see Chapter 13). Thrombocytopenia is usually most severe during the first year of life, improving subsequently. Occasionally thrombocytopenia begins in adulthood.

(b) Miscellaneous syndromic hypomegakaryocytic thrombocytopenia includes trisomy 18, trisomy 13, and radioulnar synostosis (proximal fusion of ulna and radius), among others.

(c) Congenital amegakaryocytic thrombocytopenia without skeletal or other congenital abnormalities is a rare autosomal recessive disorder involving mutations in c-mpl (thrombopoietin receptor) (see also Chapter 13).

2. **Microthrombocytopenia:**

(a) Wiskott–Aldrich syndrome (WAS) is an X-linked immunodeficiency disorder characterized by eczema, recurrent infections, increased risk of malignancy, and thrombocytopenia with small platelets caused by mutations in WAS protein (WASp). Stem cell transplantation is curative (see also Chapter 13).

(b) X-linked thrombocytopenia (variant WAS) is a less severe version of WAS also due to mutations in the WASp gene (see also Chapter 13).

3. **MYH9-associated macrothrombocytopenia** is autosomal dominant and caused by mutations in non-muscle myosin heavy-chain-9 (see Chapter 13). Platelet size is greatly increased, causing falsely-low platelet counts by electronic particle counters. Patients are often misdiagnosed as having immune (idiopathic) thrombocytopenic purpura (ITP). As the thrombocy-topenia may not be recognized until adulthood, the patient is often wrongly considered to have an acquired thrombocytopenia. Petechiae are

uncommon, whereas ecchymoses and menorrhagia often occur. Depending on the specific mutation, a variety of overlapping syndromes are recognized.

4. **Hereditary thrombocytopathic disorders** can feature thrombocytopenia, for example: gray platelet syndrome (absence of platelet α-granules) and Bernard–Soulier syndrome (absence of the GP Ib/IX/V complex) (see Chapter 13).

5. **Alcohol-induced thrombocytopenia** indicates acute, self-limited thrombocytopenia due to heavy drinking. The platelet count begins to rise 2 to 3 days after cessation of alcohol consumption, with "rebound" thrombocytosis. Bone marrow aspirate reveals reduced megakaryocyte numbers and sometimes vacuolation of normoblasts and promyelocytes.

6. **Iron depletion or repletion** can cause mild-to-moderate thrombocytopenia, either evident at presentation of severe iron deficiency anemia, or as a transient platelet count decline seen approximately one week after beginning iron replacement therapy.

7. **Acquired amegakaryocytic thrombocytopenia** features isolated thrombocytopenia with marked reduction or absence of megakaryocytes. Autoimmune mechanisms are implicated in some patients, and therapy with antithymocyte globulin, high-dose corticosteroids, and/or cyclosporine may be of benefit.

VI. Hemodilution

A. **Administration of fluid (crystalloid, colloid) and/or blood products,** usually in surgery/trauma settings, is a common explanation for thrombocytopenia. The platelet count nadir (lowest value) is reached 1 to 4 days (median, day 2) following surgery (Figure 14.1). Rebound thrombocytosis— reaching levels ~2–3 times the baseline (preoperative) platelet count— peaks at approximately day 14.

B. **Gestational thrombocytopenia.** The platelet count decreases by ~10–20% during normal pregnancy; given the ~30–50% increase in plasma volume during pregnancy, physiological hemodilution contributes to mild gestational thrombocytopenia in women with low-normal pre-pregnancy platelet counts.

VII. Sequestration (hypersplenism)

A. Hypersplenism
Hypersplenism, the reduction in one or more peripheral blood counts due to sequestration within an enlarged spleen—is a common cause of chronic thrombocytopenia. Hypersplenism arises with inflamed or congested spleen, but not with infiltrative disease such as that seen with metastatic cancer.

1. **Pathophysiology.** Usually, one-third of total body platelets reside within the spleen, even though the spleen receives only 5% of cardiac output. This discrepancy results because the splenic transit time of a platelet averages

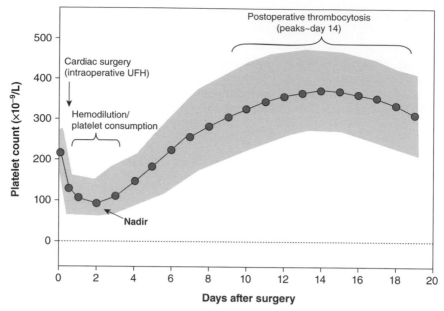

Figure 14.1 Timeline of postoperative thrombocytopenia and thrombocytosis. Intra/postoperative administration of crystalloid, colloid, and blood products results in *dilutional thrombocytopenia*, with the platelet count nadir reached between postoperative days 1 to 4, inclusive (median, day 2). Subsequently, postoperative thrombocytosis occurs, with platelet counts reaching levels approximately 2 to 3 times the preoperative baseline, and peaking usually at approximately day 14, with return to baseline over the subsequent 1 to 2 weeks. The closed circles and shaded area indicate mean ± 1 SD.

20 minutes, as opposed to ~1 minute for a platelet to return to the heart after passing through other organs. In hypersplenism, the proportion of platelets within the spleen can far exceed one-third (as high as ~90%).

2. **Clinical features** include splenomegaly and usually mild-to-moderate pancytopenia. The normal spleen is ~11 cm in length, but the spleen usually needs to be enlarged by at least 2 or 3 cm to be palpable, and thus diagnosis is most reliably made through imaging studies (e.g., ultrasound). Often, the degree of anemia is not as marked as neutropenia and thrombocytopenia. Especially severe thrombocytopenia can indicate advanced cirrhosis (with reduced thrombopoietin levels) and/or hyperfibrinolysis.

3. **Etiology** of hypersplenism in North America usually reflects primary hepatic disease (alcoholic cirrhosis, chronic viral hepatitis, etc.), whereas in some parts of the world other factors are common (e.g., schistosomiasis). Causes of hypersplenism include congestive splenomegaly (Banti's syndrome), splenic vein thrombosis, Felty's syndrome associated with rheumatoid arthritis, myeloproliferative or myelodysplastic disorders, malaria, chronic myelogenous leukemia, kala azar (leishmaniasis).

4. **Treatment** is usually not required, as thrombocytopenia rarely reaches clinically important levels, and splenectomy is not without risk.

B. Hypothermia

Hypothermia in the setting of surgery, exposure, or hypothalamic dysfunction is reported to cause thrombocytopenia in both infants and adults; platelet counts correct upon rewarming. Transient hepatosplenic sequestration was identified by platelet kinetic studies in animals.

VIII. Increased platelet consumption

Shortened platelet lifespan arising from mechanisms accelerated beyond that seen in normal physiology can be described as "consumptive" disorders. Pathologically increased thrombin generation—often called "disseminated intravascular coagulation (DIC)" or "consumptive coagulopathy"—often produces thrombocytopenia. Decreased platelet survival (with or without overt DIC) due to macrophage-mediated clearance is common in sepsis. VWF-mediated platelet clearance seen in thrombotic microangiopathy (TMA) will be classified as a platelet consumption disorder.

A. Disseminated intravascular coagulation

The central concept of DIC is dysregulated thrombin generation. DIC is not a single entity, but rather comprises several heterogeneous syndromes with many different triggers and potentiators. In order to diagnose DIC, the patient must have an underlying disorder associated with DIC, as well as laboratory evidence of generation of fibrin(ogen) degradation products, and accelerated—usually decompensated—consumption of one or more elements of the hemostatic mechanism (thrombocytopenia, hypofibrinogenemia, elevated international normalized ratio [INR] or activated partial thromboplastin time [APTT]).

1. **Acute DIC** (see also Chapter 12) has numerous causes, including:
   (a) Trauma, burns, shock (circulatory, septic) is a common cause of DIC in hospitalized patients.
   (b) Infection, most notably meningococcemia, where tissue necrosis results from acquired protein C depletion and associated microvascular thrombosis (purpura fulminans).
   (c) Obstetrical complications such as placental abruption, amniotic fluid embolism, preeclampsia/eclampsia, puerperal sepsis, and saline-induced abortion.
   (d) Malignancy, e.g., promyelocytic leukemia (see also chronic DIC).
   (e) Allergic/anaphylactic reactions.
   (f) Heparin-induced thrombocytopenia (HIT) features increased *in-vivo* thrombin generation, but in 10–15% of cases overt (decompensated) DIC with low fibrinogen and/or elevated international normalized ratio (INR) occurs.
   (g) Severe hemolysis, e.g., due to incompatible blood transfusion.
2. **Chronic DIC** (see also Chapter 12) has numerous triggers, including:
   (a) Malignancy, especially metastatic adenocarcinoma: patients often develop venous and/or arterial thrombosis, and thrombocytopenia

that improves with unfractionated heparin (UFH) or low-molecular-weight heparin (LMWH) anticoagulation; warfarin can produce micro-thrombosis due to protein C depletion (warfarin-associated venous limb gangrene).

(b) Obstetrical complications, particularly the dead fetus syndrome can cause chronic DIC and bleeding when delivery eventually occurs.

(c) Kasabach–Merritt syndrome denotes the combination of hemangioma (usually in the skin) and consumptive thrombocytopenia/coagulopathy, often presenting at birth or infancy. Although the blood picture is evocative of DIC, the disorder represents *localized* (not disseminated) consumptive coagulopathy.

(d) Abdominal aortic aneurysm often with ulcerated plaque and adherent thrombus can manifest as thrombocytopenia and consumptive coagulopathy (localized consumptive coagulopathy).

B. Sepsis from bacteremia, fungemia, or parasitemia (±DIC)

Often, microbial invasion of the bloodstream is complicated by consumptive thrombocytopenia, with or without concomitant DIC. It is for this reason why blood cultures should be performed in patients (usually hospitalized) with unexplained acute illness and thrombocytopenia. When DIC is present, thrombin likely contributes to the thrombocytopenia (thrombin is a potent platelet agonist). However, in the absence of DIC, increased macrophage-mediated platelet clearance and, perhaps, decreased platelet production occur. Thrombocytopenia that occurs after 2–3 weeks of hospitalization, especially in a patient who has received antibiotics, suggests fungemia (e.g., candidemia). World-wide, malaria is the most common parasite causing thrombocytopenia.

C. Cardiovascular disorders

Increased platelet consumption has been linked to cardiovascular disorders.

1. **Cardiopulmonary bypass (CPB).** Use of CPB ("heart–lung machine") is associated with an average 50% (range, 30–70%) decline in platelet count, although mostly due to hemodilution, with a small component of platelet consumption within the device itself. Bleeding results from thrombocytopenia, platelet dysfunction, hyperfibrinolysis, and surgical factors.

2. **Catheters and prostheses.** Platelet lifespan is somewhat reduced in patients with prosthetic heart valves, pulmonary artery and other intra-arterial catheters, and Dacron vascular grafts, but thrombocytopenia is uncommon due to compensatory increase in platelet production.

3. **Congenital heart disease.** Decreased platelet lifespan and thrombocytopenia are seen in cyanotic congenital heart disease, particularly with marked hypoxemia and polycythemia.

4. **Valvular heart disease** can evince mild thrombocytopenia due to increased platelet consumption. (However, GI bleeding from angiodysplasia associated with aortic stenosis—Heyde's syndrome—results not from

thrombocytopenia but rather from acquired deficiency of the largest VWF multimers due to increased VWF proteolysis/clearance at high shear caused by aortic stenosis; aortic valve replacement rapidly and permanently corrects the VWF multimer profile and thereby cures the GI bleeding.)
5. **Primary pulmonary hypertension** can be complicated by increased platelet consumption due to unknown mechanisms.
6. **Pulmonary embolism** occasionally features moderate or even severe thrombocytopenia, due either to DIC or because of associated HIT.

D. Thrombotic microangiopathy
Thrombocytic microangiopathy (TMA), also known as microangiopathic hemolytic anemia (MHA), is characterized by schistocytic hemolysis and thrombocytopenia (schistocytes are red cell fragments, including triangular forms and "helmet" cells) (Atlas Figures 17 and 18).
1. **Thrombotic thrombocytopenic purpura (TTP)** is characterized by TMA and organ dysfunction due to platelet-VWF aggregates within arterioles. Affected organs include brain (confusion, dysarthria, stroke), kidneys (oliguric renal failure), heart (dysrrhythmias, infarction, cardiac arrest), etc. Thrombocytopenia is often very severe (platelet count $<20,000/\mu L$).
   (a) Idiopathic TTP is most common, and often accompanied by acquired deficiency of the VWF-cleaving protease, ADAMTS13 (a disintegrin and metalloprotease with thrombospondin-like motifs-13). It rarely can also be congenital (Upshaw–Schulman syndrome) due to ADAMTS13 deletions, mutations, and missense defects. Risk factors for TTP include female sex and African-American race; most patients are middle-aged. Usually, there is little activation of coagulation (no/minimal evidence for DIC). Serum lactate dehydrogenase levels (marker of intravascular hemolysis) and platelet counts are useful parameters to judge disease activity and response to treatment. Primary therapy includes plasma exchange and high-dose corticosteroids. Rituximab (off-label indication) appears effective for refractory/recurrent TTP if the condition is acquired and there is an antibody to ADAMTS13.
   (b) Autoimmune disorders, particularly systemic lupus erythematosus (SLE), can be complicated by TTP or a TTP-mimicking disorder. This latter group of patients usually has hypertension with vasculitis and microangiopathic changes.
   (c) Pregnancy/post-partum TTP. Pregnancy is a risk factor for TTP.
   (d) Post-surgery/post-pancreatitis TTP suggests that acute inflammation rarely can trigger TTP, as affected patients develop TMA 2–7 days later.
   (e) Drug-induced and hematopoietic stem cell transplantation-associated TTP. Quinine (most often), antiplatelet agents (ticlopidine, clopidogrel), chemotherapy (e.g., gemcitabine, mitomycin C), and cyclosporine can cause TMA. Distinguishing the role of drugs versus effects of transplantation can be difficult when TMA occurs post-marrow transplantation. Whereas quinine can trigger TTP abruptly, other drugs

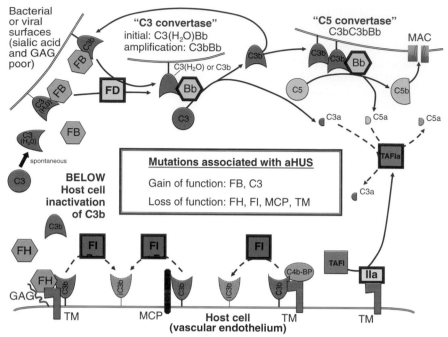

Figure 14.2 The alternative complement pathway: implications for pathogenesis of aHUS. The central molecule of the complement cascade, C3 (see far-left of figure), undergoes a continuous low level of spontaneous hydrolysis, yielding C3(H$_2$O), which is "C3b-like". When C3(H$_2$O) binds to an abnormal *activating* cell surface (i.e., lacking sialic acid and glycosaminoglycan [GAG]), such as a bacterium or virus (see top-left of Figure), the C3(H$_2$O) binds factor B (FB), forming a complex which is cleaved by factor D (FD) to form C3(H$_2$O)Bb, i.e., the "initial" C3 convertase of the alternative pathway). This initial C3 convertase cleaves C3 into C3b (the key effector molecule of the complement system) and C3a (anaphylatoxin). C3b also binds to FB, and the complex is cleaved by FD to form C3bBb, i.e., the "amplification" C3 convertase of the alternative pathway. A positive feedback loop is created, as the initial constitutive generation of low levels of C3(H$_2$O) leads to formation of much greater amounts of C3b via this process. If sufficient C3b is generated, some binds to C3bBb, forming "C5 convertase" (C3bC3bBb), which converts C5 to C5a (anaphylatoxin) and C5b; ultimately, if formed in sufficient quantities, C5b leads (via a number of steps involving C6, C7, C8, and C9, not shown) to formation of the membrane attack complex (MAC) that lyses bacteria/viruses through pore formation in their outer structures (see top-right of figure). Host cells (see bottom half of figure) have a number of fluid-phase and membrane-anchored protective regulatory mechanisms. For example, FH binds to host cells via GAG or sialic acid, and acts as a cofactor to enhance an enzyme, factor I (FI), to cleave C3b into an inactive product (iC3b), releasing a small peptide (C3f, not shown). Unlike C3b, C3bi is unable to participate in formation of C3 convertase, and thus is unable to continue the alternative complement pathway. In addition, membrane cofactor protein (MCP), which is highly expressed on renal endothelium, also acts as a cofactor to promote FI cleavage of C3 into iC3b and C3f. Another membrane-anchored protein, thrombomodulin (TM), has at least three functions relating to complement regulation: first, TM enhances inactivation of C3b by FI in the presence of FH (bottom-left of figure), as well as in the presence of C4b-binding protein (C4b-BP) (bottom-middle of figure); second, TM catalyzes activation of thrombin activatable fibrinolysis inhibitor (TAFI) by thrombin (IIa), with activated TAFI (TAFIa) degrading C3a and C5a (bottom-and middle-right of figure); and third, IIa bound to TM is unable to cleave C5 into C5a and C5b (not shown). A transmembrane protein, decay-accelerating factor (DAF; not shown), dissociates C3bBb into C3b and Bb, but C3b can bind to another FB molecule if it is not

(gemcitabine, mitomycin) require significant drug accumulation. Transplantation-associated TMA is not caused by ADAMTS13 deficiency and plasma exchange is ineffective. Clopidogrel- or ticlopidine-induced TTP is associated with reduced ADAMTS13 levels and antibodies to ADAMTS13.

2. **TTP-mimicking disorders** include:
   (a) Paravalvular leak ("macroangiopathic" hemolysis) is suggested by schistocytic hemolysis without thrombocytopenia beginning weeks or months after cardiac valve repair/replacement.
   (b) HIV infection can produce a TMA picture.
   (c) Malignant hypertension: Approximately one-quarter of patients with malignant hypertension have associated TMA.
   (d) Vasculitic disorders, e.g., systemic sclerosis and Wegener's granulomatosis, can be associated with TTP.
   (e) HELLP syndrome (**h**emolytic anemia, **e**levated **l**iver enzymes, **l**ow **p**latelets) is an obstetric TMA disorder associated with preeclampsia with increased fetal/maternal morbidity and mortality.

3. **Hemolytic-uremic syndrome (HUS)** is characterized by TMA plus prominent renal dysfunction. Despite clinical overlap with TTP, the lack of reduced ADAMTS13 levels and the unique bacterial trigger indicate a distinct etiology and pathogenesis.
   (a) Typical HUS indicates preceding bloody diarrhea (D+ HUS) triggered by certain bacteria, most often verocytotoxin-producing *Escherichia coli* O157:H7 and O104:H4, and *Shigella*. Most patients are at extremes of age (children, elderly). Compared with TTP, oliguric renal failure is more prominent, and non-renal involvement less common. The bacterial infection arises from diet (e.g., unwashed/raw spinach, contaminated/undercooked hamburger meat, bean sprouts).
   (b) Atypical HUS (aHUS) or non-enteropathic HUS (D– HUS) indicates HUS associated with complement system dysregulation, especially in the constitutively-active alternative pathway (e.g., mutations in

---

Figure 14.2 *Continued*

proteolyzed by FI (acting with one of the two cofactors, FH or MCP) in the interim. The surface carbohydrate environment to which C3b is deposited determines the relative affinity of C3b for FH or FB. On host cells (bearing sialic acid and GAG), FH binds to C3b with a higher affinity than does FB. On microbial surfaces (lacking sialic acid and GAG), however, FB binds to C3b with a higher affinity than does FH, leading to amplified cleavage of C3. "Loss of function" mutations of several proteins of the alternative complement pathway produce uncontrolled activation of complement, as C3b is not degraded efficiently, leading to excess formation of C3 and C5 convertases. This predisposes affected patients to aHUS, with the percentages in parentheses indicating the frequency by which the particular complement protein abnormality has been identified in familial and sporadic aHUS: FH (15–30%), MCP (10–15%), FI (5–10%) and TM (5%). Autoantibodies against FH have also been reported as causing aHUS (6–11%). As well, certain "gain of function" mutations in FB (1–2%) and C3 (5–10%) also predispose patients to aHUS. Solid arrows indication activation events; dashed arrows indicate inhibitory actions. Factors with heavy solid borders have enzymic activity.

complement factor H, factor I, membrane complement protein (MCP), thrombomodulin, C3, factor B) (Figure 14.2); approximately 50% of patients with aHUS have a complement factor mutation. Compared with typical HUS, there is no prodromal GI illness, and patients are at greater risk of permanent renal failure. These patients primarily present with a microangiopathic hemolytic anemia and renal failure and have less prominent thrombocytopenia. Only approximately half of the patients with these genetic abnormalities develop aHUS (50% penetrance), indicating that other factors (e.g., infection, pregnancy) are required to initiate the microangiopathic process.

IX. Increased platelet destruction

Increased platelet destruction indicates reduced platelet lifespan caused by autoantibodies, alloantibodies, or drug-dependent antibodies, which target platelet surface glycoproteins or other structures.

A. (Auto)immune thrombocytopenic purpura (ITP)

The classic 1951 report of Harrington and coworkers describing abrupt, severe thrombocytopenia following infusion of plasma from ITP patients into normal subjects proved a humoral factor—subsequently identified as platelet-reactive IgG—as the cause of ITP. The antibodies usually bind to platelet surface glycoproteins IIb/IIIa and/or GPIb/IX through their Fab "arms", producing reticuloendothelial clearance when antibody Fc bind to macrophage Fc receptors. Thrombopoietic agents in ITP increase impaired platelet production which is recognized as an additional pathogenetic factor in the disorder. The fundamental trigger for ITP is unknown. The clinical picture differs between children and adults.

1. **Acute ITP of childhood** usually follows a viral illness, and is characterized by severe, but usually transient, thrombocytopenia. Corticosteroids and/or high-dose IVIgG are given for severely symptomatic children.
2. **Chronic ITP of childhood** indicates duration >1 year, and resembles ITP in adults. But unlike adults, splenectomy is usually avoided in children (greater risk of post-splenectomy sepsis).
3. **Acute ITP in adults** usually represents the initial presentation of chronic ITP.
4. **Chronic ITP in adults** usually occurs in middle-aged or elderly patients, with female predominance. The bone marrow is normal, and splenomegaly is not found. Most ITP is "primary," but presence of other disorders (e.g., SLE, HIV, *H. pylori*, hepatitis C, lymphoma, sarcoidosis) designates the ITP as "secondary". Approximately 60–70% of patients have detectable platelet-specific autoantibodies.
   (a) First-line therapy of acute or chronic ITP includes corticosteroids, although most patients will eventually relapse during tapering.
   (b) Second-line therapy with splenectomy offers a good chance of cure (~70%) or meaningful platelet count improvement (10–20%), although

late relapse is possible. An alternative to splenectomy includes anti-CD20 therapy (rituximab), a non-FDA-approved indication.

(c) Third-line therapies are numerous (danazol, cyclosporine, cyclophosphamide, combination chemotherapy, etc.), attesting to variable benefit and toxic profiles. Non-splenectomized Rh(D)-positive patients can have platelet count increases for 1–3 weeks following treatment with anti-D, because antibody-coated red cells interfere with splenic platelet clearance. Overt hemolysis is a risk of anti-D, and this treatment is not recommended when patients have secondary ITP, are elderly, or have concomitant autoimmune hemolysis (Evan's syndrome).

(d) Emergency treatment of severe, symptomatic ITP includes high-dose corticosteroids and/or IVIgG; platelet transfusions are usually restricted to life-threatening bleeding.

(e) Newer therapies include the thrombopoietin receptor agonists, eltrombopag (oral agent) and romiplostim (administered by subcutaneous injection). How these agents are integrated into the care of these patients still needs definition, but they have been used as primary therapy with success.

5. **Drug-induced autoimmune thrombocytopenia.** Rarely, drugs (e.g., levodopa, procainamide) cause ITP by triggering platelet-reactive autoantibodies, or mimic ITP (gold) because slow elimination causes D-ITP to persist.

B. Alloimmune thrombocytopenia

Alloantigens are genetically determined molecular variations of proteins or carbohydrates that can be recognized immunologically by some normal individuals when exposed to the alloantigen(s) they lack, usually as a result of pregnancy, transfusion, or transplantation. Alloimmune thrombocytopenia results when anti-human platelet antigen (HPA) alloantibodies cause premature destruction of platelets via accelerated reticuloendothelial clearance. Five syndromes are recognized.

1. **Neonatal alloimmune thrombocytopenia (NAT)** (see Chapter 23) is a potentially severe transient alloantibody-mediated thrombocytopenia that occurs in 1/200 newborns. Passive placental transfer of anti-HPA-1a alloantibodies from an HPA-1b/b mother (2% of the population) is the most frequent cause; however, more than a dozen other platelet alloantigens have been implicated in NAT, with some alloantigen systems (HPA-5a/b, -15a/b) causing less severe thrombocytopenia. Unlike hemolytic disease of the newborn, the first born offspring is often affected by NAT. A general rule: subsequent alloantigen-positive newborns evince thrombocytopenia *at least* as severe as their previously-affected sibling(s). Treatment of unexpected NAT involves transfusion of random or (preferably) compatible platelets, whereas prenatal management of an affected fetus involves specialized care through a tertiary fetomaternal unit.

2. **Post-transfusion purpura (PTP)** is a rare disorder characterized by severe thrombocytopenia (platelet count <20,000/µL) and mucocutaneous bleeding that begins 5 to 10 days after exposure to a blood product, usually at surgery (Figure 14.3a). Most patients (>95%) are elderly parous females who are homozygous HPA-1b/b, i.e., they form high-titer anti-HPA-1a alloantibodies that somehow destroy autologous platelets. "Random" platelet transfusions (usually bearing HPA-1a alloantigens) often trigger febrile or even anaphylactoid reactions. This transient but life-threatening hemorrhagic disorder (intracranial bleeding is the most common cause of death) usually is benefited by high-dose IVIgG. Therapeutic plasma exchange can be considered if IVIgG is ineffective.

3. **Passive alloimmune thrombocytopenia (PAT)** is a rare disorder characterized by the abrupt onset of thrombocytopenia within a few hours after transfusion of a blood product containing platelet-specific alloantibodies, most often anti-HPA-1a, which will destroy the transfusion recipient's platelets if they bear the target antigen. Implicated blood donors should no longer donate blood product.

4. **Transplantation-associated alloimmune thrombocytopenia.** Rarely, thrombocytopenia that occurs weeks or even months following bone marrow transplantation (BMT) or solid organ transplantation can be caused by platelet-reactive alloantibodies generated either by residual host lymphoid cells against donor platelets (post-BMT) or from donor organ-derived "passenger" lymphocytes that destroy the organ recipient's platelets.

5. **Platelet transfusion refractoriness.** Platelet-specific alloantibodies occasionally contribute to platelet transfusion refractoriness (poor platelet count increments following platelet transfusion), but usually other mechanisms are operative (e.g., increased platelet consumption in very ill patients).

C. Classic drug-induced immune thrombocytopenic purpura (D-ITP)

1. **Quinine, etc.** Box 14.1 lists some of the drugs implicated in D-ITP. The typical picture is onset of severe thrombocytopenia (<20,000/µL) (Figure 14.4) that begins approximately one week after starting a new drug known to cause this reaction (Figure 14.3b). Petechiae are common; oral mucosal "blood blisters" and generalized GI or GU bleeding indicate more severe disease and risk of intracranial hemorrhage. Besides stopping potentially implicated drug(s), therapy includes one or more of: platelet transfusions, high-dose IVIgG, corticosteroids. When an outpatient presents with severe thrombocytopenia, it is important to inquire specifically about *quinine*, a medication used to treat "leg cramps" but also a constituent of "tonic water", and a common cause of D-ITP.

2. **Atypical D-ITP secondary to GPIIb/IIIa antagonists.** Approximately 1% of patients develop severe thrombocytopenia (usually, <20,000/µL) within a few hours of receiving a GPIIb/IIIa antagonist, even with first-time exposure, due to preexisting, naturally occurring antibodies.

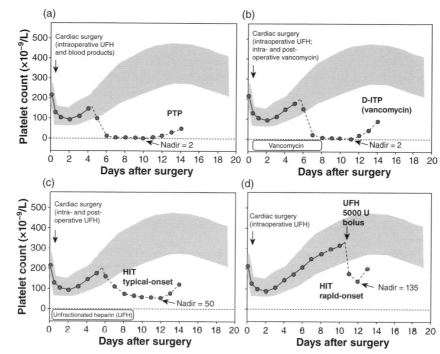

Figure 14.3 Clinical features of four different explanations for postoperative thrombocytopenia. For each example, the "background" platelet count profile is as per Figure 14.1 (post-cardiac surgery).

(a) Post-transfusion purpura (PTP) is characterized by severe thrombocytopenia (platelet nadir usually <10,000/µL) that usually begins approximately 5 to 8 days after administration of blood product.

(b) Drug-induced immune thrombocytopenia (D-ITP) is characterized by severe thrombocytopenia (platelet count nadir usually <20,000/µL) that usually begins approximately 5 to 10 days after beginning a new drug (vancomycin in the example shown).

(c) Typical-onset heparin-induced thrombocytopenia (HIT) is characterized by mild, moderate, or severe thrombocytopenia (median platelet count 60,000/µL; 90% of patients have platelet count nadirs between 15,000 to 150,000/µL) that begins 5 to 10 days after beginning an immunizing course of heparin (the remaining patients have nadirs <15,000 or >150,000/µL), in the example shown, the immunizing exposure to heparin is intraoperative administration of unfractionated heparin (UFH) during cardiac surgery. Occasionally, an identical platelet count profile can be seen even when postoperative UFH is not administered, in this case, the patient is said to have "delayed-onset HIT".

(d) Rapid-onset HIT is characterized by an abrupt decrease in platelet count after administering heparin. In the example shown, the platelet count fell immediately after a heparin bolus was given on postoperative day 18. HIT antibodies were already present at the time that the heparin bolus was given, as they were formed by the intraoperative exposure to heparin 18 days earlier at cardiac surgery. Sometimes, anaphylactoid reactions accompany rapid-onset HIT (see Box 14.2). Interestingly, because HIT antibodies are transient, a future heparin bolus given to the same patient 6 months later is very unlikely to be complicated by rapid-onset of thrombocytopenia.

> ### Box 14.1 Drug-induced ITP: implicated drugs (partial list)
>
> **Typical** (relatively common): quinine/quinidine, sulfa antibiotics, carbamazepine, vancomycin.
>
> **Typical** (less common): acetaminophen, actinomycin, amiodarone, amitriptyline, amoxicillin/ampicillin/piperacillin/nafcillin, cefalosporins (cefazolin, ceftazidime, ceftriaxone), celecoxib, ciprofloxacin, esomeprazole, ethambutol, fexofenadine, fentanyl, fucidic acid, furosemide, gold salts, haloperidol, ibuprofen, irinotecan, levofloxacin, metronidazole, naproxen, oxaliplatin, phenytoin, propoxyphene, propranolol, ranitidine, rifampin, simvastatin, suramin, trimethoprim, valproic acid.
>
> **Atypical*:** glycoprotein IIb/IIIa antagonists: abciximab, eptifibatide, tirofiban.
>
> *Usually occur in patients who have never been previously exposed to a GPIIb/IIIa antagonist.

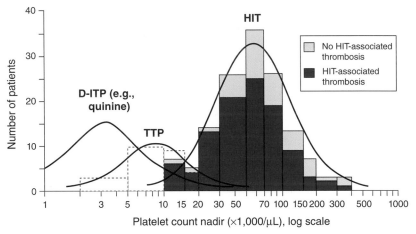

Figure 14.4 Distribution of platelet count nadirs in three different thrombocytopenic syndromes: D-ITP (quinine) vs. TTP (with absent ADAMTS13 activity) and HIT (two subgroups: with and without thrombosis). (Reprinted, with modifications, with permission, from: Warkentin TE. Think of HIT. Hematology Am Soc Hematol Educ Program 2006;408–414.)

D. Heparin-induced thrombocytopenia (HIT)

HIT is an important adverse drug reaction: it is relatively common (~1–3% of patients receiving >1 week of UFH for postoperative prophylaxis) and strongly associated with life- and limb-threatening thrombosis. It can also occur after low molecular weight heparin administration and rarely has been reported with fondaparinux.

1. **Pathophysiology.** HIT is caused by IgG that binds via Fab to multimolecular complexes of platelet factor 4 (PF4) bound to heparin; the Fc moieties bind to platelet Fc receptors, producing strong platelet activation. Formation of procoagulant platelet-derived microparticles, and activation of endothelium and monocytes, causes a prothrombotic state (*in-vivo* thrombin generation).

> **Box 14.2 Clinical sequelae of HIT**
>
> **Thrombosis**
> *Venous*: DVT (lower- and upper-limb*), PE, adrenal vein thrombosis (manifests as adrenal hemorrhage), cerebral venous (dural sinus) thrombosis, mesenteric or portal vein thrombosis.
> *Arterial*: limb artery, cerebral, myocardial, brachial, mesenteric, renal, other.
> *Intra-cardiac*: intra-atrial, intraventricular.
> *Microvascular*: usually warfarin-associated (venous limb gangrene); sometimes, overt (decompensated) DIC alone explains microvascular thrombosis.
> **Heparin-induced skin lesions** (at heparin injection sites): necrotizing and non-necrotizing.
> **Anaphylactoid reactions** (post-intravenous heparin bolus): inflammatory (fever, chills), cardiorespiratory (chest pain/tightness, tachycardia, hypertension, cardiac arrest, dyspnea, tachypnea, respiratory arrest), gastrointestinal (diarrhea), neurologic (transient global amnesia).
> *Upper-limb DVT in HIT is strongly associated with central venous catheter use.
> DIC, disseminated intravascular coagulation; DVT, deep-vein thrombosis; PE, pulmonary embolism.

2. **Clinical features.** An otherwise unexplained thrombocytopenia or a 50% drop in a normal platelet count bearing a temporal relation to a preceding immunizing exposure to UFH (usually given intra- or postoperatively) strongly suggests HIT, as this disorder is seen 10–15× more often with UFH compared with LMWH, and 3–5× more often in surgical versus medical patients. The median platelet count nadir is ~60,000/μL; for 85–90% of patients the platelet count nadir ranges between 20,000 to 150,000/μL (Figure 14.4). At least half of all patients with proven HIT develop clinically-evident sequelae, usually symptomatic thrombosis (Box 14.2).

   (a) Typical-onset HIT (~65–70% of cases) refers to a platelet count fall that begins 5 to 10 days after an immunizing exposure to heparin, and while the patient continues to receive heparin (Figure 14.3c).

   (b) Rapid-onset HIT (~25–30% of cases) refers to an abrupt drop in platelet count upon starting heparin (Figure 14.3d); almost invariably, patients were exposed to heparin within the preceding several weeks, thus explaining why thrombocytopenia begins abruptly when heparin is recommenced.

   (c) delayed-onset HIT (~3–5% of cases) resembles typical-onset HIT, except that patients are no longer receiving heparin when HIT and HIT-associated thrombosis begins. Patients have high levels of anti-PF4/heparin antibodies that also can activate platelets *in vitro* even in the absence of heparin.

   (d) spontaneous HIT (<1% of cases). Rarely, a syndrome clinically and serologically identical to HIT occurs in the absence of any preceding heparin exposure. Preceding infection or surgery is believed to trigger "spontaneous" HIT antibodies.

3. **Laboratory testing for HIT antibodies.** Anti-PF4/heparin immunoassays (e.g., enzyme-immunoassay [EIA]) and washed platelet activation assays (e.g., platelet serotonin-release assay [SRA]) detect HIT antibodies. Approximately half of EIA+ patients with clinically-suspected HIT do *not* have this diagnosis, because (more specific) platelet activation assays such as the SRA are negative, and other explanations for thrombocytopenia are evident. Although the sensitive and specific SRA is performed by only a few laboratories, the assay is nonetheless available on a referral basis. In the SRA (a "washed" platelet assay), platelets obtained from normal "pedigree" donors (known to respond well to HIT sera) are labeled with ^{14}C-serotonin and washed in buffer. A positive test is indicated when (heat-inactivated) serum from a patient with HIT causes strong platelet activation (substantial release of ^{14}C-serotonin from the washed donor platelets) in the presence of pharmacologic concentrations of heparin (0.1–0.3 U/mL) but not at high concentrations of heparin (100 U/mL). The "stronger" a positive EIA result (i.e., higher optical density [OD] units), the more likely it is the patient has platelet-activating antibodies (per the SRA) and true HIT. For example, a positive PF4/heparin EIA (normal cut-off, 0.4 OD units) with OD >2.0 units has a 90% probability of predicting for a positive SRA, whereas a weak-positive EIA result (0.4–1.0 OD units) has only a 5% probability of a positive SRA. Such a weak-positive EIA should therefore be taken as evidence *against* the diagnosis of HIT.

4. **Treatment.** For patients with serologically-confirmed or strongly-suspected HIT, whether or not complicated by thrombosis, treatment involves stopping heparin and giving an alternative, non-heparin anticoagulant, such as a direct thrombin inhibitor (recombinant hirudin [lepirudin, desirudin], argatroban, bivalirudin) or an antithrombin-dependent, factor Xa inhibitor (danaparoid [not available in the U.S.], fondaparinux). It is crucial to avoid or postpone warfarin therapy pending substantial recovery of HIT (platelet count >150,000/µL) since vitamin K antagonism is *the* major factor that explains HIT-associated limb amputation due to venous limb gangrene (limb ischemia in the setting of deep-vein thrombosis (DVT) and with palpable/Doppler-identifiable pulses). A supratherapeutic INR (>3.5) is a characteristic feature of warfarin-associated venous limb gangrene complicating HIT, and represents a surrogate marker for severe protein C depletion. Progressive microvascular thrombosis results because warfarin fails to inhibit thrombin generation in HIT, but results in failure to down-regulate thrombin due to protein C depletion. Routine duplex ultrasonography of patients with HIT is appropriate given the high frequency (~50%) of DVT in this patient population.

5. **Repeat heparin exposure.** HIT antibodies are transient (median time to non-detectability, 50 to 80 days depending upon the assay performed), are not invariably triggered by repeat heparin exposure, and (if regenerated) require at least 5 days to reach significant levels. Accordingly, for patients with a previous history of HIT, repeat heparin exposure is the favored

option for intraoperative anticoagulation when such patients need cardiac or vascular surgery.

X. Pseudothrombocytopenia

Naturally occurring antibodies that cause *ex-vivo* platelet agglutination (i.e., after collection of blood into tubes containing anticoagulant) can lead to a false diagnosis of thrombocytopenia because platelets within "clumps" are not counted by the electronic particle counter. This is why inspection of the blood film is crucial before a laboratory reports a first-occurrence of thrombocytopenia in a patient. Pseudothrombocytopenia is clinically insignificant, except when it leads to inappropriate treatment because of wrongly suspected thrombocytopenia, or makes it difficult to obtain an accurate platelet count in an affected patient who also develops true thrombocytopenia.

A. **EDTA-induced pseudothrombocytopenia** is the most common type of pseudothrombocytopenia, and results from antibody-induced agglutination in the presence of the chelating anticoagulant, ethylenediamine-tetraacetic acid (EDTA). Often, a normal platelet count result will be obtained if the blood is collected into another anticoagulant (sodium citrate, heparin) and/or collected into prewarmed tubes maintained at 37°C. before platelet enumeration. Approximately one-quarter of patients with apparent GPIIb/IIIa antagonist-induced acute thrombocytopenia have pseudothrombocytopenia.

B. **Platelet satellitism** is the phenomenon of platelet rosetting around neutrophils in EDTA-anticoagulated blood, and is caused by antibodies that make platelets adhere to neutrophils.

C. **Miscellaneous causes of pseudothrombocytopenia** include platelet cold agglutinins and paraproteinemias. As noted earlier, giant platelets as seen in MYH9-associated macrothrombocytopenia may lead to a falsely low estimate of the platelet count (See Chapter 13).

Further reading

George JN. Platelets. Lancet 2000;355:1531–9.

Noris M, Remuzzi G. Atypical hemolytic-uremic syndrome. N Engl J Med 2009;361: 1676–87.

Provan D, Stasi R, Newland AC, et al. International consensus report on the investigation and management of primary immune thrombocytopenia. Blood 2010;115:168–86.

Reese JA, Li X, Hauben M, et al. Identifying drugs that cause acute thrombocytopenia: an analysis using 3 distinct methods. Blood 2010;116:2127–33.

Warkentin TE. Drug-induced immune-mediated thrombocytopenia—from purpura to thrombosis. N Engl J Med 2007;356:891–3.

Warkentin TE. Agents for the treatment of heparin-induced thrombocytopenia. Hematol/ Oncol Clin N Am 2010;24:755–75.

Warkentin TE, Kelton JG. Temporal aspects of heparin-induced thrombocytopenia. N Engl J Med 2001;344:1286–92.

15 Thrombosis and Anticoagulation

Alvin H. Schmaier

Case Western Reserve University, University Hospitals Case Medical Center, Cleveland, OH, USA

I. Overview

Thrombosis is the most common cause of death in the world. In the United States, acute coronary syndromes and stroke, both arterial thrombotic conditions, are the number 2 and 3 killers. Combined, they kill 300,000 more individuals annually (total >850,000) than cancer. In the world, acute coronary syndromes and stroke are the number 1 and 2 killers of individuals. The presentation of thrombosis is a summation of risk factors.

A. Key concepts

1. Arterial or venous thrombosis is produced by a shift in the balance between procoagulant (i.e., thrombin generating mechanisms), profibrinolytic (i.e., clot lysing or plasmin generating mechanisms), and anticoagulation systems.
2. The genesis of thrombosis is multifactorial and can be due to vascular, cellular, protein or rheological defects or a combination of these factors.
3. Currently, we are able to recognize a molecular/protein causes for venous thrombosis in 20–40% of patients depending on the patient population. The etiologies for arterial thrombosis are more complex with a few precise causes, but most often, it is polygenic in origin. Arterial thrombosis leads to acute coronary syndrome and stroke.
4. Therapy for thrombosis is directed to prevention of future clots and lysis of existing clots.

B. Pathogenetic features

Most individuals who present with thrombosis have one or more of the following features at the time of presentation.

1. Vascular endothelial and smooth muscle dysfunction.
2. Stasis of blood.

Concise Guide to Hematology, First Edition. Edited by Alvin H. Schmaier, Hillard M. Lazarus.
© 2012 Blackwell Publishing Ltd. Published 2012 by Blackwell Publishing Ltd.

3. Platelet and leukocyte activation.
4. Activation of coagulation proteins.

C. Red (fibrin) versus white (platelet) clots
The structure of a thrombus varies as to the vessel it is found in.
1. In a high flow arterial vessel, platelet thrombi are seen. Macroscopic aggregates of platelets have a white appearance.
2. In low flow vessels (e.g., veins), the initial platelet plug, which may have started the thrombus, is often not detected. These clots result from the accumulation of red blood cells in fibrin strands and are called red thrombus.

D. Response after acute vessel injury
There are four phases that can be used to characterize vessel injury.
1. **Initial phase:** platelet thrombus formation.
2. **Acute phase:** active fibrin clot formation, initiation of the inflammatory response.
3. **Intermediate phase:** thrombus limitation, inflammatory response.
4. **Chronic phase:** re-adsorption and recanalization of the clot.

II. Arterial thrombosis

A. Overview
Arterial thrombosis can range from large vessel occlusions that result in myocardial infarction, stroke, peripheral arterial vessel occlusion, ischemic bowel syndrome to small vessels that result in digital ischemia and vasculitis.

B. Etiology
1. Arterial thrombosis is most often associated with on-going vascular disease as seen with diabetes mellitus, hyperlipidemias, hypercholestremia, or vasculitis due to connective tissue disorders or antiphospholipid antibody syndrome.
2. Hematologic conditions associated with arterial thrombosis include: sickle cell anemia, heparin-induced thrombocytopenia and thrombosis syndromes (HITTS), thrombotic thrombocytopenic purpura (TTP), hemolytic-uremic syndrome (HUS), purpura fulminans due to homozygous protein C or S deficiency, and myeloproliferative disorders (see Chapter 14).

C. Risk factors
Elevation of certain proteins or amino acids are associated with arterial thrombosis. These proteins include factor VII, fibrinogen, lipoprotein(a), plasma homocysteine, anti-phospholipid antibodies. Anti-phospholipid antibodies will be discussed in the venous thrombosis section below.
1. **Lipoprotein(a) or LP(a)** consists of LDL (low density lipoprotein) and apolipoprotein a. Apolipoprotein a has 98% sequence homology to one region on plasminogen (kringle IV). LP(a) is atherogenic, targeting LDL

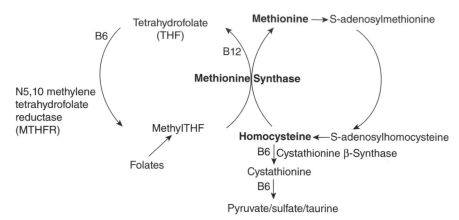

Figure 15.1 Homocysteine metabolism. Homocysteine is metabolized by two enzymes, methionine synthase and cystathionine β-synthase. N^5,N^{10} methylene tetrahydrofolate reductase makes an essential cofactor for methionine synthesis. B_{12} is a cofactor for methionine synthase and B_6 is a cofactor for cystathionine β-synthase.

away from its clearance receptor. LP(a) is also prothrombotic. It prevents plasminogen from binding to cells or fibrin, which inhibits plasminogen activation from initiating fibrinolysis. Thus, increased levels of LP(a) increase risk for both thrombosis by reduced fibrinolysis and increased atherogenesis.

2. **Homocysteine.** Elevation of plasma homocysteine is a risk factor for both arterial and venous thrombosis.

   (a) Elevation of homocysteine may arise from defective function in either of three enzymes: methionine synthase, N^5,N^{10}-methylene-tetrahydro-folate reductase (MTHFR) and cystathionine β-synthase. Homocysteine levels rise in B_{12} deficiency, a cofactor for methionine synthase, and folate deficiency, a cofactor for MTHFR, and B_6 deficiency, a cofactor for cystathionine β-synthase (Figure 15.1). N^5,N^{10}-methylene-tetrahy-drofolate reductase enzyme is present in vessel walls. Polymorphisms (e.g., C677T) in this enzyme which exist in 35% of the population in the United States do not contribute to either elevation of homocysteine or thrombosis. However, defective function of MTHFR as seen in B_{12} deficiency is associated with higher homocysteine levels and arterial thrombosis risk. Deficiency of cystathionine β-synthase results in eleva-tion of plasma homocysteine and severe arterial and venous thrombo-sis. Both arterial and venous thrombosis have been associated with homocysteine elevations (values >11 μM).

   (b) Elevation of plasma homocysteine results in endothelial cell dysfunc-tion (Figure 15.2). The normal anticoagulant surface of endothelium is converted to a prothrombotic surface manifesting by reduced protein C activation as result of reduced thrombomodulin (a receptor protein for protein C activation by thrombin on endothelium) expression,

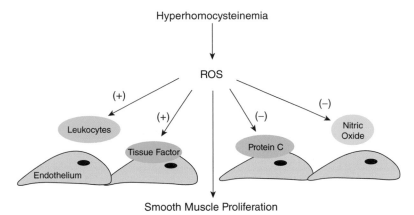

Figure 15.2 The relationship of homocysteine and endothelial dysfunction. In hyperhomo-cysteinemic states, there is increased reactive oxygen species (ROS). ROS is injurious to the anticoagulant function of endothelium. It inactivates thrombomodulin, a receptor for protein C activation by thrombin, producing reduced protein C activation and loss of a constitutive anticoagulant. Also, ROS uncouples endothelial NO synthetase allowing for reduced NO production and more ROS. Comcommittantly, ROS increases tissue factor mRNA and protein expression in endothelium. It also stimulates leukocyte migration and infiltration and smooth muscle proliferation. The sum of these activities is vascular dysfunction leading to arterial thrombosis.

reduction in tissue plasminogen activator activation of plasminogen, increased tissue factor expression, reduced nitric oxide production, increased factor V expression, and enhanced LP(a) binding to fibrin. Elevation of plasma homocysteine also results in smooth muscle cell proliferation, lipid peroxidation, and oxidation of LDL, all factors that contribute to atherogenesis and arterial thrombosis. Patients with elevated homocysteine should be treated with folate.

D. Treatment of arterial thrombosis

This area of therapy is highly specialized and resides with cardiology in the management of acute coronary syndromes, neurology in the management of stroke, or vascular surgeons in the management of peripheral arterial occlusions. However, there are certain principles to which we must adhere. In general, anticoagulant therapy is directed to limiting the amount of thrombin formation, antiplatelet therapy is directed towards limiting the degree of platelet activation. The antiplatelet agents below are used either alone in prevention studies or in combinations for acute management or in prevention studies after interventional procedure with placement of stents either in coronary, carotid, or peripheral arteries.

1. **Antiplatelet agents:**
   (a) Aspirin (acetylates platelet cyclooxygenase 1 and 2).
   (b) Thienopyridines (clopidogrel, prasugrel)—P2Y12 antagonists that block the major ADP receptor.

(c) Alpha$_{2b}$beta$_3$integrin antagonists (glycoprotein IIb/IIIa antagonists) that block fibrinogen binding to activated platelets, the final common pathway of platelet activation (see Chapter 13).

    (i)   Abciximab, a chimeric mouse-human monoclonal antibody.

    (ii) Tirofiban, a nonpeptide mimetic.

    (iii) Eptifibatide, a cyclic peptide inhibitor.

2. **Antifibrin-generating agents.** These agents are added to suppress the contribution of thrombin to an arterial thrombus either to prevent fibrin formation and to reduce thrombin's contribution to platelet activation.

  (a) Unfractionated heparin. This agent is isolated from pig intestines and partially purified.

  (b) Low-molecular weight heparin. This class of agents is 5000–15,000 molecular weight isolates from unfractionated heparin. Synthetic five saccharide forms of these gycosaminoglycans have been prepared with similar anticoagulant activity (e.g., fondapariux).

  (c) Bivalirudin. This agent, a synthetic 22 amino acid peptide, is a direct thrombin inhibitor that binds to the active site and exosite I of thrombin to block its activity.

III. Venous thrombosis

A. Overview

Venous thrombosis, unlike arterial thrombosis, occurs in low flow situations. After vessel injury, venous thrombi propagate proximally to occlude a vessel. One experimental model to create a venous thrombosis required the following: vessel injury, reduced blood flow, inhibition of an anticoagulant system, and induction of an inflammatory response. Although venous thrombi are a gelatinous material, venous thrombosis does have an inflammatory component.

B. Causes of venous thrombosis

1. **Protein defects** (Figure 15.3, Table 15.1). The numbers in parenthesis represent percent of patients seen with thrombosis.

  (a) Factor V Leiden (FVL) (20–60% of DVTs) is a "G" to "A" mutation at basepair 1691 of coagulation factor V that results in a Q^{506} amino acid instead of an R^{506}. Factor V Leiden is resistant to inactivation by activated protein C (APC) because the enzyme cleaves after arginine^{506}. As result of resistance to activated protein C inactivation, there is increased factor Va and thus increased thrombin formation. This polymorphism in factor V is a common defect in the Near East and Europe. By itself, it is a relatively low risk factor for thrombosis. However, when it is combined with other etiologies for thrombosis (e.g., estrogens in oral contraceptives) the thrombosis risk potential increases. Factor V Leiden accounts for 20% first DVTs, and 5–10 of the DVTs in the normal population. Heterozygous individuals have a 7-fold risk for thrombosis over

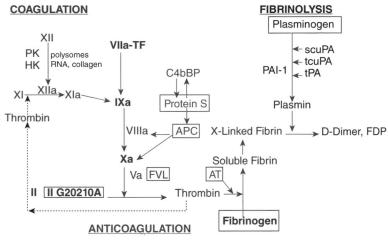

COAGULATION

FIBRINOLYSIS

Figure 15.3 Biochemistry of venous thrombosis. This figure is a juxtapositioning of the proteins involved in the coagulation (green), fibrinolytic (blue), and anticoagulation (red) systems. The proteins that are inscribed in boxes represent recognized defects that are associated with venous thrombosis. PK is prekallikrein; HK is high molecular weight kininogen; coagulations factors XII, XI, IX, X, VII and V are represented by their roman numeral alone. The presence of an "a" after the roman numeral represents an "activated" protein. TF is an abbreviation for tissue factor; FVL is an abbreviation for factor V Leiden; scuPA is single chain urokinase plasminogen activator; tcuPA is two-chain urokinase plasminogen activator; tPA is tissue plasminogen activator.

Table 15.1 Inherited procoagulant states		
Defect	Incidence in population	Percent of patients with procoagulant states
1. Factor V Leiden	5–10%	20–60%
2. Prothrombin gene mutation	2–4%	6–8%
3. Homocysteine	–	10%
4. Protein C deficiency	1:200	<5%
5. Protein S deficiency	–	<5%
6. Antithrombin deficiency	1:2000–5000	<1%
7. Dysfibrinogenemia	Unknown	~1–2%
8. Elevated lipoprotein(a)	–	

normals (0.1% annually). Oral contraceptives increase the risk of venous thromboembolism (VTE) 35-fold with heterozygous individuals. Homozygous Factor V Leiden individuals have an 80-fold increased risk.

(b) Homocysteine (10%) see above.

(c) Prothrombin 20210 (6–8%) is a single basepair mutation at position 20210 (G20210A) in the distal 3′ area of untranslated region of the prothrombin gene (factor II). This polymorphism results in an elevation of a normal prothrombin molecule. It is the third most common defect associated with thrombosis present in 2–4% of the population. By itself, it is a relatively low risk for thrombosis giving a 2.8-fold increase in heterozygous individuals. It may have a predilection for co-expression with factor V Leiden.

(d) Protein C deficiency or defect (<5%). Protein C is the zymogen of a major anticoagulant in the body, activated protein C. Activated protein C is a vitamin K-dependent enzyme whose function is to inactivate factors Va and VIIIa and stimulates fibrinolysis. In the absence of activated protein C with less inactivation of factors Va and VIIIa, there is increased thrombin formation. Deficiencies or defects in protein C are a serious risk factor for thrombosis. There are a number of clinical syndromes associated with protein C deficiency. These include:
   (i) venous thrombosis (heterozygous defect).
   (ii) coumadin skin necrosis (heterozygous defect).
   (iii) neonatal purpura fulminans (homozygous defect).
   (iv) disseminated intravascular coagulation (both).
   If one has protein C deficiency, the risk for thrombosis ranges from 0.5–2.5%/year with a 75% lifetime risk of having thrombosis and, when recognized, requires anticoagulation therapy for life. 70% of these thromboses are spontaneous and 30% are provoked by pregnancy, oral contraceptives, inflammation, infection, surgery, or trauma. Neonatal purpura fulminans at birth needs to be recognized within 3 days or it will lead to infant death.

(e) Protein S deficiency or defect (<5%). Protein S is a vitamin K dependent protein that is not an enzyme. It serves as a co-factor (i.e., binding site) for activated protein C (APC) to localize to cell surfaces. It is regulated by a complement protein, C4b binding protein. Thus in inflammatory states, free protein S can be reduced as result of binding to C4b binding protein. Pregnancy and estrogens reduce protein S. Free protein S is the form of the protein that serves as a cofactor for APC. A deficiency or defect in protein S is a serious risk factor for thrombosis that carries a 74% lifetime risk of getting thrombosis and, when recognized, requires anticoagulation therapy for life.

(f) Dysfibrinogenemias (1–2%). Some abnormal fibrinogens have the propensity for accelerated clotting. The higher the fibrinogen concentration, the greater the increased propensity for thrombosis.

(g) Antithrombin deficiency or defect (<1%). Antithrombin is a SERPIN (a serine plasma protease inhibitor) that inhibits each of the coagulation system enzymes. It is the presence of antithrombin that allows for heparin to function as an anticoagulant. It was the first protein defect recognized to be associated with venous thrombosis. All patients are heterozygous for the deficiency; homozygous antithrombin deficiency is not compatible with life. It is a severe prothrombotic defect which carries a 50% lifetime risk of getting thrombosis and, when recognized, requires anticoagulation therapy for life.

(h) Dysplasminogenemia (<1%). Dysplasminogenemia is caused by an abnormal plasminogen molecule that has reduced ability to form plasmin; thus these molecules have a reduced ability to lyse clots.

(i) Lipoprotein(a) (<1%).

(j) Elevation of factors XI, IX, VIII, VII, X, II, and plasminogen activator inhibitor-1. It is known in population studies that elevations of these factors are associated with venous thrombosis, but individual values in single patients are not helpful to understand thrombosis etiology.

2. **Hematologic diseases**

(a) Disseminated intravascular coagulation (DIC) (see Chapters 12 and 14).

(b) Heparin-induced thrombocytopenia and thrombosis syndrome (HITTS) (see Chapter 14).

(c) Antiphospholipid antibody syndrome: Antiphospholipid antibodies interfere with the anticoagulant nature of the endothelium. In particular, they bind to endothelium and interfere with the constitutive anticoagulant nature of endothelium by interfering with the anticoagulant properties of annexin V. This allows for tenase to be less regulated contributing to a prothrombotic state. Some of these patients have "lupus anticoagulants" that prolong the clot-based PT and APTT assays even though they are associated with thrombosis. Diagnosis of antiphospholipid antibody syndrome is made by finding an abnormal lupus anticoagulant assay or antibodies to cardiolipin or beta-2-glycoprotein I twice with a minimal 3 months separating the time of assay. Antiphospholipid antibody syndrome associated with thrombosis is serious and usually requires lifelong anticoagulation.

(d) Thrombotic thrombocytopenia purpura (TTP) (see Chapter 14).

(e) Hemolytic-uremic syndrome (HUS) (see Chapter 14).

(f) Atypical hemolytic uremic syndrome (aHUS) (see Chapter 14).

(g) Myeloproliferative disorders such as polycythemia vera and essential thrombocythemia (see Chapter 18).

(h) Paroxysmal nocturnal hemoglobinura (see Chapter 8).

C. Risk factors for venous thrombosis

Venous thrombosis is associated with a number of clinical risk factors. Recognizing these conditions should alert the physician to the risk of venous thrombosis.

1. **Age:** After two weeks of bed rest, the likelihood of venous thrombosis is 20% for a 20-year-old individual and 60% for a 60-year-old individual.

2. **Prolonged immobility:** An individual who is immobilized is more likely to have a venous thrombosis than one who is physically active.

3. **Obesity:** Obese individual who are more sedentary are at greater risk for venous thrombosis than individual who are not. Obesity is the single most common risk factor for venous thrombosis. >50% of patients with thrombosis are obese.

4. **Neurologic disease:** Individuals who have strokes often have thrombosis in the paretic limb, but not in the limb that is functioning.

5. **Cardiac disease:** An uncomplicated myocardial infarction has a low risk for thrombosis. However, a patient with heart failure associated with a myocardial infarction has a 25% risk for deep venous thrombosis of which 25% will have a pulmonary embolus.

6. **Pregnancy/post-partum period:** Pregnancy and the post-partum period are associated with an increased risk for thrombosis. The incidence of thrombosis in pregnancy is 1–5/1000 pregnancies (includes postpartum). In women with previous DVT, the risk is 12–35% and increases to 75% with defects like antithrombin and protein C deficiency.

7. **Oral contraceptives are associated with an increased risk for thrombosis.** Estrogens increase the relative risk 3–5-fold for venous thrombosis, but the absolute risk goes from 0.1 to 0.3–0.5. If the patient has the factor V Leiden mutation (see below), the risk is increased 28-fold.

8. **Surgery is a well-recognized risk factor for thrombosis.** It increases the relative risk for thrombosis 10–30 fold or from 0.1 to 1–3% absolute risk. It depends upon the nature of the surgery and the duration of time that the patient is under anesthesia. For example, orthopedic surgery (hip, knee) is associated with actual flexing and occlusion of the femoral and popliteal veins, respectively. The incidence of deep venous thrombosis (DVT) is 35–40% and 50%, respectively. The risk of DVT in other surgeries follows accordingly: Abdominothoracic: (14–35%); Urologic surgery: transuretheral resection (7%), suprapubic prostatectomy (35%); Gynecologic surgery: vaginal hysterectomy (7%), total abdominal hysterectomy (27%).

9. **Malignancy and thrombosis:** The incidence of occult malignancy in patients with idiopathic thrombosis is only 0.5–5.8%. However, patients with idiopathic deep venous thrombosis or pulmonary embolism (PE) will have a 3-fold higher likelihood of presenting with occult malignancy within 3 years of presentation of the clot. Further, if you have a malignancy, there is a 20% likelihood that you will have thrombosis at some time during the course of your illness.

D. Treatment for venous thrombosis

Venous thrombosis presents as deep venous thrombosis (DVT) and or pulmonary emboli. It can lead to stroke by a paradoxical embolus as result of a patent foramen ovale. Treatment is usually with anti-fibrin generating agents.

1. **Treatment principles:**
   (a) Prophylaxis: prevention of occurrence: immobile, high-risk patients.
   (b) Prevention of recurrence, propagation, embolism once thrombus has been recognized. This therapy is given upon recognition of a new thrombus.
   (c) Lysis of clots: thrombolytic therapy (tissue plasminogen activator, streptokinase, urokinase). This therapy is given upon presentation of large thrombus to decrease pain and prevent venous valve destruction as thrombus occluded vessel heals with an intravascular scarring.

2. **Anti-fibrin agents:**
   (a) Heparin and related compounds. These agents are glycosaminoglycan polymers of saccharides that bind to antithrombin to potentiate its activity mostly against thrombin and factor Xa. In the presence of heparin, antithrombin is a thousand-fold better inhibitor of thrombin. This groups of agents consists of unfractionated heparin, low molecular weight heparin that only potentiate antithrombin's inhibition of factor Xa, not thrombin, and synthetic 5 saccharide units of agent that also potentiates antithrombin's inhibition of factor Xa. These agents are administered parenterally.
   (b) Direct thrombin inhibitors. These agents directly bind to thrombin. These agents consist of argatroban—a small molecule, nonpeptide antagonist that binds the active site, bivalirudin—a peptide antagonist that binds thrombin's active and exosite I region, and lepirudin or refludan—a 6.6 kDa recombinant protein that binds thrombin's active site and exosite I. These agents are administered parenterally. Dabigatran is an oral direct thrombin inhibitor.
   (c) Warfarin. This agent is an oral vitamin K antagonist that competes with its utilization for an essential carboxylation reaction on the amino terminus of the vitamin K proteins II, VII, IX, X, protein C, and protein S. Interference of this carboxylation reaction results in reduced binding of these proteins to cell membranes with less activation. Warfarin treatment makes abnormal proteins that function as inhibitors and reduces the amount of protein made.

Further reading

Bauer KA. Hypercoagulable states. In: Hematology: Basic Principles and Practice. Hoffman R, Benz EJ, Shattil SJ, Furie B, Silberstein LE, McGlave P, Heslop H, eds. Philadelphia, PA: Churchill Livingstone, 2009:2021–41.

Krakow EF, Ginsberg JS, Crowther MA. Arterial thromboembolism. In: Hoffman R, Benz EJ, Shattil SJ, Furie B, Silberstein LE, McGlave P, Heslop H, eds. Hematology: Basic Principles and Practice. Philadelphia, PA: Churchill Livingstone, 2009:2055 65.

Lim W, Crowther MA, Ginsberg JS. Venous thromboembolism. In: Hoffman R, Benz EJ, Shattil SJ, Furie B, Silberstein LE, McGlave P, Heslop H, eds. Hematology: Basic Principles and Practice. Philadelphia, PA: Churchill Livingstone, 2009:2043–54.

Weitz J. Antithrombotic drugs. In: Hematology: Basic Principles and Practice. Hoffman R, Benz EJ, Shattil SJ, Furie B, Silberstein LE, McGlave P, Heslop H, eds. Philadelphia, PA: Churchill Livingstone, 2009:2067–82.

16 Myeloid Cell Physiology and Disorders

Alvin H. Schmaier[1], Lilli M. Petruzzelli[2], Niels Borregaard[3] and Laurence A. Boxer[4]

[1]Case Western Reserve University, University Hospitals Case Medical Center, Cleveland, OH, USA
[2]Novartis Institutes for BioMedical Research, Inc., Cambridge, MA, USA
[3]University of Copenhagen, Copenhagen, Denmark
[4]University of Michigan, Ann Arbor, MI, USA

I. Myeloid cells

Myeloid cells are a subset of white blood cells, or leukocytes. This subset includes neutrophils, eosinophils, monocytes, and basophils. These cells mediate host defense against infection and modulate the immune response. All of these cells contain granules and are derived from a common pluripotent myeloid stem cell precursor (see Figure 16.2).

II. Laboratory studies

An automated cell counter is used to determine the number of white blood cells (WBCs) in each microliter (µL) or cubic millimeter (mm^3) of blood. The cells are further analyzed to determine the percentage of each subtype, or the *relative proportion* of each type of cell. The enumeration is known as the *differential cell count*.

The *absolute number* of each circulating component of WBCs is determined by multiplying the percentage of each type of cell by the total number of white blood cells. When used to determine the absolute number of neutrophils this value is called the "ANC"—absolute neutrophil count. Table 16.1 defines the terms that are used to describe variations in the white blood cell differential. Tables 16.2 and 16.3 show white blood cell differential counts at various ages and the relative proportion of each type of cell in various clinical situations.

III. Subsets of myeloid cells

A. Neutrophils
Neutrophils have a central role in host defense to infection. They are normally the major component of circulating white blood cells. Neutrophils act by

---

Concise Guide to Hematology, First Edition. Edited by Alvin H. Schmaier, Hillard M. Lazarus.
© 2012 Blackwell Publishing Ltd. Published 2012 by Blackwell Publishing Ltd.

Table 16.1 Terms used to describe variations of the white blood cell differential

Term	Definition	Example
Absolute	Actual number of a specific type of white blood cells WBC/mm³ or µL of blood	ANC (number/µL) = total WBC count × % of neutrophils and bands in the differential; if the WBC count is 5000/µL and the percentage of neutrophils are 20%, ANC is 1000/µL
Relative	Relation of the number of a specific type of WBC to the total WBC count (the percentage shown in the WBC differential)	If the WBC count is 5000/µL and the differential shows that 90% of these cells are neutrophils, neutrophils are described as relatively increased (relative neutrophilia); "normal," or reference, neutrophil percentage is 50–80%
– Philia, – cytosis	Indicate increased levels in the blood: – philia is used for granulocytes oytosis is used for lymphocytes and monocytes	Neutrophilia, eosinophilia, monocytosis, lymphocytosis
– Penia	Suffix indicating decreased level in the blood; applicable to any WBC, to platelets, and to many non-hematologic substances that are normally present in blood	Neutropenia, thrombocytopenia, insullnopenia

ANC, absolute neutrophil count; WBC, white blood cell.

Table 16.2 Age-related white blood cell differential counts

Age	WBC (per µL)	PMN (%)	Band (%)	Lympocytes (%)	Monocytes (%)	Eosinophils (%)	Basophils (%)
Birth	22,000	60	2	30	5	2	1
1 to 4 years	11,000	35	3	55	5	3	1
6 to teens	9,000	50	3	40	4	2	1
Adult	8,000	70	2	20	5	2	1

WBC, white blood cell; PMN, polymorphonuclear.

ingesting (i.e., phagocytizing) offending organisms and releasing toxic oxygen metabolites and antimicrobial proteins/peptides into the surrounding tissue. Neutrophils are needed continuously, and turnover is constant. 100 billion (10^{11}) neutrophils are produced every day. These cells proliferate from early promyelocytes through myelocytes and then mature to metamyelocytes, and band stages to segmented neutrophils in the bone marrow over approximately 5–6 days, then they enter the circulation, where they remain for approximately 0.5–5 days. Granulocyte colony stimulating factor (G-CSF) stimulates their production. Finally, they are recruited to the tissue where they

Table 16.3 White blood cell counts in various disease states

Condition	WBCs (per μL)	PMN (%)	Band (%)	Lymphocytes (%)	Monocytes (%)	Eosinophils (%)	Basophils (%)
Bacterial infection	16,000	78	8	9	3	1	1
Viremia	3500	5	1	81	10	2	1
Chemotherapy	2800	10	0	85	2	2	1
Steroid therapy[a]	12,000	78	4	14	2	0	0
Splenectomy[b]	13,000	50	2	40	5	2	1

PMN, polymorphonuclear leukocytes; WBC, white blood cell.
a WBC counts also reveal 2% metamyelocytes.
b Nucleated red blood cells and target cell are also seen after splenectomy.

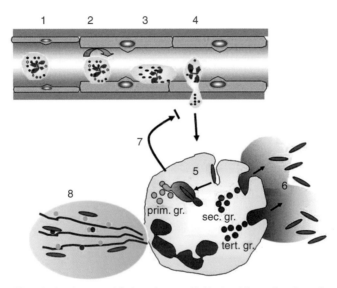

Figure 16.1 Diapedesis of neutrophils into tissues. (1) Neutrophil passing through normal post-capillary venules. (2) Neutrophil rolling along activated endothelium during inflammation. (3) Neutrophil adhering firmly to activated endothelium. (4) Neutrophil migrating through the endothelial lining. (5) Uptake of microorganisms in a phagocytic vacuole. (6) Exocytosis of gelatinase granules and specific granules. (7) Negative feed back to dampen neutrophil diapedesis by secretion of resolvins. (8) Extrusion of DNA and formation of neutrophil extracellular traps that bind and kill microorganisms.

perform their specified function for approximately 1–2 days. Neutrophils are recruited to areas of inflammation where they ingest (phagocytize) microorganisms to kill them by their granule contents and ability to generate high levels of reactive oxygen spcies (ROS) (Figure 16.1). Blood cells develop in the bone marrow, and the earliest cells (progenitor cells) become committed to a specific type of blood cell. As they develop, the blood cells become restricted

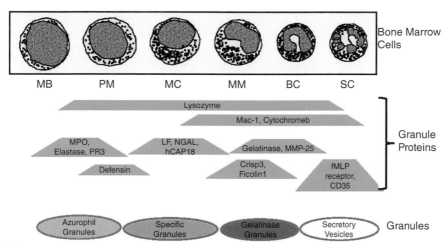

Figure 16.2 Formation of granules during maturation of neutrophils in the bone marrow. Transcription profiles for granule proteins are depicted during maturation of neutrophils from myeloblasts (MB) through promyelocytes (PM), myelocytes (MC), metamyelocytes (MM), bands cells (BC) and segmented cells (SC). Four kinds of granules are seen in neutrophils: azurophilic, specific, gelatinous, and secretory vesicles. The contents of each of these granules are indicated on the figure.

in their ability to proliferate; this occurs at various points for the different WBC types. Commitment begins in the bone marrow at the myeloblast stage, and proliferation occurs through the promyelocyte and myelocyte stages. Metamyelocytes, band forms, and mature neutrophils no longer divide. Proliferation and maturation depend on the presence of colony-stimulating factors (CSF), such as granulocyte CSF and granulocyte–macrophage CSF, in combination with other factors. Each stage is defined by characteristic granules. Classes of granules include primary or azurophilic; secondary or specific; and tertiary (Figure 16.2). All three classes of granules have specific enzymes as well as different staining characteristics on blood smears.

Neutrophil adhesion which is essential for neutrophils getting to an inflammatory site is mediated by L-selectin and the $\alpha M\beta 2$ integrin (CD11b/CD18). The $\beta 2$ integrin is CD18. CD11b/CD18 is also a receptor for C3bi (a proteolytic fragment of C3). Neutrophils ingest bacterial by phagocytosis and kill them through the development of NADPH oxidase, a multiprotein assembly consisting of $gp91^{phox}$, $p22^{phox}$, $p67^{phox}$, $p47^{phox}$, $p40^{phox}$ and others, which creates hydrogen peroxide (H_2O_2) and other reactive oxygen species (ROS) necessary for killing injested organisms. Primary granules of neutrophil (azurophilic granules) contain elastase, myeloperoxidase, defensins, and a variety of other proteins (Figure 16.2). Secondary granules are secretory granules acquired at the transition to the myelocyte stage. Secondary granules (specific granules) contain lactoferrins, transcobalamin 1, and metalloproteinases. Tertiary granules (Gelatinase granules) contain gelatinase and are formed during later stages of neutrophil development. Secretory vesicles are generated by endocytosis and contain plasma proteinases.

B. Eosinophils

Eosinophils are distinguished from neutrophils at the early myelocyte stage. They contain large, bright-staining orange-red granules that are composed of major basic protein, peroxidase, and other lysosomal enzymes (Atlas Figure 6). After these cells spend approximately 9–10 days maturing in the bone marrow and 12 hours in the circulation, they cross the endothelial barrier in areas exposed to the external environment, such as the tracheobronchial tree, gastrointestinal tract, mammary glands, cervix, and vagina. Eosinophilia are also found in connective tissue below the epithelial layer. These cells contain immunoglobulin E receptors on their surface. These receptors, which are not found in neutrophils, play a role in killing parasites. In nonallergic people, the blood eosinophil count is usually less than 400/µL, and averages 120/µL. Eosinophils have a major role in mediating IgE-mediated allergic reactions. Interleukin 5 (IL-5) stimulates eosinophil production.

C. Basophils and mast cells

Basophils and mast cells are the circulating and tissue-bound forms of cells, respectively, that are related but develop from separate precursor cells. Basophils are easily identified by their dark, dense granularity on Wright–Giemsa stain (Atlas Figure 7). These cells are present in the blood in very small numbers. Mast cells arise from CD34+/c-Kit+/CD13+ pluripotent hematopietic cells in bone marrow. They share cytoplasmic basophilic granules, high affinity IgE receptors, and histamine release upon stimulation like basophils, but are considered distinct. Mast cells reside in connective tissue. Both types of cells are believed to play a critical role in host defense against parasites and participate in atopic processes. Basophils increase in myeloproliferative disorders.

D. Monocytes

Once monocytes reach the tissue, they differentiate into macrophages and remove microorganisms and noxious agents. Like neutrophils, these cells phagocytize pathogens. They also generate toxic oxygen metabolites that play a role in killing microorganisms. Monocytes have an essential role in the presentation of antigen to T-lymphocytes. They are essential for tissue repair and remodeling. An increase in monocytes (monocytosis) occurs in tuberculosis and neoplasms.

IV. Neutrophil disorders

A. Overview

Neutrophil disorders may be acquired or inherited. They may occur in the production of white cells, in the maturation of granules, in the expression of proteins that are necessary for critical function, or in the recruitment of cells from the circulation.

B. Disorders in the numbers of circulating neutrophils

Evaluation of these disorders includes a complete blood count and determination of the percentage of each class of white blood cells. Because underlying disease or medication may affect the neutrophil count, this information must be linked to the clinical evaluation. Neutrophil counts vary with age, sex, and race (Table 16.2). For example, the lower limit of the normal blood neutrophil count is 1500/µL in most populations; African Americans have a lower neutrophil limit, approximately 1000/µL.

1. **Neutrophilia** is present when the neutrophil count exceeds the upper limit of the normal range by two standard deviations from the mean value for normal individuals. The value is higher in children than in adults, and the percentage can be higher than normal even if the total count is within the normal range. Neutrophilia is caused by both chronic and acute conditions.
   (a) Chronic stimulation and expansion of the number of neutrophils occurs in a number of conditions. Including:
      (i) infection—toxic granulation (Atlas Figure 31) and Döhle bodies (Atlas Figure 30) are signs of infection in review of neutrophils on the peripheral smear
      (ii) cancer (breast, gastric, lung)
      (iii) myeloproliferative disorders
      (iv) pregnancy and lactation
      (v) eclampsia
      (vi) chronic acidosis
      (vii) anxiety
      (viii) Down syndrome
      (ix) heavy metal poisoning
      (x) metastatic infiltration of the bone marrow
      (xi) proliferation of immature circulating forms (e.g., with leukemia)
      (xii) during recovery of the bone marrow from a toxic incident.
   (b) An acute rise in the neutrophil count in the peripheral blood may occur after the following events:
      (i) during exercise
      (ii) epinephrine administration
      (iii) episodes of hypoxia and stress
      (iv) in response to corticosteroid administration.
2. **Neutropenia** is present if the blood neutrophil count is below 1500/µL. Mild neutropenia is present when the neutrophil count is 1000–1800/µL. Complications rarely develop in this situation. A neutrophil count of 500–1000/µL is associated with increased risk of infection. When the neutrophil count is ≤500/µL, the patient has considerable susceptibility to infection with endogenous organisms in the skin, oropharynx, and intestine. Infections with Gram-positive cocci, especially *Staphylococcus aureus*, are common in these patients. If the patient has been receiving antibacterial agents for a long period while neutropenic, suppression of

bacterial flora facilitates fungal overgrowth and infections due to *Candida* or *Aspergillus* species arise. Neutropenia is caused by decreased production or increased use of neutrophils.

(a) **Conditions that cause decreased production of neutrophils to result in neutropenia:**

    (i)   Medication is the major cause of neutropenia. Medications can have a specific effect on myeloid production producing isolated neutropenia (agranulocytosis) or general bone marrow suppression of all three cell lines; granulocytes, red cells, and platelets. Granulocytes colony stimulating factor (G-CSF), a growth factor stimulating neutrophil production from progenitors, is used as a therapeutic agent to stimulate neutrophil production, particularly in patients undergoing chemotherapy. Medications associated with neutropenia include:

        • Chemotherapeutic agents.
        • Anti-inflammatory agents (e.g., sulindac [Clinoril]).
        • Antibiotics (e.g., sulfonamides, high-dose penicillins).
        • Phenothiazines.
        • Antithyroid drugs (e.g., methimazole, propylthiouracil).

    (ii)   Autoimmune diseases:

        • Rheumatoid arthritis and Felty syndrome due to hypersplenism.
        • Systemic lupus erythematosus due antibody-mediated reduced bone marrow release or agranulocytosis.

    (iii)   Neutropenia may also be a component of *lymphoid diseases* (e.g., Hodgkin lymphoma, non-Hodgkin lymphoma, chronic lymphocytic leukemia), and viral illnesses (e.g., Epstein–Barr virus, human immunodeficiency virus, hepatitis). Antibodies directed against neutrophils may be associated with these conditions. In these patients, neutropenia may be caused in part by decreased neutrophil production in the bone marrow.

(b) **Enhanced removal of neutrophils from the circulation is seen with:**

    (i)   Hemodialysis and cardiopulmonary bypass due to sticking in the apparatus.

    (ii)   Endotoxin release associated with overwhelming bacterial sepsis.

(c) **Neutropenia** is a major clinical feature of severe idiopathic chronic neutropenia, severe congenital neutropenia and cyclic neutropenia. In cyclic neutropenia, neutrophils disappear from the circulation at regular 3-week intervals. Levels of other blood components, especially monocytes, can also fluctuate. Several congenital neutropenia are associated with mutations in the neutrophil elastase gene. The cyclic, congenital and idiopathic neutropenias are usually amenable to treatment with recombinant G-CSF.

Table 16.4 Structural and functional defects in neutrophils

Step	Disease	Molecular defect
Rolling	Leukocyte adhesion deficiency (LAD-2)	Sialyl Lewis^x carbohydrate abnormalities due to a fucosylation defect due to a defective protein necessary for transport of GDP-fucose in Golgi. Generalized loss of expression of fucosylated glycans on cell surfaces.
Tight adhesion and phagocytosis	LAD-1	Loss or diminished β_2 integrin (CD18) expression
Defective neutrophil and platelet activation	LAD-3	Defection activation pathway of β2 integrin due to mutations in kindlin-3, an integrin binding protein
Migration and Degranulation	Specific granule deficiency	Deficiency of the myeloid specific transcription factor C/EBPε
Degranulation	Chediak-Higashi syndrome	Lysosomal trafficking regulator protein CHS1 (LYST) gene leading to a defect in granule morphogenesis
Oxidative burst	Chronic granulomatous disease	NADPH oxidase activation defect due to deficiencies in gp91^{phox} (65%), p22^{phox} (5%), p67^{phox} (5%), p47^{phox} (25%) or p40^{phox} (rare).
	Myeloperoxidase deficiency	Loss of HOCl production; defective posttranslational processing of MPO

NADPH, reduced nicotinamide adenine dinucleotide phosphate.

C. Structural and functional defects in neutrophils

Neutrophils are recruited from the circulation in response to chemotactic agents that are released at the site of infection. Chemotactic agents are peptides and proteins that diffuse from the site of tissue injury, bind to specific receptors on the cell surface, and stimulate neutrophils to attach (adhere and roll) and migrate though the blood vessel wall (Figure 16.1). After neutrophils move from the circulation and cross the endothelial cell barrier, they phagocytize invading organisms, and with the help of granules, destroy them. Disorders of neutrophil function impair the ability of neutrophils to move from the circulation, phagocytize particles, or degranulate. The net result is impaired neutrophil function. Several inherited disorders have been defined at the molecular level, and these disorder have shed light on critical steps of neutrophil function (Table 16.4).

1. **Leukocyte adhesion deficiency** are a group of rare diseases that have led to the understanding that recruitment across the endothelial cell barrier occurs as a result of specific protein-protein or protein-carbohydrate interactions and neutrophil activation is mediated by integrin action. Three types have been recognized:LAD-1, LAD-2, and LAD-3. These disorders are characterized by recurrent bacterial and fungal infections as well as by neutrophilia. The neutrophil count is often 20,000–90,000/μL.

    (a) LAD-1 is caused by a deficiency or defect in the cell surface proteins of the β_2 integrin (CD18). This defect limits or prevents expression of alpha integrins (CD11a, CD11b, CD11c, and CD11d) with CD18 on cell surfaces. Patients who lack CD18 have markedly decreased or absent neutrophils at the site of inflammation because these cells cannot adhere to the endothelial cell wall.

       (i) The severity of the disease is related to the level of expression of the β_2 integrin (CD18).

       (ii) Manifestations of LAD-1 include delayed separation of the umbilical cord in infants, skin infections, chronic leg ulcers, and gingivitis. *Staphylococcus aureus*, Gram-negative organisms (e.g., *Escherichia coli*), and fungal agents are usually responsible.

       (iii) Diagnosis is made by flow cytometry on activated neutrophils with an antibody to the β_2 integrin subunit or CD11b.

       (iv) Treatment includes antibiotics if the condition is mild and bone marrow transplant if it is severe.

    (b) LAD-2 is a complex disease that is associated with leukocyte adhesion defects, neurologic defects, craniofacial defects, and the rare Bombay (hh) erythrocyte phenotype. The Bombay erythrocyte phenotype is the expression of a nonfucosylated form of the H antigen of red cells. This antigenic variant represents the failure to form certain fucose carbohydrate linkage. These patients have an impaired ability to form sialyl Lewis^x carbohydrate structures on neutrophils and other cells. The basic defect is in Golgi and their inability to transport GDP-fucose into Golgi. This leads to improper sialylated selectins which are not able to tether by-passing neutrophils to endothelium and promote their rolling. along the endothelial cell wall. This rolling is the initial step in the recruitment of neutrophils from the circulation. If this action does not occur, then neutrophils do not cross the endothelium and cannot localize to the site of infection.

    (c) LAD-3 is a mutation in *kindlin 3*, a β-integrin binding protein that is essential for neutrophil and platelet activation. Affected individuals have reduced neutrophil and platelet activation.

2. **Chronic granulomatous disease** (CGD) is a rare ($4–5/10^6$ people) disease that is characterized by recurrent life-threatening bacterial and fungal infections. These infections occur because of an impaired ability to kill bacteria after they are phagocytized. CGD neutrophils are unable to develop reduced nicotinamide adenine dinucleotide phosphate (NADPH) oxidase to kill intracellular bacteria. Several proteins [gp91^{phox} (65%), p22^{phox} (~5%), p67^{phox} (~5%) p47^{phox} (~25%)] or p40^{phox} (rare) that participate in the assembly of NADPH oxidase are known to be defective in individuals with CGD. The numbers in parenthesis indicate the frequency of defects seen in the proteins of the multiprotein assembly of NADPH oxidase in patients with CGD. NADPH oxidase is responsible for the production of superoxides leading to ingested bacterial killing.

    (a) Catalase-positive bacteria and fungi pose a major risk of infection in patients who have CGD.

        (i) Ingested bacteria are contained in the phagosome, and myeloperoxidase is delivered by degranulation.

        (ii) Hydrogen peroxidase (H_2O_2) is produced in the neutrophil and converted to oxygen species that kill microorganisms by NADPH oxidase.

        (iii) Normal neutrophils produce sufficient H_2O_2 to overcome the H_2O_2 that is catabolized by the catalase that is produced by bacteria. In CGD, because of the defects in the subunits of NADPH, little or no H_2O_2 is formed.

        (iv) Therefore, the catalase that is produced by the microorganism removes any residual H_2O_2.

        (v) In this situation, *S. aureus*, *Serratia*, *Salmonella*, *Candida*, and *Aspergillus* pose an infectious risk.

    (b) Clinically, the disease varies in severity and time of presentation (childhood to adulthood). Microabscesses and granulomas point to the diagnosis.

    (c) The diagnosis is made by examining the colorless to blue-black change of a dye nitroblue tetrazolium (NBT) placed in neutrophil phagosomes. Patients with CGD have markedly diminished conversion of the dye to the blue-black color.

3. **Specific granule deficiency** is a rare autosomal recessive inherited disorder. These patients have a relative deficiency of specific granules that contain the enzymes that are necessary for the migration and delivery of receptors to the cell surface. These receptors are needed for complete neutrophil function. As a result, patients with this disease have impaired migration of neutrophils and recurrent infections of the skin, sinuses, and lungs. The basic defect in this condition is a deficiency of the myeloid specific transcription factor C/EBPε. This transcription factor regulates expression of certain genes activated during granulocyte differentiation. The defect can also effect granules of eosinophils.

4. **Chediak–Higashi syndrome (CHS)** is a rare autosomal recessive disorder that is associated with immune deficiency.

    (a) Neutrophils from patients who have CHS show a defect in the formation of granules. Defects in lysosomes and vesicular structures are also seen in other cells.

    (b) The underlying defect is a defect in granule morphogenesis in multiple tissues resulting from mutations in the CHS1 (LYST-lysosomal trafficking regulatory protein) gene encoding a lysosomal trafficking regulator protein. This abnormality results in a giant coalesced azurophil/specific granules in neutrophils resulting in ineffective neutrophil production, neutropenia, and impaired chemotaxis and killing of microorganisms.

(c) Patients who have CHS are susceptible to infection and hemophago-cytic lymphohistiocytosis. These patients also have oculo-cutaneous albinism and cranial and peripheral neuropathy. Natural killer cell activity is absent, and moderate neutropenia occurs. The only real treatment of this disorder is bone marrow transplantation.

5. **Hereditary myeloperoxidase syndrome** occurs at a rate of approximately 1:2000 to 1:4000. The disorder is produced by variable expression of the myeloperoxidase (MPO) gene due to defective post-translational process-ing of an abnormal MPO precursor polypeptide. Partial or complete MPO deficiency produces diminished production of hypochlorous acid (HOCl) or HOCl-derived chloramines. HOCl activates metalloproteinases and inactivates antiproteinases like alpha-1-antrypsin which contribute to bacterial killing. This syndrome is usually found incidentally on morpho-logic examination of neutrophils. The major finding is intact phagocytosis of bacteria and fungi, but impaired ability to kill fungi such as *Candida* and *Aspergillus*. Some patients with concurrent diabetes have recurrent visceral fungal infections.

V. Disorders of eosinophils

A. Eosinopenia

Eosinopenia is less well characterized than neutropenia. The average eosi-nophil count is 200 cells/μL and can range from 0–400 cells/μL. The eosi-nophil count can decrease as a result of infection or administration of corticosteroids, prostaglandins, or epinephrine. However, unlike neutrope-nia, this condition is usually transient and is not associated with a significant risk of infection.

B. Eosinophilia

Eosinophilia is characterized by an absolute eosinophil count of greater than 500 cells/μL. Secondary causes of eosinophila are as follows:

1. Allergic reactions to certain drugs (e.g., aspirin, sulfonamides, penicillins, nitrofurantoin) or to iodide-containing substances are the most common cause.
2. Allergies to environmental agents (e.g., grass, trees, dust) and allergic diseases.
3. Asthma and various respiratory tract disorders.
4. Dermatitis and cutaneous disorders e.g., eczema, psoriasis.
5. Connective tissue disorders and vasculitis.
6. Ulcerative colitis and inflammatory bowel disease.
7. Malignancy (e.g., Hodgkin lymphoma, non-Hodgkin lymphoma, brain and skin tumors, acute leukemia).
8. Serum sickness also is associated with an elevated blood eosinophil count.
9. Infection with parasites, both protozoan e.g., pneumocytes, toxoplasmo-sis, malaria, and metazoan e.g., ascariasis, trichinosis, schistosomiasis., is common.

10. Addison disease.
11. Immunodeficiency disorders.

C. Idiopathic hypereosinophilic syndrome or hypereosinophilic syndrome (HES)

HES is associated with an elevation (>1500 cells/μL) of the circulating eosinophil count for at least 6 months without another explanation. These patients have to have organ infiltration by eosinophils leading to dysfunction of the heart, central nervous system, kidney, lungs, gastrointestinal tract, and skin. They may or may not have evidence of a clonal disorder as seen in patients with chronic eosinophilic leukemia (CEL), acute eosinophilic leukemia (AEL), chronic myelogenous leukemia (CML), polycythemia rubra vera (PRV), and essential thrombocytosis (ET). Some patients with CEL have an interstitial chromosomal deletion of the *CHIC2* domain on chromosome 4q12 producing an activated tyrosine kinase fusion protein *FIP1L1-PDGFRA* (gene FIP1-like-1—platelet-derived growth factor receptor-α gene). Patients with HES and this fusion gene often respond to treatment with the tyrosine kinase inhibitor imatinib. Most eosinophil function is associated with degranulation and release of major basic protein. This protein kills parasites, but is also toxic to the skin, intestine, tracheal epithelial cells, and other mononuclear cells.

VI. Disorders of basophils

1. A low basophil count is associated with glucocorticoid treatment and hypersensitivity reactions.
2. The basophil count is increased in patients who have allergic conditions, infection, endocrinopathy, and myeloproliferative disorders (e.g., cell-mediated lymphotoxicity, polycythemia rubra vera, myeloid metaplasia, essential thrombocythemia).
3. Systemic mastocytosis is a disorder associated with mast cell infiltration of the skin or other organs also occurs. Systemic mastocytosis, a mast cell infiltrative disorder, is associated with symptoms related to excess histamine and include urticaria, hives, and dizziness. It is due to a gain-of-function mutation in *c-Kit*, Kit D816V. Two other mutations *FIP1L1-PDGFRA* and Kit F522C have been associated with the disorder. *FIP1L1-PDGFRA* (platelet-derived growth factor receptor A) which has tyrosine kinase activity also is associated with eosinophilia as described above.

VII. Disorders of monocytes parallel those seen with neutrophils

1. The average circulating monocyte count is 300/μL and can range from 0 to 800 cells/μL.
2. Monocytopenia occurs in response to stress, endotoxemia and after glucocorticoid administration.

3. Monocytosis is present when the absolute monocyte count exceeds 800/μL. It occurs chronic inflammatory states such as in:
    (a) Myelodysplastic syndromes.
    (b) neutropenic states (e.g., cyclic neutropenia).
    (c) During the recovery phase of agranulocytosis.
    (d) Exacerbations of lymphoma.
    (e) Patients who have undergone splenectomy.
    (f) Subtypes of leukemia.
    (g) Response to infection (e.g., acute bacterial, tuberculosis, listeria, cytomegalovirus, tuberculosis, subacute bacterial endocarditis, syphilis, fever of unknown origin).
    (h) Patients who have underlying inflammatory disease, such as systemic lupus erythematosis, rheumatoid arthritis, temporal arteritis, polyarteritis, gout, ulcerative colitis, regional enteritis, sarcoidosis.

VIII. Summary

Each of the members of the myeloid series—neutrophils, eosinophils, basophils, and monocytes—has a critical role in host defense against pathogenic organisms. Some of the roles overlap and others are unique to each class of cells. The members of this series exhibit variations in number in response to disease or infection. An understanding of the regulation of their blood levels and functions aids in understanding the clinical picture of a patient. Although the information provided appears exhaustive, a considerable amount about the function of each of these cells has yet to be uncovered.

Further reading

Ackerman SJ, Butterfield JH. Eosinophilia, eosinophil-associated diseases, chronic eosinophil leukemia, and the hypereosinophilic syndromes. In: Hoffman R, Benz EJ, Shattil SJ, Furie B, Silberstein LE, McGlave P, Heslop HE, Anastasi J, eds. Hematology Basic Principles and Practice. Philadelphia: Churchill Livingstone, Elsevier, 2009:1167–86.

Borregaard N, Boxer LA. Disorders of neutrophil function. In: Lichtman MA, Beutler E, Kipps TJ, Seligsohn U, Kaushansky K, Prchal JF, eds. Williams Hematology. New York: McGraw-Hill, 2006:921–57.

Dinauer MC, Coates TD. Disorders of phagocyte function and number. In: Hoffman R, Benz EJ, Shattil SJ, Furie B, Silberstein LE, McGlave P, Heslop HE, Anastasi J, eds. Hematology Basic Principles and Practice. Philadelphia: Churchill Livingstone, Elsevier. 2009:687–720.

17 Bone Marrow Structure and Diagnostic Testing

Howard J. Meyerson and Hillard M. Lazarus

Case Western Reserve University and University Hospitals Case Medical Center, Cleveland, OH, USA

I. Bone marrow structure

A. Overview
Bone marrow is a semi-solid gelatinous tissue which resides within the bony cavities of the axial skeleton. It contains hematopoeitic cells (red marrow), stromal cells, and fat (yellow marrow).

B. Bone
The bone that surrounds the marrow is composed of a thick layer of compact bony material referred to as *cortical bone*. This bone is covered by fibrocartilaginous tissue (*periosteum*). The space inside the cortical bone is called the *medullary cavity*. The medullary cavity itself contains a lattice-like network of thin bone referred to as *trabecular* or *cancellous* bone. Hematopoietic cells reside in the intervening spaces of trabecular bone.

1. Structure of bone
(a) Woven bone is tissue in which the normal parallel fibrillar structure of the bone has not been fully created. It is the pattern seen in newly formed bone.
(b) Lamellar bone is mature bone in which there is a microscopically visible parallel structure referred to as *cement lines.*

2. Cellular components of bone
(a) Osteoblasts:
    (i)   Osteoblasts are bone forming cells of mesenchymal origin that synthesize glycosoaminoglycans and collagen fibers (*osteoid* or non-mineralized bone) forming the basis of bone structure.

Concise Guide to Hematology, First Edition. Edited by Alvin H. Schmaier, Hillard M. Lazarus.
© 2012 Blackwell Publishing Ltd. Published 2012 by Blackwell Publishing Ltd.

(ii)   On tissue biopsy sections the cells are flat to slightly rounded and line the bony trabeculae and cortical bone particularly in areas of new bone formation.

(iii)   On aspirate smears the cells resemble plasma cells although the nucleus appears to be falling out of the cell. The cells commonly occur in small loose collections.

(iv)   Osteoblasts are not generally encountered in bone marrow aspirated from normal adults but may be seen in growing children, sites of bony injury, or hyperparathyroidism.

(b) Osteoclasts:

(i)   Osteoclasts are bone resorbing/remodeling multinucleated cells derived from the monocyte/macrophage lineage.

(ii)   The cells reside in scooped out areas of trabecular bone referred to as *Howship's lacunae.*

(iii)   Osteoclasts like osteoblasts are not normally encountered on an aspirated bone marrow smear unless bone remodeling changes are present or bone growth is occurring.

(iv)   Osteoclasts resemble megakaryocytes due to their large size and multi-nucleation but differ from megakaryocytes as their nuclei are separate and distinct rather than overlapping.

3. Biology of bone

(a) The skeleton undergoes continuous remodeling during life. The remodeling is carried out by osteoclasts resorbing bone followed by osteoblasts producing osteoid, which then becomes mineralized.

(b) Osteoblastic and osteoclastic activity is coupled together.

(i)   Osteoclastic activity is stimulated by the action of osteoblasts which are activated by various environmental signals.

(ii)   Bone resorption by osteoclasts requires *RANKL,* a member of the TNF ligand protein family expressed by osteoblasts. RANKL stimulates osteoclastic differentiation, cellular fusion generating multinucleated cells, and activation resulting in bone resorption.

(iii)   Osteoclasts subsequently direct the differentiation and activation of osteoblasts to synthesize new bone through the action of both membrane-bound and secreted signaling molecules.

(c) *Osteocytes* are cells that are encased by bone and appear as small nuclei within trabecular or cortical bone. They are terminally differentiated osteoblasts.

C. Components of bone marrow

1. Bone marrow stroma

(a) The bone marrow stroma is the supporting matrix for hematopoietic cells.

(b) The bone marrow stroma is composed primarily of:

(i)   Macrophages.

(ii)   Specialized bone marrow stromal cells:

- Bone marrow stromal cells have the important ability to differentiate into other mesenchymal tissues such as bone, cartilage and fat.
- Stromal cells also provide important micro-anatomical niches supporting hematopoiesis and hematopoietic stem cells.

(iii) Fat cells (adipose tissue):
- The function of marrow adipose tissue in regulating hematopoiesis or osteogenesis is unclear. Marrow fat secretes cytokines that can influence granulopoiesis and T cell and monocyte function.
- There is an inverse relationship between amount of marrow fat and erythropoiesis and bone density not seen with subcutaneous adipose tissue.
- Marrow adipose tissue also differs from peripheral adipose tissue in that it is not lost in starvation.

2. Vasculature

(a) The marrow vasculature consists of a *nutrient artery* that penetrates the bone and branches into smaller and smaller divisions (arterioles) ultimately forming open vascular channels, a *sinusoidal network*, in the medullary cavity.

(b) Sinusoids are dilated thin walled channels at the capillary-venous junction.

(i) Adventitial cells:
- Sinusoids are lined on the outside by adventitial cells.
- Adventitial cells serve as an additional niche supporting hematopoiesis.
- Adventitial cells likely make *reticulin*, a form of collagen, which can increase in disease states.

(ii) Morphologically, on tissue sections, sinusoids are generally not apparent since they are often collapsed.

(iii) Sinuoids drain into venous sinuses which connect to ultimately form the *comitant* vein.

(c) The comitant vein exits the marrow through the same channel as the nutrient artery.

3. Hematopoietic cells

(a) Hematopoietic cells lie in groups or cords in the inter-trabecular spaces and enter the circulation by migrating through the sinusoidal endothelium.

(b) Hematopoietic cells are not randomly distributed through the marrow but are present in small niches. On histologic sections these zones are not always evident:

(i) Erythroid progenitors localize in small collections around marrow macrophages.

(ii) Granulocytes generally reside adjacent to adipose cells with immature granulocytes near bony trabeculae and adventitial cells.

(iii) Megakaryocytes lie abutting marrow sinusoids.

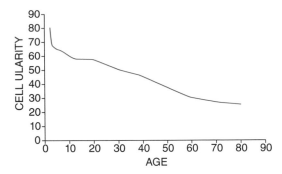

Figure 17.1 Relationship of bone marrow cellularity with age.

(c) Marrow cellularity:
  (i)   The ratio of marrow space occupied by hematopoietic cells to the total available marrow space is referred to as the *marrow cellularity*.
  (ii) Marrow hematopoietic cellularity varies with age (Figure 17.1). As a rule of thumb marrow cellularity is equivalent to 100 minus the patient's age in years. In reality, marrow cellularity decreases to roughly 50% by age 30 and declines slowly thereafter until late adulthood.
  (iii) Marrow cellularity may change rapidly in response to a peripheral cytopenia, infection, or growth factors.

II. Bone marrow diagnostic testing

A. Overview
Clinical reasons to evaluate the bone marrow are given in Box 17.1. In general a bone marrow examination should be done for an unexplained cytopenia, evaluation for a lymphoproliferative process or suspected hematopoietic disorder. A thorough examination of a suspected marrow process consists of a review of the blood cell counts and indices and microscopic review of the peripheral blood smear. Medical history is important and the reason for the marrow biopsy needs to be transmitted to the pathologist to help focus the evaluation. Bone marrow morphology changes dramatically in the face of chemotherapy. Therefore the timing of the marrow biopsy in relation to therapy needs to be known. A bone marrow performed 14 days after initiating chemotherapy has a significantly different appearance than a marrow examined 35 days later. A history of recent treatment with growth factors is especially relevant.

B. Bone marrow aspirate and biopsy procedure
1. Overview
The diagnostic bone marrow aspiration and biopsy procedure is an essential tool in the evaluation of patients who have a suspected hematologic disorder.

Box 17.1 Clinical reasons to perform a bone marrow examination

Unexplained cytopenia (anemia, thrombocytopenia, neutropenia)

Staging for non-Hodgkin or Hodgkin lymphoma

Suspected acute leukemia or recurrence of acute leukemia

Suspected myeloproliferative disorder

Suspected myelodysplastic syndrome

Suspected metastatic carcinoma

Suspected plasma cell neoplasm (monoclonal immunoglobulin present in serum)

Evaluation of lymphoproliferative disorder

Staging of small cell tumors of childhood

Follow-up and treatment response in patients with hematopoietic neoplasms

Assessment of bone marrow after hematopoietic progenitor cell transplantation

Unexplained leukoerythroblastic blood smear

Fever of unknown origin

Evaluation of suspected macrophage disorder (storage disease, hemophagocytosis)

This technique can provide tissues that are analyzed by morphologic methods for cellularity and cellular characteristics, flow cytometry for immunophenotyping and cytogenetic and fluorescent *in situ* hybridization (FISH) studies as well as for molecular markers. A variety of disorders can be diagnosed including bone marrow failure states, hematologic malignancies, metastatic cancers, enzymatic and congenital storage diseases and other conditions.

2. Personnel and equipment

(a) **Medical practitioner.** The bone marrow aspirate and biopsy procedure has been part of the stock-and-trade of the hematology–oncology physician for decades. With proper training this technique can be undertaken successfully in most patients by medical practitioners such as internists, house officers in-training and depending on the state in which a person practices, mid-level care providers (licensed nurse practitioners and physician assistants) as well. Procedures in very young children, however, should be restricted to individuals highly experienced in this patient subpopulation. In general, there are no absolute contraindications to performing this test. Caution, however, must be exercised in seriously ill patients or in those subjects with bleeding disorders (see below: Complications). Untrained medical personnel must be supervised extremely closely when performing this procedure and must not be permitted to undertake this testing without having fulfilled all local institutional policies and procedural regulations. Further, only very highly trained professionals should be performing diagnostic bone marrow examinations from the sternum due to the danger of penetration into critical structures in the chest cavity; nearly all procedures should be undertaken at the posterior superior iliac crest site (see below).

(b) **Additional personnel and necessary equipment:**

   (i)   **A trained laboratory assistant.** This person takes the specimens, prepares the slides for morphologic evaluation, and submits the bone marrow clot and biopsy in containers with appropriate media.

   (ii) **Chlorhexidine swabs** unless contraindicated due to a serious adverse reaction, in which case povodine-iodine can be used for sterilization purposes.

   (iii) **Sterile gloves.**

   (iv) **Pre-packed bone marrow diagnostic kit** containing sterile drapes, ampoules of local anesthetic (1% plain lidocaine or 0.25%/0.5% bupivacaine), disposable needles and syringes, disposable sterile bone marrow aspiration and biopsy needles.

3. Consenting process

The patient must be identified as the appropriately intended person and the subject (or guardian) must furnish consent for this procedure. Further, although extremely rare, the patient must be made aware of potential complications that have been reported to occur at a rate of 0.12 to 0.30% (Bain 2003 and 2006). Always verify that the patient is not allergic to either the local anesthetic or any other agents used for sedation.

4. Complications

In survey reports (Bain 2003; Bain 2006) of 20,323 procedures, hemorrhage was the most frequent and most serious adverse event, necessitating rare blood transfusions and leading to death in a single patient. Potential risk factors most often associated with bleeding were a diagnosis of a myeloproliferative disorder, aspirin therapy or both, use of other anticoagulant treatment, disseminated intravascular coagulation and obesity. Other complications have included trauma such as lacerations to tissues in the region, local infection and hemorrhage. Other very rare, serious adverse events include retroperitoneal hematomas due to puncture of the a branch of the iliac artery that runs on the inner surface of the hip (Arellano-Rodrigo; Wahid) and fractures of the bone that has been penetrated, especially in those individuals who have underlying bone disorders.

5. Sedation

Prior to the bone marrow aspirate and biopsy procedure, the patient may experience significant anxiety and during and after the procedure, pain may be a prominent feature. The patient should be re-assured that the test is indicated at the time this person is giving consent. Some patients may require use of minor tranquilizing or sedating agents. During the procedure itself, the patient should be given a judicious amount of local anesthesia but not exceeding local institutional guidelines. In those patients in whom their anxiety is excessive, possibly due to problems during a previous procedure, or in pediatric patients, conscious sedation administered by an anesthesiologist or other qualified health-care professional should be used.

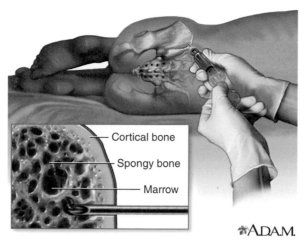

Cortical bone

Spongy bone

Marrow

✻A.D.A.M.

Figure 17.2 Bone marrow biopsy. (Reproduced with permission from adamimages.com.)

6. Preparation for the procedure

(a) **Site.** One of the most important aspects of the procedure is identifying the appropriate site for aspirate and biopsy. The patient can be in the prone or ventral supine position, or in the lateral decubitus position. Many physicians mark the posterior superior iliac crest with a marking pen or use a coin to make an impression. The posterior superior iliac crest is lateral to the sacroiliac joint and can be palpated easily even in moderately obese patients. In more obese patients, identify the anterior iliac crest and use the same latitude to identify the posterior superior iliac crest (see Figure 17.2).

(b) **Sterilization and anesthesia.** The site is sterilized with chlorhexidine and a sterile (windowed) drape is placed over the area prior to administering local anesthesia. An injection wheal is raised by injecting subcutaneously with a 25-gauge needle. Then, the anesthetic is infiltrated into the subcutaneous tissues by slowly advancing the needle to the periosteal tissues. Sufficient time should be made to allow for the local anesthetic to take effect.

7. Bone marrow aspiration and biopsy

(a) **Overview.** Many clinical personnel prefer to perform the aspirate and biopsy using the same instrument although two separate instruments can be used. Further, many persons prefer to enter the skin directly with the instrument rather than use a lance to create a small skin incision (and as such may leave a scar).

(b) **Bone marrow aspiration:**

    (i)   Some bone marrow aspiration needles have a guard to limit the degree of penetration and prevent the needle from passing all the way through the bone. The guard is removed from the instrument except for sternal procedures (see above; use of sternal sites is to be discouraged except in rare circumstances and only by highly-qualified and experienced health-care providers).

(ii) The angle of entry is important and the needle should be positioned so that at the start of insertion, the instrument is perpendicular to the posterior superior iliac crest prominence (see Figure 17.2).

(iii) The needle is slowly advanced through the bone cortex using a semi-circular motion with care to note the degree of penetration, usually only a few centimeters. Practitioners use different ways to define depth of insertion; one simple method is to put the index finger about one centimeter above the skin and stop advancing when this distance is achieved. Once inside the medullary area of the bone, the needle will feel fixed solidly within bone.

(iv) At this juncture, the stylet is removed and a syringe is affixed to withdraw/aspirate approximately 0.5–1 mL of liquid bone marrow into the syringe. The syringe is removed and passed to the laboratory assistant to prepare the microscopic slides. An adequate marrow aspirate will have visible particles. If no particles have been obtained, reasons include either failure to adequately penetrate the bone marrow cavity, or the patient may have a hypoplastic or aplastic marrow space with limited or no hematopoietic tissue. In such instances, the person performing the procedure may withdraw the instrument and begin again using the same skin site but re-directing the needle in a slightly different position. Failure to obtain a marrow aspirate is referred to as a "dry tap".

(c) **Bone marrow biopsy:**

(i) Usually the same skin site used for the aspirate is used for the biopsy, although the direction and bone insertion site may differ slightly. As noted above, many practitioners use the biopsy needle to collect both an aspirate and biopsy, separated in time.

(ii) The instrument is inserted slowly into bone using a semi-circular motion of the hand but with gentle pressure. Bones may vary in composition from extremely hard to extremely soft and caution is urged when initiating this maneuver. The needle is inserted into the bone until it appears fixed and stable (usually after about one-half to one centimeter of depth).

(iii) The stylet is withdrawn and the needle is slowly advanced a minimum of 1.5 centimeters using the semi-circular motion.

(iv) The needle is removed with the specimen in place. This is accomplished by gently rocking the needle back and forth in various directions while also twisting/rotating the needle clockwise and counter-clockwise. Failure to initiate these actions often results in the bone marrow biopsy (or "core") being left within the patient when the needle is removed.

(v)   Upon removal of the needle, the core is extracted from the sharp end of the needle by pushing a thin stylet into the needle until the biopsy has been pushed out of the proximal end (the contact point used for the syringe while performing the aspiration).

(vi)   The biopsy or core should be pushed onto a small sterile gauze pad so that touch-preparations of the slide can be made by the laboratory assistant, especially if an aspirate was not obtained as in the case of a "dry tap".

(vii)   Upon completion of the biopsy portion of the procedure, pressure is applied to obtain adequate hemostasis; such will take longer in the setting of a patient who has a coagulopathy or thrombocytopenic state. The area is cleaned with a disinfectant and a sterile bandage; the latter can be removed after 24 hours. Enhanced pressure and hemostasis can be accomplished by having the patient lie supine on a small towel rolled up into a flat ball using the person's own weight to apply the needed pressure.

(viii) The bone marrow aspiration and biopsy site should be inspected for delayed bleeding or infection over the next several days.

(d) Post-procedure issues. Patients and those who accompany the patient to the procedure should be instructed to watch for signs of bleeding at the biopsy site. If significant problems arise such as light-headedness, severe pain, altered mental status or other adverse events, the patient should immediately seek medical attention.

C. Morphologic examination of the bone marrow
1. Overview
Bone marrow aspirate smears are performed primarily to evaluate the cytological features of marrow hematopoietic cells whereas the bone marrow tissue core biopsy is used to determine global changes such as marrow cellularity or infiltration of the marrow by mass lesions such as lymphoma or metastatic tumor. Smears are routinely stained with a Romanowsky stain such as Wright–Giemsa whereas bone marrow biopsies are stained with hematoxylin and eosin similar to other surgical biopsy specimens. To further aid in the diagnosis and evaluation of hematopoietic disorders ancillary studies are necessary such as histochemical and immunohistochemical stains, flow cytometry and cytogenetics.

2. Bone marrow aspirate
(a) **Adequacy.** Adequacy of the marrow aspirate smear can be determined by the presence of visible marrow particles or *spicules* (Figure 17.3). The unfortunate use of the term spicule leaves the erroneous impression that small bone fragments are present on the aspirate smear. In fact, the particles are mini-pieces of bone marrow aspirated into the syringe maintained as small tissue fragments. Actual bony fragments are not present.

(a) (b)

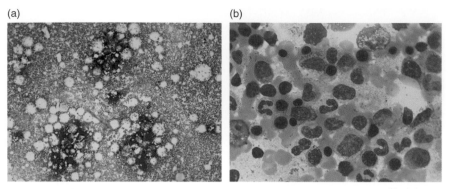

Figure 17.3 Normal bone marrow aspirate, Wright–Giemsa stain. Low power magnification (40×), (a), showing three spicules, or bone marrow fragments, an indication of good marrow sampling. High power examination (1000×), (b), allows for the evaluation of the cytologic features of marrow hematopoietic elements, primarily granulocyte and erythroid precursors. Cell differential counts are routinely performed on bone marrow aspirate smears.

A good quality aspirate smear should contain one or more marrow particles.

(b) Low-power examination (40× or 100×).
    (i)   The bone marrow aspirate smear should first be viewed under low-power magnification to determine the number of particles. One also assesses the quality of the aspirate to determine the adequacy of the sample.
    (ii)   Megakaryocytes, metastatic tumor cells and other rare elements are best scanned for at low power since they are not abundant.
    (iii)   Low-power examination is a necessary first step. Jumping to a high power examination results in the morphologist overlooking items to examine.

(c) High-power examination (400×, 500× or 1000×).
    (i)   Areas to review:
- Areas of well-preserved cells near the edges of bone marrow particles should be identified at low power and used for high-power examination.
- An oil immersion lens (500× or1000×) should be used liberally.
- Examining cells within particles is difficult due to overlapping cells and the presence of many broken cells. Additionally, the thickness of the smears in the spicules often prevents the Romanowsky stain from fully penetrating the cells leading to an artificially pale stain.
- Examination of the smear far away from particles is also to be avoided since these areas are significantly diluted by peripheral blood.

    (ii)   Bone marrow differential:
- A minimum of 200 cells are generally counted and classified to determine a *bone marrow differential* count (Table 17.1).

Table 17.1 Normal bone marrow differential count	
	Normal range (%)
Promyelocyte	1–5
Myelocyte	5–10
Metamyelocyte	10–25
Band	10–20
Segmented neutrophil	5–30
Eosinophil	2–4
Basophil	0–1
Blast	0–1
Lymphocyte	5–25
Monocyte	0–2
Plasma cell	0–2
Erythroid cell	17–35
Myeloid/erythroid	1.5–3

- All neutrophil granulocyte precursor stages are enumerated (promyelocyte, myelocyte, metamyelocyte, band, segmented neutrophils) as well as eosinophils, basophils, erythroid progenitors, monocytes, lymphocytes and plasma cells.
- The various stages of erythroid maturation are not usually specifically distinguished in the marrow differential.

(iii) Myeloid/erythroid ratio (M/E ratio).
- The cell count includes only hematopoietic elements and is used to determine the *myeloid/erythroid ratio* (M/E ratio)
- The normal M/E ratio is the ratio of the number of all granulocytic elements to the number of erythroid cells.
- It is normally 1.5–3 to 1 and remains fairly steady throughout life. Only the relative distribution of granulocytes to erythroid cells can be determined on aspirate smears.
- The M/E ratio can be affected by the quality of the smear and areas of the smear examined:
  - A bone marrow smear devoid of particles and diluted by peripheral blood generates a high M/E ratio with many mature segmented neutrophils due to the inclusion of peripheral blood elements.
  - Enumerating cells away from marrow particles will also lead to an overestimation of the M/E ratio due to inclusion of peripheral blood cells in these areas.

(d) Cell distribution:
(i) Cellular elements do not distribute evenly on the aspirate smear.
(ii) Larger cells, primarily granulocyte precursors, tend to be dragged to the edges.
(iii) Plasma cells, mast cells and megakaryocytes often remain close to the marrow particles.

(iv) Lymphoid collections may be found focally on aspirate smears due to aspiration of a lymphoid aggregate.

(v) All areas of the smear should be examined to generate an estimate of the relative distribution of cell types and the zones chosen for cell counts should sample the most representative areas.

(e) Adequacy of megakaryocytes:

(i) Counting megakaryocytes on aspirate smears is not considered reliable.

(ii) Megakaryocytes tend to reside in or near marrow particles and can get caught up in small clots during the aspiration procedure making them difficult to detect.

(iii) A general sense of the relative abundance of megakaryocytes can be assessed in a good quality, unclotted aspirate to at least determine whether a thrombocytopenia is the result of peripheral destruction (many megakaryocytes) or marrow failure (few megakaryocytes). The best method to assess the adequacy of megakaryocytes, however, is the bone marrow core biopsy.

3. Bone marrow core biopsy

(a) Adequacy:

(i) Bone marrow core biopsies should be 1.5 cm in length and contain at least five inter-trabecular spaces (Figure 17.4).

(ii) The likelihood of detecting metastatic tumor or marrow involvement by lymphoma is dependent on the length of the marrow biopsy. Marrow biopsies shorter than 1.5 cm are less sensitive for the detection of solid tumors. Minimal additional sensitivity is gained above this length. In children, biopsies are shorter by necessity requiring bilateral cores for the evaluation of metastatic disease.

(iii) It is debatable whether bilateral biopsies add significantly to an otherwise adequate 1.5 cm unilateral biopsy in adults for the staging of lymphoma or detection of metastatic tumor.

(b) Processing:

(i) Biopsy specimens are handled much like other tissue biopsies although the hardness of the bone requires removing calcium with a weak acid during the fixation process to allow microtome sectioning.

(ii) The specimen is fixed in formalin or similar fixative, processed, and embedded in paraffin blocks. Several shavings of the block are taken and laid onto glass slides whereupon they are stained with hematoxylin and eosin (H&E).

(iii) Additional stains such as a reticulin are performed for specific indications. Iron stains are not reliable on core biopsies since iron may leech out during the decalcification process.

(c) Low power examination (40×, 100×):

(a)

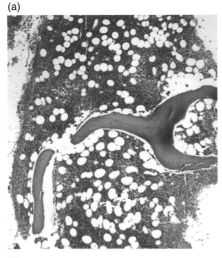

(b)

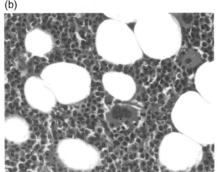

Figure 17.4 Normal bone marrow biopsy, hematoxylin and eosin stain. Low power magnification (40×), (a), helps to assess the cellularity of the bone marrow biopsy, adequacy of megakaryocytes and evaluate for infiltrative processes. High power examination (400×), (b), allows for determination of megakaryocyte morphology and cytologic assessment of other marrow elements and infiltrative processes, if present.

(i)   As for bone marrow aspirate smears, bone marrow biopsy specimens should first be scanned at low power prior to examining at higher power magnification.

(ii)   Evaluation of biopsy sections with an oil immersion lens is not necessary.

(iii)   A general scan at low power is helpful to determine the adequacy of the specimen, assess marrow cellularity and identify focal processes such as granulomas, lymphoid aggregates and metastatic tumor.

(iv)   Adequacy of megakaryocyte numbers is best determined on the core biopsy at low power magnification.

(d) High power examination (200×, 400×):

(i)   Higher power magnification is useful to assess the distribution and nature of the hematopoietic cellular elements, bone structure, and to evaluate the details of infiltrative processes, if any.

(e) **Assessment of cells and cellular structures:**

(i)   A judgment of the increase or decrease of the granulocyte or erythroid cells can be made from the core biopsy in conjunction with the aspirate smear cell counts. A hypocellular core biopsy with a decreased M/E ratio indicates a granulocytic hypoplasia whereas a hypercellular core biopsy with a low M/E ratio reflects an erythroid hyperplasia.

(ii)   Bony trabeculae should be evaluated for evidence of increased bony remodeling and trabecular thickness. Increase in bony remodeling may indicate hyperparathyroidism due to renal disease, a previous injury or biopsy, or a solid malignancy inducing reactive bony changes. Lymphomas have a predilection for growing adjacent to the bony trabeculae, especially follicular lymphoma.

(iii)   Marrow sinuses should be collapsed. Dilated or drawn open sinusoids suggest a pathologic increase in reticulin fibrosis.

(iv)   Hematopoietic cells in the normal bone marrow will demonstrate some zonation with erythroid progenitors and granulocyte progenitors remaining in loose ill-defined collections. This zonation is enhanced in the recovery phase after chemotherapy or hematopoietic stem cell transplant. Cells should be arranged in large cords. "Lining up" of the hematopoietic cells in parallel streams is an indication of marrow reticulin fibrosis.

(v)   All stages of hematopoiesis should be evident although this is best judged on the aspirate smears:

- Erythroid progenitors contain very dark "ink dot" nuclei that are round. Erythroid cytoplasm has distinct cell borders under high power magnification.
- Granulocytes progenitor nuclei are irregular to oval, depending on the stage of development, and are pale. Cytoplasm is granular, slightly refractile, and pink to red.
- Eosinophil cytoplasm is strikingly orange to orange-red with strongly refractile granules. The number of eosinophils is easy to overestimate on a core biopsy since their color attracts the morphologist's eye.

(vi)   Megakaryocytes:

- Megakaryocytes are generally scattered, perisinusoidal and easily recognized based on their increased size compared to other hematopoietic cells.
- Between 7 to 15 megakaryocytes per mm^2 should be present on marrow sections. However adequacy is most often assessed subjectively. Megakaryocyte numbers should mirror overall cellularity.
- Large, focal collections of megakaryocytes is pathologic.
- Megakaryocyte nuclei should have multiple overlapping nuclear lobes. However, not all lobes of the megakaryocyte are

visible in the plain of sectioning on an H and E section. Therefore assessing megakaryocytes for small hypolobated nuclei can be difficult.

4. Bone marrow aspirate clot

(a) **Overview.** Aspirated marrow left in the aspirating syringe not used to generate smears is an additional source of material that can be used for morphologic examination. This aspirated material is left to clot (*aspirate clot*) and can be fixed and sectioned similar to the core biopsy allowing review of supplementary marrow tissue fragments (particles) caught up in the clot.

(b) **Use.** The morphologic features of the clot are similar to that of the core biopsy but clot sections lack bony fragments. Most laboratories will use clot sections to maximize morphologic examination of the bone marrow. Additionally, Perl's Prussian blue stain for iron stores can be performed on the clot sections since hemosiderin is not lost during processing.

5. Bone marrow touch imprint

(a) **Overview.** Occasionally bone marrow cannot be aspirated from a patient (see above) due to hypocellularity, fibrosis or extensive infiltration of the marrow by a neoplastic process. This is referred to as a *"dry tap"*. To view the individual cellular elements of the marrow, a *touch imprint* or *touch prep* can be performed.

(b) **Method.** A fresh core biopsy specimen is physically touched to a slide depositing cells from the marrow on the glass. Multiple light imprints should be performed as the first touches will contain adsorbed peripheral blood elements. Touch imprints, if performed correctly, give the most representative distribution of marrow cellular elements.

(c) **The evaluation** of touch preps is identical to that of the aspirate smear.

(d) **Artifacts.** The pressure of imprinting cells on a slide can distort cell morphology leading to artifacts. The force of touching a core biopsy to glass leads to spreading of a cell over a slightly larger area on the slide compared to that on the aspirate smear. As a result cells and cell structures on a touch imprint appear paler and larger than on an aspirate. A benign lymphocyte, appearing larger with a pale nucleus can easily be misinterpreted for a blast in such circumstances.

6. Iron stain

(a) **Overview.** Due to the importance of iron for erythropoiesis, stains for iron stores are routinely performed on bone marrow specimens. Microscopic examination of bone marrow stained for iron is considered the gold standard for determining iron depleted states. Iron stains can be done on the bone marrow aspirate smear or a bone marrow clot section or both.

(b) **Method. Perl's Prussian blue stain** is the method of choice for iron staining. The stain generates a blue color when *hemosiderin* is present. Sections
are often counter-stained with safranin, a red dye, to enhance the visuali-
zation of the stained iron.

(c) **Evaluation:**

   (i)   Iron stores are evaluated by examining several particles on the
          aspirate smear or clot section. A marrow specimen lacking particles
          is insufficient to determine iron stores.

   (ii)   Marrow iron is present within macrophages and erythroid
          progenitors:
          • Erythroid cells containing iron are referred to as *sideroblasts*. Iron
            in sideroblasts is present as one or two fine siderotic granules best
            visualized with an oil immersion lens (1000×).
          • Siderotic granules in macrophages should be small, few to
            moderate in number, and visible under low power magnification
            (100×).

   (iii) Stainable iron is in the form of *hemosiderin*, a macromolecule complex
          of *ferritin* and iron.

   (iv)   Iron stores are assessed subjectively, as a practical matter, as absent,
          reduced, normal, or increased. Iron visible only in a few cells under
          high power magnification (1000×) is decreased whereas iron in
          many cells aggregating in clumps is an indication of iron
          overload.

   (v)   *Ring sideroblasts* are defined as erythroid cells that contain five or
          more siderotic granules encircling one third or more of the nucleus.
          These cells are seen only in pathologic states and are an indication
          of abnormal iron accumulation in the mitochondria.

(d) **Clinical relevance:**

   (i)   Stainable iron is increased post-transfusion, in thalassemia, hemo-
          chromatosis, and in sites of previous hemorrhage.

   (ii)   Macrophage iron may be increased in anemia of chronic disease but
          is associated with decreased iron in sideroblasts.

   (iii) Decreased stainable iron is present in iron deficiency and is nor-
          mally difficult to identify in growing children.

7. **Ancillary tests**

(a) **Histochemical stains:**

   (i)   **Overview.** Stains that use a chemical to impart color to subset of
          cells, identify organisms, or highlight specific tissue or cellular com-
          ponents are referred to as *histochemical stains*. Perl's Prussian blue
          stain is one type of histochemical stain. Histochemical stains can be
          performed on the bone marrow aspirate smear or core biopsy.

   (ii)   **Reticulin.** Reticulin is visualized using a silver impregnation tech-
          nique. The stain is only used on tissue sections. Reticulin should be
          assessed in marrow biopsies in which there was a "dry tap", in

(a) (b)

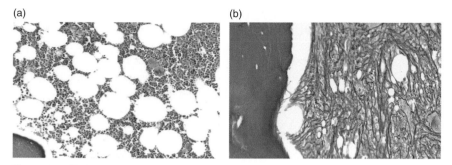

Figure 17.5 Reticulin staining of bone marrow. (a) Normal bone marrow reticulin stain. Only a few fine wisps of fine reticulin fibers are seen. (b) Abnormal reticulin deposition. Coarse reticulin fibers are present encircling nearly all hematopoeitic cells.

disease states known to be accompanied by increased reticulin fibrosis, and where the H and E sections suggest increased reticulin formation (Figure 17.5).

(iii) **Special stains for acute leukemia.** These stains include myeloperoxidase, sudan black B, butyl esterase (with and without fluoride), chloracetate esterase (leder), and periodic acid Schiff (PAS). The stains are used on aspirate smears mostly to highlight the differentiation state of blasts. They are primarily of historical interest since most have been replaced by more specific antibody stains and flow cytometry.

(iv) **Stains for microorganisms.** These stains are used on tissue biopsy sections and should be considered when there is a granuloma or other evidence to suggest an infection. The most commonly used stains are *Grocott's methenamine silver (GMS)* stain to highlight yeast and fungi and the *Ziehl–Neelsen (AFB)* stain to locate mycobacteria.

(v) **Stains for amyloid.** Amyloid is an extracellular deposition of proteins in tissue into an insoluble beta pleated sheet structure. It has a waxy, homogeneous and eosinophilic appearance on an H and E stain. Amyloid may accompany plasma cell diseases. The *Congo red stain* is most often used to identify amyloid inducing an apple green color under polarized light.

(vi) **Others.** Additional stains such as toluidine blue and giemsa for mast cells, trichrome for collagen deposition are used when there is a specific indication.

(b) Immunohistochemical stains:

(i) **Overview.** Immunohistochemical stains use antibodies to direct a chromogen (colored compound) to specific cells. This is carried out by adding an antibody of known specificity to a cut section of tissue on a glass slide. The site of antibody deposition is made visible through conjugation of the antibody to an enzyme, most often horseradish peroxidase or alkaline phosphatase, which can convert a chemical into a colored substance. Evaluation of the bone marrow is enhanced through the judicious use of immunohistochemical stains, a full discussion of which is beyond the scope of this book. Immunohistochemical stains allow for an assessment of the phenotype of cells while maintaining cellular morphology. The stains are used to determine the location and nature of specific cell subsets in the bone marrow. Immunohistochemistry is complimentary to flow cytometry for assessing cell antigen expression. Table 17.2 lists commonly used antibodies and cells they detect.

(ii) **Use:**
- Lymphoid aggregates. One of the more common uses of antibody stains is to determine the cellular composition of lymphoid aggregates in the bone marrow. Focal collections of lymphocytes in the bone marrow are common and deciphering the nature of such aggregates (reactive versus neoplastic) requires phenotypic analysis including antibody stains. The relative distribution of T and B lymphoid cells within the aggregate can be examined using B and T cell specific antibodies.
- Plasma cells. Immunohistochemical stains are also useful to evaluate for clonality of plasma cells by demonstrating a skewed ratio of kappa expressing to lambda expressing plasma cells.
- Other. Antibody stains are utilized to evaluate metastatic foci, examine for residual leukemia or lymphoma cells, and to bring out cellular elements that may be difficult to perceive on H and E stained slides (mast cells, small megakaryocytes, blasts etc.). Antibody stains should be used when the result will change the diagnostic interpretation or medical management.

(iii) **Flow cytometry:**
- Overview. Flow cytometric analysis has become an integral part of a bone marrow examination. A *flow cytometer* is an instrument that analyzes fluorescence emitted from cells as they are excited by a laser in a flow stream. The detection of specific cellular elements is made possible by adding fluorochrome-conjugated monoclonal antibodies to cells prior to evaluation on the machine. Cells expressing a particular antigen are tagged by an antigen-specific fluorescent antibody and then analyzed. Hydrodynamic focusing ensures that only one cell traverses the path of the laser light at a time allowing for linkage of the fluorescent signal with a particular cell. The fluorescence emitted is recorded as fluorescent intensity per cell with the degree of fluorescence roughly correlated with the amount of antigen expressed. Cells need to be dispersed, unclumped, and viable when analyzed. Therefore specimens must be procured in an anticoagulant, received fresh

Table 17.2 Typical markers used to assess bone marrow cells

Antigen	Method	Detects	Use
CD3	FC or IHC	T cells	Assess lymphoid aggregates, evaluate for T cell infiltrates
CD7	FC	T cells	Lineage of acute leukemia, assess lymphoid aggregates, evaluate for T cell infiltrates
CD10	FC or IHC	Precursor B cells, germinal center B cells	Lineage of blasts and B cell lymphomas
CD13	FC	Granulocytes and monocytes	Identify granulocytes and monocytes, lineage assignment of acute leukemia
CD14	FC	Monocytes	Identify monocytes, lineage assignment of acute leukemia
CD19	FC	B cells	Lineage of acute leukemia, assess lymphoid aggregates, evaluate for B cell infiltrates
CD20	FC or IHC	B cells	Assess lymphoid aggregates, evaluate for B cell infiltrates
CD33	FC	Granulocytes and monocytes	Identify granulocytes and monocytes, lineage assignment of acute leukemia
CD34	FC or IHC	Stem cells/blasts	Assess for blasts
CD45	FC or IHC	Hematopoietic cells except erythroid cells and platelets	Identify hematopoietic cells
CD41/CD61	FC or IHC	Platelets/ megakarycoytes	Identify megakaryocytes, lineage assignment of acute leukemia
CD117	FC or IHC	Myeloid blasts, mast cells	Lineage assignment of acute leukemia, identify mast cells
CD138	FC or IHC	plasma cells	Identify plasma cells
Kappa or lambda	FC or IHC	B cells/plasma cells	Assess for clonality
Myeloperoxidase	FC or IHC	Granulocytes, myeloid blasts	Lineage assessment of blasts and hematopoietic cells
TDT	FC or IHC	Lymphoid blasts	Lineage assessment of blasts
Glycophorin A	FC or IHC	Red cells/red cell progenitors	Identify red cell progenitors, lineage assignment of acute leukemia

FC, flow cytometry; IHC, immunohistochemistry.

without fixatives, and delivered in a timely fashion to the laboratory; easily accomplished with bone marrow and peripheral
blood samples.

- Applicability. The strength of flow cytometry resides in its sensitivity and multi-parametric ability:
  - Multi-parametric ability. Most flow cytometers in use today are
    capable of detecting four or more fluorescent tags (colors)
    simultaneously enabling the identification of an abnormal cell
    population within complex cell mixtures such as bone marrow
    specimens. For example, the simultaneous assessment of "n"
    antigens segregates cells into 2^n non-overlapping cell subsets.
    For a four color instrument (n = 4) 16 separate cell populations
    can be resolved. Immunohistochemical stains also detect
    expressed antigens on cells; however immunohistochemistry is
    limited to evaluating one antigen at a time impeding the ability
    to determine the relationship of the antigens detected. Different
    cells of bone marrow separate on flow cytometric studies
    (Figure 17.6).
  - Sensitivity. Flow cytometers can detect less than 200 molecules
    per cells making them significantly more sensitive than immu-
    nohistochemical stains on an antigen per cell basis.

(iii) **Data collection and representation.** Flow cytometry data is usually
presented as two-dimensional "dot plots" in which the expression
of one antigen is compared with another (see Figure 17.6). The main
cell subsets (granulocyte, monocytes, blasts, red cells and lymphocytes) can be resolved by plotting the expression of cells stained
with CD45 (leukocyte common antigen) versus the scatter of light
off of cells at a 90° angle (*side scatter*). The individual cell subsets
(CD4(+) T cells for example) in these regions can then be probed
more specifically with additional antibodies.

(iv) **Use:**
- Aspirated marrow should be sent for flow cytometry in most
  instances. It is not necessary when the clinical indication for the
  bone marrow is Hodgkin lymphoma staging, metastatic disease
  evaluation, or routine monitoring of a myeloproliferative
  disorder.
- Flow cytometry is particularly useful for the enumeration of
  blasts in leukemia and pre-leukemic (myelodysplastic) states,
  documenting clonality of lymphoid cells, determining cell lineage
  of acute leukemia and subtyping a lymphoma or lymphoproliferative disorder. Plasma cells are readily identified but the number
  of cells detected is often far less than that seen morphologically.
  Nonetheless, flow cytometry is useful to document a plasma cell
  neoplasm and studies have shown that flow cytometry is adept
  at monitoring disease after therapy.

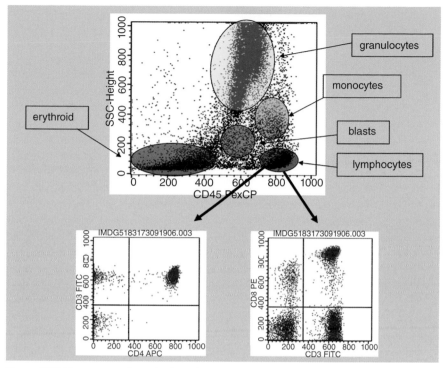

Figure 17.6 Flow cytometric evaluation of bone marrow. The phenotype of marrow hematopoietic elements can be determined using multi-color flow cytometry. Top, cellular expression of CD45 (x-axis) and light scatter off cells (y-axis) can be used to separate the main groups of hematopoietic cells. The expression of antigens on cells within these regions can then be further probed. In the example shown, lymphocytes are evaluated for the expression of CD3, CD4 and CD8, bottom. Morphologically CD4 and CD8 T cell subsets cannot be differentiated. Flow cytometry is useful for the enumeration of cell subsets, identifying abnormal cell elements and documenting clonality.

- Minimal residual disease. The morphologic detection limit for neoplastic cells is roughly 2–5%. The presence of detectable disease below which can be visually identified is referred to as *minimal residual disease*. Additional techniques are required for this degree of sensitivity. Flow cytometry can identify neoplastic cells from acute leukemia and other disorders down to 0.01% making it an excellent method to monitor minimal residual disease. Flow cytometry is used to identify high risk acute lymphoblastic leukemia patients needing additional treatment based on minimal residual disease after the initial phase of therapy.

(v) **Limitations:**
- Flow cytometry is not particularly useful for the detection of solid, non-lymphoid neoplasms since cells need to be dispersed

when analyzed. Carcinoma cells contain tight junctions between cells preventing adequate cellular dispersal.

- Large cells and cells adherent to other elements, such as carcinoma cells, Reed–Sternberg cells in Hodgkin lymphoma and plasma cells usually are poorly identified by this technique. Otherwise, the relative cell numbers seen by flow cytometry are roughly equivalent to that on marrow aspirate smears.
- Elements that may not aspirate well, such as cells in lymphoid aggregates, are equally poorly recovered on flow cytometry. The actual extent of marrow involvement by these processes is therefore best determined on the bone marrow core biopsy.
- Flow cytometry does not incorporate visual data and therefore should be considered complementary to and not used in place of morphology.

(d) **Cytogenetics:**

    (i)   **Overview.** Cytogenetics is the study of the structure and number of chromosomes in cells in disease states.

    (ii)   **Karyotype.** A karyotype is the overall chromosomal make-up of a tumor. It is determined by arresting the neoplastic cells in metaphase, staining the chromosomes, and analyzing the chromosomal structure and number under high power magnification (1000×). A fresh heparinized sample is needed since cells are cultured prior to processing and analyzing. Individual chromosomes can be recognized by their size and specific *banding pattern* (light and dark staining regions). Cytogeneticists have expertise in recognizing the specific chromosomes and structural chromosomal abnormalities.

- **Aneuploidy** is the presence of an abnormal number of chromosomes other than the expected 46.
  - Hyperdiploid—increased number of chromosomes.
  - Hypodiploid—decreased number of chromosomes.
- **Translocation** is the shuffling and re-annealing of one chromosomal segment onto another segment. Translocations may be balanced (without loss of genetic material) or unbalanced (loss of some genetic material). The nomenclature for a translocation includes the letter "t" followed by parenthesis enclosing the translocating chromosomes followed by a second parenthesis encompassing the arm and band site of the corresponding translocated chromosomes. The long arm of a chromosome is designated the "q" arm and the short arm the "p" arm. A reciprocal translocation involving the long arms of chromosome 9 at band 3 sub-region 4 and chromosome 22 at band 1 sub-region 1 as seen in chronic myelogenous leukemia is designated t(9;22)(q34;q11). Translocations are common in hematopoietic neoplasms.
- **Fluorescent *in-situ* hybridization (FISH)** is commonly performed on bone marrow samples. This technique uses fluorescent

tagged DNA probes to specific chromosomal regions to identify chromosomal translocations or alterations.
  - FISH studies can be performed on fixed cells and tissue blocks.
  - FISH probes are used for disease specific indications such as probing with bcr and abl to examine for the t(9;22)(q34;q11) translocation in chronic myelogenous leukemia.
- Use. Visible structural and numerical alterations of chromosomes are common in cancers and recurrent abnormalities are important for classification and prognosis of hematopoeitic neoplasms. A full review is beyond the scope of this book. Aspirated bone marrow should be sent for cytogenetic evaluation whenever a hematologic malignancy is suspected or to evaluate for persistent disease in a patient with a neoplasm with a known cytogenetic or FISH abnormality.

Further reading

Arellano-Rodrigo E, Real MI, Muntañola A, Burrel M, Rozman M, Fraire GV, Cervantes F. Successful treatment by selective arterial embolization of severe retroperitoneal hemorrhage secondary to bone marrow biopsy in post-polycythemic myelofibrosis. Ann Hematol 2004;83:67 70.

Bain BJ. Bone marrow aspiration. J Clin Pathol 2001;54:657–63.

Bain BJ. Bone marrow trephine biopsy. J Clin Pathol 2001;54:737–42.

Bain BJ. Bone marrow biopsy morbidity and mortality. Br J Haematol 2003;121:949–51.

Bain BJ. Morbidity associated with bone marrow aspiration and trephine biopsy—a review of UK data for 2004 (letter). Haematologica 2006;91:1293–4.

Bain BJ, Clark DM, Lampert IA, Wilkins BS. Bone Marrow Pathology, 3rd edn. Malden, MA: Blackwell Science, 2001.

Boyce BF, Xing L. Biology of RANK, RANKL, and osteoprotegerin. Arthritis Res Ther. 2007; 9(Suppl 1): S1.

Farhi D. Pathology of Bone Marrow and Blood Cells, 2nd edn. Baltimore, MD: Lippincott Williams and Wilkins, 2009.

Hasserjian RP. Reactive versus neoplastic bone marrow: problems and pitfalls. Arch Pathol Lab Med 2008;132:587–94.

Lee S-H, Erber WH, Porwit A, Tomonaga M, Peterson LC. ISCH Guidelines for the standardization of bone marrow specimens and reports. Int J Lab Hem 2008;30:349–64.

Meyerson H. Flow cytometry as a tool for the diagnosis of cutaneous T-cell lymphoma. J Clin Derm 2010;1:31–42.

Riley R.S, Williams D, Ross M, Zhao S. Bone marrow aspirate and biopsy: a pathologist's perspective. II. Interpretation of the bone marrow aspirate and biopsy. J Clin Lab Anal 2009;23:259–307.

Wahid SF, Md-Anshar F, Mukari SA, Rahmat R. Massive retroperitoneal hematoma with secondary hemothorax complicating bone marrow trephine biopsy in polycythemia vera (letter). Am J Hematol 2007;82:943–44.

18 Myeloproliferative Neoplasms and Myelodysplastic Syndromes

Gabriela Motyckova and Richard M. Stone

Dana-Farber Cancer Institute, Boston, MA, USA

I. Chronic myeloid disorders

The chronic myeloid disorders can be divided into myeloproliferative neo-plasms (MPN), myeloid and lymphoid neoplasms associated with eosi-nophilia and abnormalities of the genes *PDGFRA*, *PDGFRB* or *FGFR1*, overlap myelodysplastic/myeloproliferative neoplasms (MDS/MPN), and myelo-dysplastic syndromes (Box 18.1).

II. Myeloproliferative neoplasms

Myeloproliferative neoplasms (MPN) are clonal disorders of progenitor cells. Signs and symptoms of MPNs include arterial and venous thromboses and hemorrhages especially in patients with essential thrombocythemia (ET) and polycythemia vera (PV), microcirculatory problems including erythromelal-gia, and neurologic and visual disturbances. Erythromelalgia is a red, painful region on distal extremities due to ischemia from reduced blood flow from polycythemic red blood cells and/or thrombocytosis. Bleeding complications in the setting of high platelet count and platelet dysfunction can also occur. Constitutional symptoms including weight loss, fatigue, and pruritus, fever, night sweats and bone pain can accompany these disorders. Patients with MPNs are at risk of transformation to acute myelogenous leukemia (AML). Without treatment, the risk of transformation is highest in chronic myelo-genous leukemia (CML) (up to 90%) and lowest in ET. Recently, the molecular underpinnings of MPNs have been described. For summary of disease catego-ries, molecular and cytogenetic aberrations, please see Table 18.1.

A. Polycythemia vera

Polycythemia vera (PV) is a chronic clonal disorder with increased hematocrit, elevated red blood cell mass, and erythropoietin levels below the normal

---

Box 18.1 2008 World Health Organization Classification of Chronic Myeloid Neoplasms. From Swerdlow et al., 2008.

Myeloproliferative neoplasms
Chronic myelogenous leukemia (CML, *BCR-ABL* positive)
Polycythemia vera (PV)
Essential thrombocythemia (ET)
Primary myelofibrosis (PMF)
Chronic neutrophilic leukemia (CNL)
Chronic eosinophilic leukemia, not otherwise specified (CEL, NOS)
Mastocytosis
Myeloproliferative neoplasm, unclassifiable (MPN, unclassifiable)
Myeloid and lymphoid neoplasms associated with eosinophilia and abnormalities of *PDGFRA, PDGFRB,* or *FGFR1*
Myelodysplastic/myeloproliferative neoplasms
Chronic myelomonocytic leukemia (CMML)
Juvenile myelomonocytic leukemia (JMML)
Atypical chronic myelogenous leukemia (aCML)
Refractory anemia with ringed sideroblasts associated with thrombocytosis (RARS-T)
Myelodysplastic syndromes
See Table 18.3

---

reference range. Splenomegaly, leukocytosis (in 75% of patients) and thrombocytosis (in 50% of cases) can also be present. Patients may develop skin pruritus, abdominal pain from splenomegaly, and are at risk for hemorrhage and thrombosis. The diagnosis of PV requires the presence of two major criteria (increased red cell mass or hemoglobin values of >18.5 g/dL in men and 16.5 g/dL in women, and the presence of JAK2 (JANUS kinase 2) mutation JAK2V617F, or other JAK2 mutations such as exon 12 mutation causing constitutive activation of the tyrosine kinase and downstream signaling pathways) and one of the following minor criteria: bone marrow hypercellularity with trilineage hyperplasia, low serum erythropoietin level, or endogenous colony formation *in vitro*.

Complications of PV include arterial and venous thromboses, myocardial infarctions, strokes, transient ischemic attacks, and other thrombotic events due to markedly sluggish blood flow and hyperviscosity of a blood with high hematocrit. The risk of transformation into AML is around 5%. While there are no widely used prognostic criteria in PV, serious complications can be prevented if blood counts are well controlled.

Phlebotomy should be used to decrease hematocrit to 45% or lower in men and 42% or lower in women. Moreover, in low-risk and asymptomatic patients less than 60 years of age and with no prior history of thrombosis, low dose aspirin (81 mg daily) without cytoreductive therapy is appropriate. Aspirin

Table 18.1 Molecular and cytogenetic aberrations of myeloproliferative neoplasm

MPN	Disease incidence	Mutations	Cytogenetics
CML, BCR-ABL positive	1–2/100,000	BCR-ABL fusion protein 100%	BCR-ABL fusion protein resulting from t(9;22) in 100% of cases
PV	2–2.8/100,000	JAK2V617F 95–97% JAK2 exon 12 3% TET2 16%	Gain of 9p, 1p, del 20q, del13, trisomy 8
ET	1.5–2.4/100,000	JAK2V617F 50% MPL 4–5% TET2 5%	Abnormalities in 5.3% patients, no consistent findings
PMF	0.5–1.3/100,000	JAK2V617F 43–57% MPL 5–10% TET2 17%	Unbalanced translocations between chromosome 1 and 6; 12q-, 20q-, partial trisomy 1q, trisomy 8, gains of 2q, 3p, 4, 9p, 12q, 13q
CNL	Rare, about 150 cases reported	JAK2 rare CBL <1%	Rare BCR-ABL p230 from t(9;22)
CEL, NOS	Rare	CBL rare	FIP1L1-PDGFRA; trisomy 1, t(5;12); t(5;15) t(8;21) and others
Mastocytosis	Unclear	c-KIT mutations in almost all patients, KIT816V most common KITF522C and others TET2 29%	FIP1L1-PDGFRA rearrangements

CBL, Casitas B-lineage lymphoma oncogene; CEL, NOS, chronic eosinophilic leukemia, not otherwise specified; CML, chronic myeloid leukemia; CNL, chronic neutrophilic leukemia; ET, essential thrombocythemia; MPL, myeloproliferative leukemia virus oncogene, functions as thrombopoietin receptor; MPN, myeloproliferative neoplasm; PMF, primary myelofibrosis; PV, polycythemia vera; TET2, TET oncogene family member 2.

should not be used in patients with platelets over $1500 \times 10^9/L$ due to bleeding risk, or in patients with a history of bleeding or with acquired von Willebrand's syndrome. As PV symptoms develop, treatment with pegylated interferon or hydroxyurea are recommended. In patients over 60 years of age and/or those with a history of thrombosis, hydroxyurea should be added. To better control platelet counts in some patients, anagrelide that interferes with the development of megakaryocytes can be used, especially with a history of bleeding or thrombotic complications in patients who do not respond to hydroxyurea. Anagrelide has ionotropic and vasodilatory effects, therefore side effects such as palpitations, high output heart failure, headache and dizziness can occur.

B. Essential thrombocythemia (Atlas Figure 37)

Essential thrombocythemia (ET) is a clonal disorder of the hematopoietic stem cell. The diagnosis of ET is made in patients who have each of the following four criteria: (i) sustained platelet count $\geq 450 \times 10^9/L$; (ii) bone narrow biopsy showing increased proliferation of megakaryocytes, with increased number of enlarged, mature megakaryocytes; (iii) clinical presentation not meeting diagnostic criteria for other myeloid disorders; (iv) the presence of the JAK2V617F mutation (or other clonal marker) or no evidence of reactive thrombocytosis in the absence of JAK2V617F mutation.

Although many patients are asymptomatic at the time of diagnosis, symptoms and complications of ET include splenomegaly, bleeding and thromboses especially with platelet counts above $1000 \times 10^9/L$, neurologic symptoms such as headache, paresthesias, and transient ischemic attacks, erythromelalgia or digital ischemia. Platelets in ET have a qualitative defect and show abnormalities in platelet aggregation studies and acquired von Willebrand's syndrome can occur with extremely high platelet counts.

The risk of leukemia transformation is 1.4% and myelofibrosis occurs in 3.8% of patients in first decade of the disease duration. The survival of patients with ET appears comparable to the general population in the first 10 years of diagnosis, but decreases with longer duration of the disease as the risk of leukemia transformation and development of myelofibrosis increases. Secondary myelofibrosis can occur in patients with other MPNs such as PV and ET, in patients with other malignancies, such as lymphoma, metastatic breast, prostate, lung, and stomach carcinomas, or with infections including disseminated tuberculosis or histoplasmosis.

The goal of therapy is to control platelet count to decrease the risk of thromboses and bleeding. Low-dose aspirin is recommended for young asymptomatic (low-risk) patients except for patients with platelet counts above $1500 \times 10^9/L$ (due to risk of bleeding from qualitative platelet defect) or with acquired von Willebrand syndrome. Hydroxyurea is usually started in asymptomatic patients with platelet counts above $1500 \times 10^9/L$, but there are no clear guidelines on management of extreme thrombocytosis in asymptomatic low-risk patients.

Treatment is indicated in high-risk (age over age 60 or prior history of thrombosis) and in symptomatic patients. Acute treatment with platelet pheresis to rapidly decrease platelet count can be used in the setting of serious thrombotic events, acute coronary syndrome, stroke, transient ischemic attack, or life-threatening hemorrhages. Hydroxyurea as the first line cytoreductive therapy to decrease platelets to below $600 \times 10^9/L$ can be used in addition to low dose aspirin for chronic treatment of ET to control thrombocythemia and decrease the thrombotic and bleeding risks. The side effects of hydroxyurea include neutropenia, nausea, lower extremity and oral ulceration, nail discoloration, and hair loss. Interferon-α does not cross the placenta and is therefore the agent of choice in symptomatic pregnant women, but carries significant side effects such as flu-like symptoms, fatigue, bone and muscle pain, or fever. Anagrelide can be used in ET to control platelet count in patients not responding to or intolerant of hydroxyurea.

C. Primary myelofibrosis (PMF)

The bone marrow fibrosis in PMF develops as a reaction of polyclonal stroma to clonal malignant hematopoietic cells and their cytokines. Up to 25% of patients may be asymptomatic at the time of diagnosis when their enlarged spleen is noted on exam. Most patients with PMF present with enlarged spleen, fatigue and constitutional symptoms such as fevers, sweats, weight loss. Peripheral blood analysis of patients with PMF can show tear drop cells, nucleated red blood cells, and immature myeloid cells, megathrombocytes and fragments of megakaryocytes. Bone marrow aspirate is usually difficult to obtain due to marrow fibrosis. The bone marrow biopsy specimen usually shows hypercellular bone marrow, increased number of megakaryocytes, varying number of reticulin, and increased vascularity.

Patients with PMF have problems due to cytopenias and/or and extramedullary hematopoiesis. Thrombotic and bleeding complications (from thrombocytopenia, dysfunctional platelets or DIC) can also occur. Extramedullary hematopoiesis can cause organ damage including CNS sites and organ failure.

The diagnosis of PMF is made in patients fitting three major criteria: (i) presence of megakaryocyte proliferation and atypia, accompanied by either reticulin or collagen fibrosis or, in the absence of significant reticulin fibrosis, megakaryocyte changes accompanied by increased marrow cellularity with granulocytic proliferation and often decreased erythropoiesis; (ii) disease not meeting WHO criteria for PV, MDS, CML or other myeloid disorders; (iii) presence of JAK2V617F or other clonal markers (such as MPLW515K/L) or no evidence of secondary myelofibrosis in the absence of clonal markers; and two of the following four minor criteria: leukoerythroblastosis, increased serum lactate dehydrogenase level, anemia and/or splenomegaly.

The median survival of patients with PMF from the time of diagnosis is about 5 years, but there is a wide range of reported survival data (1–30 years). Several prognostic scoring systems have been used to risk stratify patients with myelofibrosis. For example, the Lille score identifies three prognostic categories (low, intermediate and high-risk) according to hemoglobin level and leukocyte count with median survivals of 93, 26 and 13 months respectively. Moreover, the Mayo clinic score added thrombocytopenia (platelet count <100 × 10^9/L) and monocytosis (>1 × 10^9/L) to the adverse risk factors. The International Working Group prognostic scoring system uses age greater than 65 years, presence of constitutional symptoms, hemoglobin less than 10 g/dL, leukocyte count above 25 × 10^9/L, and 1% or greater circulating blasts as predictors of shortened survival, stratifying patients into low-risk (0 risk factors), intermediate-1 (one risk factor), intermediate-2 (two risk factors) and high-risk (three or more risk factors) groups with median survivals of 135, 95, 48, and 27 months, respectively.

Low-risk patients with PMF are usually observed. Therapy for PMF is indicated when symptoms develop including constitutional symptoms, complications related to anemia, thrombocytopenia, bleeding, hyperuricemia, portal hypertension, or bone pain. Many treatment strategies (including lenalidomide, hydroxyurea, busulfan, 6-thioguanine, chlorambucil with prednisone, interferon-α, low-dose melphalan, corticosteroids, IVIG) have been used in patients with PMF. Hydroxyurea remains the most commonly used treatment for symptomatic PMF. Erythroid stimulating agents and androgens play a limited role and are only occasionally used.

Patients in high-risk groups with poor prognosis are considered for allogeneic hematopoietic cell transplantation (HCT). This modality has been used as a possibly curative therapy resulting in gradual resolution of myelofibrosis. Allogeneic HCT recipients can have a 5-year survival of 47–58%. In early clinical trials with PMF patients, JAK2 inhibitors decreased spleen size, improved transfusion requirement and cytopenias, but not the extent of myelofibrosis.

The role of splenectomy in patients with PMF is controversial. Splenic enlargement in PMF can cause abdominal discomfort and bowel complications, hemolytic anemia or life-threatening thrombocytopenia, splenic pain from enlargement or infarct, or portal hypertension. Splenectomy is currently performed in only select patients given its high post-procedure morbidity and mortality of about 10%.

D. Chronic myeloid leukemia (Atlas Figure 36)

Chronic myeloid leukemia (CML) is a clonal expansion of hematopoietic elements caused by the *BCR-ABL* fusion gene (Philadelphia chromosome) created by chromosomal translocation t(9;22) (q34;q11). The resulting fusion gene is comprised of a 5′ portion of the *BCR* signaling gene with multiple domains on chromosone 22 and a 3′ portion of the non-receptor tyrosine kinase *ABL* gene from chromosome 9, giving rise to a 210-kd constitutively active tyrosine kinase.

While many patients with CML are asymptomatic at presentation, symptoms of CML may include fatigue, sweats, weight loss and splenomegaly causing abdominal discomfort. Patients' peripheral blood analysis usually reveals leukocytosis with left shifted differential, basophilia, and thrombocytosis. The bone marrow analysis shows a hypercellular marrow with increased granulopoiesis and decreased erythropoiesis. Basophils and eosinophils may also be increased. Megakaryocytes may appear hypolobated and smaller compared to normal bone marrow. Reticulin stain shows increased fibrosis in up to 50% of patients.

Bone marrow blast percentage in the chronic phase is less than 5%, compared to 6–19% in the accelerated phase and 20% or more in the blast phase of CML. Most patients present in the chronic phase of CML. The accelerated phase of CML can present with systemic symptoms of weight loss, fever, fatigue, rising blood counts and is characterized by an increase bone marrow or peripheral blood blasts (to 6–19%), peripheral blood basophils above 20%,

Table 18.2 Treatment response milestones in patients with CML

Duration of treatment with imatinib	3 months	6 months	12 months	18 months
Optimal treatment response	CHR	MCR	CCR	MMR

CHR, complete hematologic response occurs when wbc, platelet count and wbc differential normalize, and all symptoms attributable to CML disappear. CCR, a complete cytogenetic (CCR) response is achieved when no Philadelphia chromosome positive metaphases are identified in the bone marrow. MCR, major cytogenetic response occurs when bone marrow biopsy has <36% Ph-positive metaphases. MMR, a major molecular response occurs when there is a three-log or more reduction of the *BCR-ABL* mRNA. CMR, complete molecular response (CMR) occurs when there is no detectable *BCR-ABL* mRNA in the peripheral blood. Ph, Philadelphia chromosome.
(Based on data from Deininger MW. Milestones and monitoring in patients with CML treated with imatinib. Hematology Am Soc Hematol Educ Program: 2008;419–26.)

persistent thrombocytopenia (less that $100 \times 10^9/L$), persistent thrombocytosis (above $1000 \times 10^9/L$), increased white blood cell (wbc) count and spleen size. CML blast crisis is defined as bone marrow or peripheral blood blast percentage above 20% or when extramedullary disease develops in other organs (skin, spleen, lymph nodes, CNS or other sites) and is associated with shortened survival.

The disease burden and response to therapy in patients with CML can be assessed by hematologic, cytogenetic and molecular responses (Table 18.2).

Current therapy for CML involves the use of targeted tyrosine kinase inhibitors (TKI) which have changed the prognosis of CML patients. The most widely used initial TKI in CML treatment is imatinib, but recently second generation TKIs (nilotinib and dasatinib) were also approved for the first line treatment of CML. The TKIs inhibit the BCR-ABL fusion protein and also other tyrosine kinases such as c-KIT and platelet-derived growth factor receptor. The usual initial dose of imatinib is 400 mg orally daily. Side effects of imatinib treatment include myelosupression, neutropenia, thrombocytopenia, bleeding (in patients with thrombocytopenia), nausea, diarrhea, fatigue, muscle cramps, musculoskeletal pain, and fluid retention. The dose of nilotinib is 300–400 mg PO BID, and dasatinib is dosed at 100 mg PO daily for the initial treatment of CML. The side effect profile of the second generation TKIs overlaps with imatinib, but unique side effects such as QTc prolongation and risk of arrhythmias have been reported with nilotinib (requiring EKG monitoring), and the development of pleural effusions has been observed with dasatinib.

Achievement of responses in CML predicts progression free survival. Treatment with imatinib in the chronic phase CML maintains CCR in 63% of patients at 6 years and results in overall survival of 88%. Interestingly, even with long-term treatment with TKIs, sensitive PCR assays are able to detect the *BCR-ABL* transcript and there still appear to be residual cells with leukemogenic potential. Therefore continuing treatment with TKIs as long as they are effective remains the current approach.

Unfortunately, about half of *de novo* and acquired imatinib resistance occurs in CML due to either point mutations in the tyrosine kinase domain of the *BCR-ABL* gene or by amplification of the fusion transcript. Tyrosine kinase inhibitors (TKIs) including dasatinib and nilotinib have been used in patients with imatinib resistance or treatment failure with good responses. The BCR-ABL T315I mutation causes resistance to all three TKIs (imatinib, dasatinib and nilotinib). Clinical trials with a specific T315I inhibitor are underway for CML patients. Allogeneic SCT is reserved for very young patients or those who do not respond to TKIs.

E. Mastocytosis

Mastocytosis is a rare and heterogenous clonal disorder of mast cells which includes cutaneous mastocytosis, indolent systemic mastocytosis, systemic mastocytosis with associated clonal hematological non-mast cell lineage disease, aggressive systemic mastocytosis, mast cell leukemia, mast cell sarcoma, and extracutaneous mastocytoma. Cutaneous mastocytosis includes three major forms of the disease: maculopapular cutaneous mastocytosis, diffuse mastocytosis, and solitary skin mastocytoma. The lesions present as yellow to reddish brown plaques or nodules and commonly have urticarial reaction to mechanical stimulation. Patients with systemic mastocytosis may present with rash or other symptoms of mast cell degranulation in other organs. In systemic mastocytosis, the bone marrow or other extracutaneous organs contains multifocal infiltrates of mast cells. The diagnosis of systemic mastocytosis is made when one major criterion is present: multifocal aggregates of mast cells in bone marrow confirmed by tryptase or other stains, and three of the following minor criteria are present: (i) more then 25% of mast cells appear atypical in bone marrow biopsy or 25% mast cells the aspirate are atypical or immature; (ii) mast cells coexpress CD117 with CD2 and/or CD25; (iii) c-KIT816 mutation in bone marrow, blood or other extracutaneous organs; (iv) serum total tryptase >20 ng/mL.

The main approach in the treatment of systemic mastocytosis is management of symptoms from mast cell degranulation and prevention of degranulation. Exposure to alcohol, emotional or physical stress, or extreme temperatures can trigger mast cell degranulation. Treatment of mastocytosis and associated symptoms include H-1 and H-2 antihistamines for management of pruritis and peptic ulcer symptoms, cromolyn for nausea, abdominal pain and diarrhea due to mast cell disease, corticosteroids, interferon, chemotherapy (such as 2CdA/Cladribine) and the small molecule c-KIT inhibitors.

III. Myeloid and lymphoid neoplasms associated with eosinophilia and abnormalities of *PDGFRA*, *PDGFRB* or *FGFR1*

This category of MPNs includes three groups of rare clonal disorders with rearrangements of *PDGFRA* (4q12 translocations), *PDGFRB* (5q33 translocations) and *FGFR1*(8p11.2 translocations), causing the formation of aberrant fusion genes coding for tyrosine kinases. The disorders can present as myeloid or lymphoid neoplasms. There is a heterogeneity of clinical presentations of the diseases depending on the fusion gene partner. Interestingly, some of the neoplasms with abnormalities in the *PDGFRA* and *PDGFRB* genes have responded to imatinib. The *FIPL1-PDGFRA* mutation, which results from a cytogenetically invisible deletion on 4q12, was detected in this disease category, but also in chronic eosinophilic leukemia and systemic mastocytosis. Patients with the *FIPL1-PDGFRA* mutation usually respond to imatinib, but mutations in the *FIPL1-PDGFRA* gene causing imatinib resistance have been reported.

IV. Myelodysplastic/myeloproliferative neoplasms (MDS/MPN)

Myelodysplastic/myeloproliferative neoplasms category (MDS/MPN) includes myelodysplastic/myeloproliferative neoplasms, unclassifiable, MDS/MPN-U; provisional category of refractory anemia with ringed sideroblasts associated with marked thrombocytosis, RARS-T; chronic myelomonocytic leukemia, CMML; juvenile myelomonocytic leukemia, JMML; and atypical chronic myeloid leukemia *BCR-ABL* negative, aCML.

A. Chronic myelomonocytic leukemia (CMML)
CMML has components of both MDS and MPD. Patients with CMML usually undergo treatment when systemic symptoms develop or when there is worsening of peripheral blood counts (cytopenia, leukocytosis, or increased blast percentage). Treatment options for patients with CMML include supportive care, hydroxyurea, chemotherapy with azacitidine or decitabine, higher intensity chemotherapy such as cytarabine, topotecan, and etoposide, or SCT in select patients. Some patients with CMML contain a fusion gene with platelet derived growth factor receptor beta on 5q33 and respond to imatinib.

B. Atypical CML, BCR-ABL negative (aCML)
The aCML is a rare disease with myelodysplastic and myeloproliferative features, without the presence of the *BCR-ABL* fusion gene. Patients usually present with leukocytosis with dysplastic neutrophils and precursors. About 30% of patients have activating mutations in *NRAS* and *KRAS*. Patients with aCML usually carry poor prognosis with 15–40% risk of AML transformation and high incidence of bone marrow failure.

C. Juvenile myelomonocytic leukemia (JMML)
JMML is characterized as proliferation of granulocytic and monocytic lineages with <20% blasts in the bone marrow of peripheral blood. Patients can present with constitutional symptoms, splenomegaly, and lymphadenopathy. There is increased synthesis of hemoglobin F in many young patients of CMML.

About 65% of patients have normal karyotype and 25% have monosomy 7. The median survival without treatment with allogeneic SCT is 1 year. The risk of developing into acute leukemia is low.

D. Myelodysplastic/myeloproliferative neoplasm unclassifiable (MDS/MPN-U)

The MDS/MPN-U category includes disease with clinical and morphological features of overlap between MDS and MPN without falling into other specific MPN disease categories.

E. Refractory anemia with ring sideroblasts associated with marked thrombocytosis (RARS-T)

The RARS-T disease is a provisional category including patients with clinical and morphological characteristics of a myelodysplastic syndrome and thrombocytosis. Up to 60% of cases have the JAK2V617F mutation and less commonly MPLW515K/L mutation.

V. Myelodysplastic disorders

The myelodysplastic disorders (MDS) include a group of clonal stem cell disorders (Table 18.3) characterized by hypercellular marrow, but ineffective blood production resulting in cytopenias, increased risk of infections, frequent need for transfusions, and varying rate of progression into acute myeloid leukemia. MDS occurs *de novo* or can be acquired as a complication of prior treatments with chemotherapy or radiation, or exposure to toxins. In addition, a group of disorders falling into the category of treatment-related myeloid neoplasm has been proposed by the WHO and includes treatment related MDS and AML (acute myelogenous leukemia).

A. MDS presentation

MDS is a disease of older patients with a median age of onset of 71 years. The presentation of MDS can vary dramatically among patients. Some cases are asymptomatic and detected only on routine complete blood count (CBC). Other patients may present with symptomatic anemia such as fatigue, dizziness, increased exercise intolerance, or angina. In other patients increased bruising, petechiae and bleeding due to decreased platelets, or infections due to low white blood cells lead to further workup. Infection is one of the most serious sequelae of MDS and the most common cause of death in patients with MDS. Infections occur due to neutropenia but also due to granulocyte dysfunction with defective phagocytosis, adhesion, chemotaxis and bactericidal activity.

B. Workup of MDS and differential diagnosis

Myelodysplastic syndrome should be suspected in patients with progressive cytopenias. The initial workup should include of complete blood count,

Table 18.3 2008 WHO Classification System for *de novo* MDS

MDS subtype	Peripheral blood cytopenia	Peripheral blood blasts	Peripheral blood monocytes/ microliter	Bone marrow blasts (%) and RS (%)	Bone marrow dysplasias
RCUD	Anemia or neutropenia or thrombocytopenia, or bicytopenia	None or rare		<5% blasts <15% RS	Unilineage
RARS	Anemia	None		<5% blasts ≥15% RS	Erythroid
RCMD	Cytopenia(s)	None or rare (<1%), no Auer rods	<1000	<5% blasts, no Auer rods ±15% RS	In ≥10% of cells in two or more myeloid cells lines
RAEB-1	Cytopenias	<5% blasts, no Auer rods	<1000	5–9% blasts, no Auer rods	Unilineage or multilineage
RAEB-2	Cytopenias	5–19% blasts, Auer rods ±	<1000	10–19% blasts, Auer rods ±	Unilineage or multilineage
MDS-U	Cytopenias	None or rare <1%, no Auer rods		<5% blasts, no Auer rods	Dysplasia in <10% cells in one or more myeloid cell lines with cytogenetic abnormality of MDS
MDS with isolated del(5q)	Anemia (platelets normal or increased)	No or rare <1% blasts		<5% blasts, no Auer rods	Normal to increased megakaryocytes with hypolobated nuclei

MDS-U, myelodysplastic syndrome, unclassified; RAEB-1, refractory anemia with excess blasts-1; RAEB-2 refractory anemia with excess blasts-2; RARS, refractory anemia with ring sideroblasts; RCMD, refractory anemia with multilineage dysplasia; RCMD-RS, refractory cytopenia with multilineage dysplasia and ring sideroblasts; RCUD, refractory cytopenia with unilineage dysplasia (includes RA, refractory anemia; RN, refractory neutropenia; and RT, refractory thrombocytopenia); RS, ring sideroblast.
(Based on data from Swerdlow et al. WHO Classification of tumours of haematopoietic and lymphoid tissues. Lyon: IARC Press, 2008.)

peripheral smear, reticulocyte count, erythropoietin levels, folate and B_{12} levels, copper, zinc, ferritin, iron and total iron binding capacity. The analysis of bone marrow in MDS patients usually shows hypercellular bone marrow and single- or multi-lineage dysplasia. Some patients with MDS develop myelofibrosis which carries poor prognosis.

Causes of secondary bone marrow dysplasia include HIV infection causing dysplastic hematopoiesis, erythrodysplasia due to drugs (valproic acid, mycofenolate mofetil, ganciclovir, alemtuzumab, or nucleoside analogs such as cytarabine and fludarabine), methotrexate, or mercaptopurine. Acquired dysplastic changes can be also seen in patients with nutritional deficiencies of B_{12}, folate or copper, or in patients with increased zinc level.

C. Morphological features of MDS

Bone marrow of MDS patients can reveal diminished normal myeloid maturation with increased myeloid precursors but decreased mature granulocytes. Megakaryocyte number is normal or increased, and there are abnormal megakaryocyte forms including micromegakaryocytes, cells with multiple dispersed nuclei (also called Pawn ball changes), and large mononuclear or hypogranular cells.

Peripheral blood smear often shows granulocytes with decreased segmentation, called pseudo Pelger–Huet abnormality (Atlas Figure 33). Absolute neutropenia occurs in up to 50% of MDS patients. Thrombocytopenia is present in about 25–50% of patients with MDS. Thrombocytosis is less common but can be seen in low-risk disease and in some cases of 5q- and 3q21q26 abnormality, and refractory anemia with ringed sideroblasts with thrombocytosis. Red blood cells (rbc) abnormalities, including ovalocytes, teardrop cells, stomatocytes or acanthocytes due to changes in rbc cytoskeletal proteins can also be present. Howell–Jolly bodies (Atlas Figure 15), nucleated red blood cells, and basophilic stippling (Atlas Figure 14) can occur due to dyserythropoiesis.

D. Cytogenetic and molecular changes in MDS

Approximately 50% of patients with primary MDS have normal karyotype, compared to 20% of therapy related MDS. The most common cytogenetic changes include trisomy 8, monosomy 5 or 7, loss of the Y chromosome, and deletions in the long arms of chromosomes 5, 7, 11, 13, and 20. Up to 15% of cases have complex karyotype with three or more cytogenetic aberrations. Therapy related MDS after exposure to alkylator chemotherapy often carries partial or complete loss of chromosomes 5 or 7. Other therapy related cytogenetic abnormalities include 3p14-21, 6p12, 12p11-17, or 19p13, and mutations in chromosome 17p in the p53 gene. The karyotype changes affecting prognosis are incorporated into the International Prognostic Scoring System (IPSS) and help predict patient's prognosis.

E. International Prognostic Scoring System (IPSS)

The MDS subgroups have been divided into the FAB or WHO morphological categories, but the IPSS has been useful in predicting a patient's prognosis and in guiding therapeutic decisions. The IPSS (Table 18.4) takes into account bone marrow blast percentage, number of cytopenias and types of cytogenetic aberrations and divides MDS into prognostic categories with low-risk (IPSS

Table 18.4 International Prognostic Scoring System (IPSS) for MDS				
Bone marrow blasts (%)	<5	5–10		11–20	21–30
Karyotype	Good	Intermediate	Poor	
Cytopenias	0–1	2–3		
Score	0	0.5	1.0	1.5	2.0

MDS risk group	IPSS	Survival age ≤60	Survival age >60	Survival age >70
Low	0	11.8	4.8	3.9
Intermediate-1	0.5–1.0	5.2	2.7	2.4
Intermediate-2	1.5–2.0	1.8	1.1	1.2
High	2.5–3.5	0.3	0.5	0.4

Cytopenias are defined as hemoglobin <10 g/dL, neutrophil count <1800/microliter, and platelets <100,000/microliter.
(Based on data from Greenberg P. International scoring system for evaluating prognosis in myelodysplastic syndromes. Blood 1997;89(6): 2079–88.)

score 0), intermediate-1 risk (IPSS score 0.5–1), intermediate-2 risk (IPSS score 1.5–2) and high-risk (IPSS score 2.5–3.5) disease, with overall median survival of 5.7, 3.5, 1.2, and 0.4 years, respectively. A patient's karyotype is divided into good (normal karyotype, -Y, del(5q), del(20q)), poor (complex karyotype with ≥3 aberrations, and chromosome 7 abnormality), and intermediate cytogenetic groups. WHO classification based Prognostic Scoring System has modified the IPSS based on need for transfusions which predicts worse prognosis.

F. Treatment of MDS

The decisions about treatment of MDS take into account patients IPSS score, age, and performance status in the setting of other comorbidities. It is important to define therapeutic goal, whether it is control of symptoms, prolongation of life or potentially curative therapy with HCT. The types of MDS treatments include supportive care (transfusions, antibiotics), low intensity therapy (growth factors, immunomodulatory agents such as lenalidomide, immunosuppressive treatment, demethylating agents such as azacitidine or decitabine, and low intensity chemotherapy with cytarabine) and high intensity treatment with chemotherapy and allogeneic HCT.

Immunosuppresive therapy is one of the approaches to MDS treatment since cytopenias in some patients may arise from immune suppression of stem cells. Some patients, especially with HLA D15 or with hypocellular bone marrow and low IPSS score can derive benefit from treatment with immunosuppressive therapy such as cyclosporine or ATG (anti-thymocyte globulin).

Patients with the 5q minus clonal abnormality and low-risk or intermediate-1 risk MDS can have very good responses to treatment with lenalidomide, including improvement in transfusion dependence, and complete or partial cytogenetic response that translates to improved survival. On the other hand, compared to good or intermediate-1 MDS, the response to lenalidomide in 5q minus MDS with intermediate-2 or high-risk MDS is much less.

Low-risk MDS patients are usually treated with supportive care. The level of serum erythropoietin is important in guiding erythropoietin supplementation since patients with MDS and low erythropoietin levels may respond to erythropoietin injections (alone or in combination with G-CSF) and have improved survival. If no response is achieved with growth factor support, and low-risk patients have severe transfusion requirement, hypomethylating agents (azacitidine or decitabine) or HCT can be considered. Treatment with azacitidine results in improved survival of patients with higher risk MDS of 24.5 months versus 15 months without azacitidine. In addition to supportive therapy, treatment options for high-risk patients include hypomethylating agents followed by HCT which is the only potentially curative therapy.

The risk of evolution of MDS into AML varies among the MDS subgroups, with 5–15% risk in RA and RARS, up to 40–50% risk in refractory anemia with excess blasts. Patients with higher ferritin concentration as a reflection of iron overload due to frequent rbc transfusions tend to have worse prognosis; it is unclear whether iron chelation treatment in such patients improves their outcome.

Further reading

Barzi A, Sekeres MA. Myelodysplastic syndromes: a practical approach to diagnosis and treatment. Cleve Clin J Med 2010;77(1):37–44.

Beer PA, Green AR. Pathogenesis and management of essential thrombocythemia hematology. Am Soc Hematol Educ Program 2009;621 8.

Campbell PJ, Green AR. The myeloproliferative disorders. N Engl J Med 2006;355(23): 2452–66.

Cervantes F, Dupriez B, Pereira A, et al. New prognostic scoring system for primary myelofibrosis based on a study of the International Working Group for myelofibrosis research and treatment. Blood 2009;113(13):2895–901.

Cutler CS, Lee SJ, Greenberg P, et al. A decision analysis of allogeneic bone marrow transplantation for the myelodysplastic syndromes: delayed transplantation for low-risk myelodysplasia is associated with improved outcome. Blood 2004;104(2):579–85.

Deininger MW. Milestones and monitoring in patients with CML treated with imatinib. Am Soc Hematol Educ Program 2008;419–26.

Fenaux P, Mufti GJ, Hellstrom-Lindberg E, et al. Efficacy of azacitidine compared with that of conventional care regimens in the treatment of higher-risk myelodysplastic syndromes: a randomised, open-label, Phase III study. Lancet Oncol 2009;10(3):223–32.

Gotlib J, Cools J. Five years since the discovery of Fip1l1-Pdgfra: what we have learned about the fusion and other molecularly defined eosinophilias. Leukemia 2008;22(11):1999–2010.

Greenberg P, Cox C, LeBeau MM, et al. International Scoring System for Evaluating Prognosis in Myelodysplastic Syndromes. Blood 1997;89(6):2079–88.

Hochhaus A, O'Brien SG, Guilhot F, et al. Six-year follow-up of patients receiving imatinib for the first-line treatment of chronic myeloid leukemia. Leukemia 2009;23(6): 1054–61.

Hoffman R, Benz EJ Jr, Shattil SJ, et al., eds. Hematology: Basic Principles and Practice. Edinburgh: Churchill Livingstone, 2009.

Kantarjian H, Shah NP, Hochhaus A, et al. Dasatinib versus imatinib in newly diagnosed chronic-phase chronic myeloid leukemia. N Engl J Med 2010;362(24):2260–70.

List A, Dewald G, Bennett J, et al. Lenalidomide in the myelodysplastic syndrome with chromosome 5q deletion. N Engl J Med 2006;355(14):1456–65.

Malcovati L, Della Porta MG, Cazzola M. Predicting survival and leukemic evolution in patients with myelodysplastic syndrome. Haematologica 2006;91(12):1588–90.

Pardanani A, Tefferi A. Systemic mastocytosis in adults: a review on prognosis and treatment based on 342 Mayo Clinic patients and current literature. Curr Opin Hematol 2010;17(2):125–32.

Saglio G, Kim DW, Issaragrisil S, et al. Nilotinib versus imatinib for newly diagnosed chronic myeloid leukemia. N Engl J Med 2010;362(24):2251–9.

Stone RM. How I treat patients with myelodysplastic syndromes. Blood 2009;113(25): 6296–6303.

Swerdlow SH, Campo E, Harris NL et al., eds. Who Classification of Tumours of Haematopoietic and Lymphoid Tissues. Lyon: International Agency for Research on Cancer (IARC), 2008.

Tefferi A. Essential thrombocythemia, polycythemia vera, and myelofibrosis: current management and the prospect of targeted therapy. Am J Hematol 2008;83(6):491–7.

Tefferi A. Novel mutations and their functional and clinical relevance in myeloproliferative neoplasms: Jak2, Mpl, Tet2, Asxl1, Cbl, Idh and Ikzf1. Leukemia 2010;24(6):1128–38.

Tefferi A, Gotlib J, Pardanani A. Hypereosinophilic syndrome and clonal eosinophilia: point-of-care diagnostic algorithm and treatment update. Mayo Clin Proc 2010;85(2):158–64.

19 Acute Leukemia

Tsila Zuckerman and Jacob M. Rowe

*Rambam Medical Center and Bruce Rappaport Faculty of Medicine, Technion—
Israel Institute of Technology, Haifa, Israel*

Leukemias are an uncommon and heterogeneous group of diseases characterized by infiltration of the bone marrow, blood and visceral organs by neoplastic cells of the hematopoietic system. Acute leukemia is broadly divided into
acute myeloid leukemia (AML) and acute lymphoblastic leukemia (ALL).
With the advances in laboratory techniques and knowledge regarding the
biological basis of the diseases, these leukemias have been further classified
into different subgroups enabling investigators and practitioners to categorize
them into different prognostic entities with the aim of individualizing the
treatment.

Acute leukemia results from two broad complementation groups of mutations: mutations conferring a proliferative and/or survival advantage to
hematopoietic progenitors and those mutations that impair hematopoietic
differentiation. These processes result in accumulation of blast cells in bone
marrow (BM) and/or peripheral blood (PB).

The diagnosis of acute leukemia is arbitrarily defined as the presence of
≥20% blasts in BM or PB, although, in practice, the biology of the disease
cannot be defined by such a cut-off. The classification is based on integrated
results of morphology, immunohistochemistry, immunophenotyping, cytogenetic and molecular studies.

I. Acute myeloid leukemia (AML)

AML, arising from hematopoietic precursors of the non-lymphoid compartment, is the most common acute leukemia in adults, with an annual incidence
of 3/100,000. The frequency increases with age (median 70 years) with
the incidence of 3.5/100,000 at age 50 and almost 10 times higher at the age
70–80 years.

Concise Guide to Hematology, First Edition. Edited by Alvin H. Schmaier, Hillard M. Lazarus.
© 2012 Blackwell Publishing Ltd. Published 2012 by Blackwell Publishing Ltd.

A. Pathogenesis

AML is a genotypically heterogeneous disease resulting from multistep cooperating mutations in hematopoietic precursors. Class I mutations confer a proliferative and/or survival advantage usually as a consequence of aberrant activation of signal transduction pathways such as mutation in *fms-like tyrosine kinase 3* (FLT3) and RAS signaling pathways. Class II mutations impair hematopoietic differentiation usually resulting from mutations in transcription factors or co-activators important for normal hematopoietic development. Sometimes such mutations include chromosome translocations caused by rearrangement of parts between non-homologous *chromosomes*, creating a gene fusion between the two otherwise separated genes, and conferring properties such as impairment of differentiation or enhanced proliferative capacity. Examples of such translocation occur in the so-called core binding factor (CBF) leukemias involving t(8;21) and inv(16)/t(16;16). These two changes result in increased number of clonal malignant cells and suppression of normal elements.

B. Etiology

Largely unknown, although some predisposing factors are associated with the disease.
* Hereditary:
    – Chromosome aneuploidy: Down syndrome (trisomy 21).
    – Defective DNA repair: Fanconi anemia, Bloom syndrome, ataxia telangiectasia.
    – Congenital neutropenia (Kostmann syndrome).
* Ionizing radiation: therapeutic or non-therapeutic (accidental).
* Chemicals: benzene, petroleum, smoking.
* Prior cytotoxic therapy:
    – Topoisomerase II inhibitors (anthracyclines, mitoxantrone, epipodophyllotoxins): often associated with chromosome 11q23 aberrations. Typically with a short latency from exposure (1–3 years).
    – Alkylating agents: associated with chromosome 5 and 7 aberrations (usually a longer latency period of 4–5 years).

C. Classification

The French-American-British (FAB) classification (Table 19.1) is based on morphologic evaluation of blasts and their differentiation level, although prognostically this is currently unimportant.

The recent World Health Organization (WHO) classification incorporates morphological, biological and clinical features to classify cases of AML into unique groups (Table 19.2).

1. Immunophenotyping

Immunophenotyping of samples of BM or PB with monoclonal antibodies for cell surface antigens, using multiparameter flow cytometry is employed to

Table 19.1 FAB Classification of AML

FAB subtype	Name	Percentage of adult AML patients
M0	AML with minimal differentiation	5%
M1	AML without maturation	15%
M2	AML with maturation. Associated with t(8;21)	25%
M3	Acute promyelocytic leukemia >30% promyelocytes. Associated with t(15;17).	10%
M3V	Microgranular variant. Associated with t(15;17) and high WBC	
M4	Acute myelomonocytic leukemia, >20% monocytes	20%
M4 eos	Acute myelomonocytic leukemia with eosinophilia (5–30% eosinophils)	5%
M5	Acute monocytic leukemia	10%
M6	Acute erythroid leukemia	5%
M7	Acute megakaryoblastic leukemia	5%

Table 19.2 WHO Classification of AML

1. **Acute myeloid leukemia with recurrent genetic abnormalities**
   - AML with t(8;21)(q22;q22); *RUNX1-RUNX1T1*
   - AML with inv(16)(p13.1q22) or t(16;16)(p13.1;q22); *CBFB-MYH11*
   - APL with t(15;17)(q22;q12); *PML-RARA*
   - AML with t(9;11)(p22;q23); *MLLT3-MLL*
   - AML with t(6;9)(p23;q34); *DEK-NUP214*
   - AML with inv(3)(q21q26.2) or t(3;3)(q21;q26.2); *RPN1-EVI1*
   - AML (megakaryoblastic) with t(1;22)(p13;q13); *RBM15-MKL1*
   Provisional entity: AML with mutated NPM1
   Provisional entity: AML with mutated CEBPA
2. **Acute myeloid leukemia with myelodysplasia-related changes**
3. **Therapy-related myeloid neoplasms**
4. **Acute myeloid leukemia, not otherwise specified**
   - AML with minimal differentiation
   - AML without maturation
   - AML with maturation
   - Acute myelomonocytic leukemia
   - Acute monoblastic/monocytic leukemia
   - Acute erythroid leukemia
     - Pure erythroid leukemia
     - Erythroleukemia, erythroid/myeloid
   - Acute megakaryoblastic leukemia
   - Acute basophilic leukemia
   - Acute panmyelosis with myelofibrosis
5. **Myeloid sarcoma**
6. **Myeloid proliferations related to Down syndrome**
   - Transient abnormal myelopoiesis
   - Myeloid leukemia associated with Down syndrome
7. **Blastic plasmacytoid dendritic cell neoplasm**

determine lineage involvement of a newly diagnosed AML. For most markers ≥20% of the cells expressing a marker is considered as diagnostic. . The most common markers in AML are CD13, CD14, CD33, CD34 and CD117. They reliably differentiate AML from ALL and are increasingly used in the evaluation of post-remission minimal residual disease (MRD), the situation in which the PB and BM are grossly free of disease but leukemia cells persist at hard to detect levels.

2. Cytogenetic and molecular analysis

Chromosomal abnormalities such as translocations, inversions and deletions are detected in approximately 55% of adult AML. Cytogenetic as well as molecular markers are the most powerful predictors of prognosis in AML patients.

Numerous genetic abnormalities, undetectable under conventional karyotypic analyses (e.g., gene mutations, gene expression abnormalities), have been recently discovered allowing further dissection of AML into molecular subtypes with distinctive prognosis. Relatively favorable genotypes of AML (i.e., those forms that are more responsive to therapy), for example, involve mutations in the genes of the transcription factor *CEBPA* (CCAAT enhancer binding factor alpha) or *nucleophosmin-1* (*NPM1*), whereas unfavorable genotypes (i.e., those forms that are less responsive to therapy) may include AML with partial tandem duplications of the *MLL* gene (*MLL*-PTD), internal tandem duplications of the gene of *fms-like tyrosine kinase 3* (*FLT3*-ITDs), mutations in *Wilms' tumor 1* gene (*WT1*), neuroblastoma RAS (NRAS) gene and KIT gene (Figure 19.1). Currently known cytogenetic and molecular risk groups are summarized in Table 19.3.

D. Clinical features

- Acute presentation with signs and symptoms related to: (i) increased clonal malignant populations and internal organ dysfunction due to leukemia cell infiltration; (ii) decreased normal blood cell elements; (iii) other associated

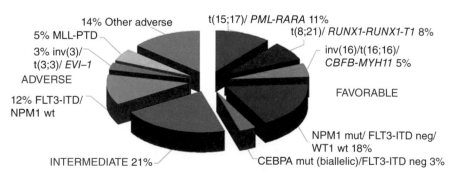

Figure 19.1 Frequency of prognostically relevant molecular and cytogenetic subgroups of AML arising in younger adults. (Reproduced with permission from Grimwade D, Hills RK. Independent prognostic factors for AML outcome. Hematology Am Soc Hematol Educ Program. 2009:385–395.)

Table 19.3 Pre-treatment cytogenetic and molecular entities shown to predict disease outcome in multivariable analysis studies conducted in younger adults

	Cytogenetic/molecular abnormality	Comments
Favorable	t(15;17)(q22;q12–21)/*PML-RARA* t(8;21)(q22;q22)/*RUNX1-RUNX1T1* inv(16)(p13q22)/t(16;16)(p13;q22)/*CBFB-MYH11* NPM1 mutant/FLT3-ITD⁻, WT1 wild type CEBPA mutant (biallelic, FLT3-ITD⁻)	Remain favorable irrespective of additional cytogenetic abnormalities
Intermediate	Entities not classified as favorable or adverse	
Adverse	abn(3q) [excluding t(3;5)(q21~25;q31~35)], inv(3)(q21q26)/t(3;3)(q21;q26)/*EVI-1* expression add(5q), del(5q), −5, −7, add(7q), t(6;11) (q27;q23), t(10;11)(p11~13;q23), t(9;22) (q34;q11), −17, abn(17p) with other changes Complex (>3 unrelated abnormalities)	Excluding cases with favorable karyotype
	FLT3-ITD	In absence of favorable karyotype. Particularly poor prognosis with high level FLT3-ITD mutant ratio or if FLT3-ITD accompanied by *WT1* mutation
	MLL-PTD	

Reproduced with permission from Grimwade D, Hills RK. Independent prognostic factors for AML outcome. Hematology Am Soc Hematol Educ Program. 2009:385–395.

factors such as disseminated intravascular coagulation (DIC) discussed later.
- Anemia: weakness, lethargy, shortness of breath and palpitations.
- Neutropenia: fever, infection (usually with Gram-negative organisms or *Staphylococcus* species).
- Thrombocytopenia: purpura, menorrhagia, mucosal bleeding (epistaxis, gingival), retinal hemorrhage.
- Gum hypertrophy and skin infiltration (FAB subtypes M4, M5).
- Extramedullary chloromas, also called granulocytic sarcomas, are collections of blasts in sites outside the PB or BM. Chloromas may precede the development of AML and are more common in the undifferentiated and minimally differentiated AML (M2 with t(8;21)) subtypes.
- Hyperleukocytosis is defined as a blast count greater than 100,000/µL, although the clinical manifestations may occur at lower WBC counts, especially in the monocytic variants or in an AML with a very rapid proliferation rate. Hyperleukocytosis may be accompanied by leukostasis with clinical manifestation of microcirculatory dysfunction with slugging of leukemic cells in capillary vessels, especially in the lungs, CNS and retina that may present as hypoxemia, confusion and retinal hemorrhage.

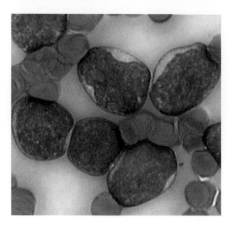

Figure 19.2 Myeloid blasts in bone marrow.

- DIC: hemorrhage, thrombosis or the combination.
- CNS involvement: headache, confusion, cranial nerve palsy. Occurs rarely at presentation and during follow up in 5% of patients.
- Bone pain caused by expansion of medullary bone marrow space, involving long bones, ribs and sternum, is the initial manifestation in 25% of patients.

E. Leukemia workup
- CBC and peripheral blood smear (search for Auer rod which are reddish rod-like filaments of aggregated primary granules) (Figure 19.2) (Atlas Figure 38).
- BM aspirate or biopsy.
- Immunohistochemistry of PB or BM is performed if immunophenotyping is not available. It identifies granules present in normal myeloid and mono-cytic populations and in the leukemic cells; such include myeloperoxidase (MPO), nonspecific esterase (NSE) and PAS.
- Immunophenotype using flow cytometry of PB and /or BM.
- Cytogenetic analysis of BM.
- Molecular analysis of PB or BM to identify special abnormalities such as Flt3 or nucleophosmin-1, discussed later.

F. Differential diagnosis
- Severe sepsis with leukemoid reaction which presents with leukocytosis exceeding 50,000/μL, which is often characterized by a significant increase in early neutrophil precursors usually due to infection.
- ALL.
- Chronic myeloid leukemia (CML)—blast crisis which is usually associated with basophilia. Cytogenetic and molecular studies reveal the presence of Philadelphia chromosome, t(9;22), i.e., the translocation between chromosomes 9 and 22.

G. Treatment

1. Supportive treatment

- Instruction regarding the disease treatment course.
- Hydration (aim for urine output >100 mL/hour) to prevent renal failure from tumor lysis. Tumor lysis syndrome (TLS) is caused by massive destruction of cells, occurring either spontaneously due to high proliferation rate or following chemotherapy. In this syndrome, the leukemia cells release large quantities of intracellular substances such as electrolytes and nuclear material. Clinically it is manifested as hyperkalemia, hyperphosphatemia and hyperuricemia, the latter due to breakdown of DNA.
- Allopurinol, a xanthine oxidase inhibitor, to be given for prevention of hyperuricemia. Rasburicase, a recombinant urate oxidase, which converts uric acid to a soluble metabolite of uric acid and hence prevents renal obstruction and renal failure associated with established hyperuricemia.
- Hydroxyurea is an orally administered antimetabolite which selectively inhibits ribonucleotide diphosphate reductase preventing the conversion of ribonucleotides to deoxyribonucleotide, thus halting cell cycle at the G1/S phase and reducing WBC. It may be given to control high WBC count until the start of chemotherapy.
- RBC transfusions for anemia and platelet transfusion support for thrombocytopenia. Prophylactic platelet transfusion is recommended to keep a platelet count above the threshold of 10×10^9/L. Filtered and irradiated blood products (with WBC removed and lymphocytes inactivated, respectively) are recommended for prevention of alloimmunization and transfusion-associated graft-versus-host disease (inadvertent engraftment of viable lymphocytes present in the blood component), respectively.
- Antibiotic prophylaxis with quinolone antibacterials is recommended. For febrile neutropenia use of broad spectrum antibacterials is recommended.
- Antifungal (anti-mold) prophylaxis.
- Leukopheresis (mechanical removal of WBC) for WBC count >100,000/µL or for symptoms of leukostasis.
- DIC which is an activated blood coagulation and clot lysing state that present as extensive bleeding or blood clotting and requires urgent intervention with replacement blood coagulation factors and platelets (see Chapter 12)—replacement therapy with fresh frozen plasma, cryoprecipitate or fibrinogen and platelet transfusions.
- Fertility consultation. Male patients should be offered the possibility of sperm cryopreservation. Fertile female patients should be offered gonadotropin agonists to prevent menstrual bleeding during thrombocytopenia given the evidence supporting the gonadal protection with these agents.
- Non-invasive cardiac evaluation in older patients, including echocardiogram, MUGA scan and echocardiogram, as many chemotherapeutic agents are cardiotoxic.

2. Definitive treatment in patients aged 18–60 years

Treatment of newly diagnosed AML is divided into two phases—induction and post-remission. The goal of induction treatment is to induce prompt reduction in leukemia cells and eliminate gross evidence of leukemia on repeat diagnostic BM examination, termed a complete remission (CR). Leukemic cells, however, persist in sub-microscopic concentrations and without subsequent therapy will re-populate the patient within months. Thus, additional treatment is necessary, termed post-remission therapy, given with the goal to eradicate residual leukemic cells, prevent relapse and prolong survival. CR is strictly defined as <5% blasts in BM, absence of blasts with Auer rods, absence of extramedullary disease, absolute blood neutrophil count $>1.0 \times 10^9$/L, platelet count >100,000/μL and RBC transfusion independence.

(a) Induction therapy

The initial management of AML depends on whether the leukemia is the most common AML, or a less common sub-type, termed acute promyelocytic leukemia (APL). The approach to APL is fundamentally different as this disorder is characterized predominantly by a block in differentiation and a significantly greater tendency for severe spontaneous bleeding. Early suspicion and intervention to reduce complications of consumption coagulopathy (DIC) are critical in APL and to immediately start differentiating agent and apoptotic therapy is mandatory (see below). Most other AML patients require a combination of cytotoxic drug therapies as these disorders are the result of excessive proliferation of leukemia cells, rather than a differentiation block.

For non-APL adults (aged 18–60 years), standard induction treatment consists of 3 days of anthracycline (daunorubicin 60–90 mg/m^2, idarubicin 10–12 mg/m^2 or mitoxantrone 10–12 mg/m^2) and 7 days of cytarabine (100 mg/m^2 i.v. continuous infusion), the so-called "3 + 7" protocol. There is no evidence for superiority of idarubicin or mitoxantrone over daunorubicin. A higher dose of daunorubicin, up to 90 mg/m^2, is safe and may become standard of care. CR is achieved in 60–80% of patients. Addition of a third cytotoxic agent (etoposide, fludarabine, thioguanine or high dose cytarabine) leads to increased toxicity without significantly improving efficacy.

(b) Post-remission therapy

At diagnosis, leukemic tumor burden exceeds 10^{12} cells. After successful induction chemotherapy and attainment of complete remission (CR), the body tumor cell burden decreases to less than 10^9 cells. If no additional therapy is given, relapse within months is inevitable. Hence, consolidation is directed against the sub-microscopic residual disease state.

Various post-remission strategies include repetitive cycles of intensive conventional chemotherapy and high dose chemotherapy followed by either autologous or allogeneic hematopoietic cell transplantation. The selection of treatment is based on individual patient risk stratification as determined by cytogenetic and molecular analysis at diagnosis.

High-dose cytarabine ($3 \, g/m^2$ every 12 hours on days 1, 3, 5) was found to be superior to intermediate or standard dose ($400 \, mg/m^2$ or $100 \, mg/m^2$ continuous IV for 5 days). This result was most pronounced in patients with favorable cytogenetics.

Autologous hematopoietic cell transplantation (HCT) is considered an alternative option for post-remission therapy in patients with favorable and intermediate cytogenetic risk groups. The outcome after autologous HCT is at least as good as with the use of chemotherapy alone as post-remission treatment and is associated with a lower rate of relapse.

Allogeneic HCT is associated with the lowest risk of relapse mainly due to the potent graft-versus-leukemia effect, i.e., an effect beyond chemotherapy-killing of cells via an immunologic effect of donor T cells destroying residual leukemia cells in the patient. This treatment is mostly beneficial in patients with intermediate and unfavorable cytogenetics. However, due to significant toxicity, the treatment is limited to patients with good performance status without considerable co-morbidities (other diseases antedating the onset of leukemia that have resulted in internal organ dysfunction) and with an HLA-matched sibling. The recent introduction of reduced intensity conditioning (RIC), i.e., use of less intense bone marrow ablative treatment, and improved supportive care have decreased the toxicity of this modality. Furthermore, use of an alternative donor (matched unrelated, cord blood and haploidentical) has increased the availability of HCT (see Chapter 26 for a full description of hematopoietic stem cell transplantation).

Suggested algorithm for treatment of AML patients aged 18–60 years is shown in Figure 19.3.

3. Management of patients aged ≥60 years

Increasing age is associated with a higher incidence of adverse factors resulting in decreased ability to tolerate therapy (poor performance status, co-morbidities) and biologically more resistant leukemia reflected by unfavorable cytogenetics, secondary AML and therapy resistance. The overall CR rate with standard induction therapy in the 60–80-year group is 50%, being ≤30% for a subset with adverse cytogenetics. For fit older patients, the dose of "3 + 7" should not be attenuated. Post-remission therapy is still controversial due to inherent bias in patient selection for clinical trials, although recent data from the international registries (collecting data on treatment of consecutive patients, have less bias in results of treatment outcome) suggest that repetitive cycles of modest dose consolidation are associated with a longer survival compared with lower doses. Application of reduced intensity conditioning (RIC) allogeneic HCT (which employs decreased doses of chemotherapy and increased immunosuppression) enables the use of this modality in older patients with acceptable toxicity.

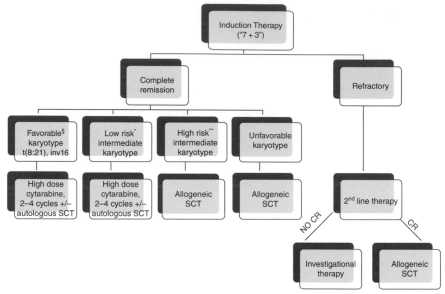

Figure 19.3 Algorithm for treatment of AML patients aged 18–60 years. SCT, stem cell transplantation (HCT); CR, complete remission.

§Patients with favorable karyotype and *c-kit* mutations have an adverse prognosis and should be offered allogeneic HCT. Patients with molecular evidence of disease persistence may also be considered for intensive treatment.

*Low risk intermediate karyotype includes patients with mutated NPM1, biallelic CEBPA.

**High risk intermediate karyotype includes patients with mutated FLT-ITD, MLL-PTD and other unfavorable mutations as well as patients with other poor risk factors (antecedent hematologic disorder, failure to attain remission with conventional induction).

Patients aged ≥75–80 years may be offered induction therapy, if fit, or only supportive treatment with hydroxyurea or low dose cytarabine (20 mg daily subcutaneously for 10 days) to control WBC count.

H. Acute promyelocytic leukemia (APL)

APL (FAB M3) accounts for about 10–15% of AML cases (Atlas Figure 40). Patients tend to be younger (median age 40 years), have a low WBC count, high incidence of consumption coagulopathy and a higher survival compared with other AMLs. The disease is associated with balanced translocation involving the retinoic acid receptor alpha (RAR-α) gene on chromosome 17 and PML gene on chromosome 15, i.e., t (15;17). Retinoic acid is a critical ligand in the differentiation pathway of hematopoietic cells, mediated through binding to a retinoic acid receptor alpha (RAR-α). The fusion protein, PML-RARα, interacts with nuclear repressor protein complex which attracts histone deacetylase altering chromatin conformation and therefore inhibiting transcription; these events ultimately lead to blocking differentiation to mature cells. Treatment of APL includes aggressive control of DIC coupled with induction with high dose anthracycline (daunorubicin 50 mg/m^2/d × 4 days) and oral all-*trans* retinoic acid (ATRA) at 45 mg/m^2/d, an orally administered Vitamin A-like agent that "relieves" the block to differentiation until remission is documented. ATRA treatment is critical to be started with the first suspicion of APL to prevent coagulopathy. Post-remission therapy consists of repeat cycles of anthracyclines. It is unclear whether there is a role for cytarabine in induction or consolidation. In addition, maintenance therapy with ATRA ± chemotherapy is superior to observation. Arsenic trioxide (ATO) (a parenterally administered agent that induces apoptosis) also has a role in treating APL both in induction and relapse.

I. Prognostic factors

Factors adversely influencing the likelihood of entering CR, the length of CR and curability of AML include:

- Age >60 years.
- Unfavorable cytogenetic and molecular markers as discussed above.
- Failure to achieve CR after induction therapy.
- Presence of minimal residual disease (MRD) after induction. MRD is detected by flow cytometry or FISH (fluorescence *in situ* hybridization) analysis if a marker has been identified at diagnosis. MRD positivity post-induction can suggest an increased risk of relapse and necessity for a more aggressive treatment.
- AML arising in a patient with a pre-existing myelodysplasia (MDS) that has occurred spontaneously or is treatment-related; such situations are often associated with unfavorable cytogenetics.
- WBC >100,000/μL at presentation (hyperleukocytosis) results in seeding sanctuary sites in the brain and testis that are resistant to standard treatment and may be a source for relapse.

J. Prognosis

Induction therapy is associated with CR in 60–90% of patients aged <60 years and ~50% of older patients. Long-term survival is 65–70% in the favorable group, 35–40% in the intermediate and 3–10% in the unfavorable cytogenetic group.

K. Conclusion

Diagnosis and treatment of AML is a complex task and it should be performed by clinicians and institutions experienced in these disorders. Its management is rapidly evolving towards segregation into different biological entities and patients' specific risk. Whenever possible, patients should be treated within clinical trials in order to promote knowledge of this disease. Allogeneic HCT in intermediate and high risk groups offers the best option for cure.

II. Acute lymphoblastic leukemia

ALL is a leukemia arising from the hematopoietic precursors of the lymphoid lineage. It is the commonest malignancy in childhood (3–4/100,000) with the majority of cases in the 2–10-year age group. The incidence of adult ALL is much lower (0.7–1.8/100,000 annually).

A. Pathogenesis

ALL is characterized by gross numerical and structural chromosomal abnormalities, including hyperdiploidy (>50 chromosomes), hypodiploidy (<46 chromosomes), translocations (t(12;22),(1;19),(9;22),(4;11), rearrangements (MYC, MLL) as well as complex karyotypes (≥5 separate cytogenetics abnormalities). However, several observations indicate that these lesions alone are insufficient to induce leukemia and cooperating lesions are required.

B. Etiology

Although unknown, several predisposing factors have been described:
- Ionizing radiation.
- Radon exposure.
- Hereditary syndromes—Down, Bloom, Klinefelter, Fanconi.

C. Classification

The WHO Classification of ALL (2008) integrates immunophenotyping with genetic and molecular data and segregates to B and T type and unique genetic alterations (Box 19.1 and Table 19.4).

1. Cytogenetics

Abnormal cytogenetics are present in up to 85% of ALL patients and serve for risk stratification.

Translocations:
- **t(12;21)** is associated with TEL-AML1. It is the most common genetic aberration in childhood (≈25%) and is associated with good prognosis.
- **t(4;11)** is associated with refractory disease and early relapse. Occurs in 80% of infant and 6% of adult ALL.

Box 19.1 WHO Classification of ALL

B lymphoblastic leukemia/lymphoma

B lymphoblastic leukemia/lymphoma, NOS

B lymphoblastic leukemia/lymphoma with recurrent genetic abnormalities

B lymphoblastic leukemia/lymphoma with t(9;22)(q34;q11.2);*BCR-ABL 1*

B lymphoblastic leukemia/lymphoma with t(v;11q23);*MLL* rearranged

B lymphoblastic leukemia/lymphoma with t(12;21)(p13;q22) *TEL-AML1 (ETV6-RUNX1)*

B lymphoblastic leukemia/lymphoma with hyperdiploidy

B lymphoblastic leukemia/lymphoma with hypodiploidy

B lymphoblastic leukemia/lymphoma with t(5;14)(q31;q32) *IL3-IGH*

B lymphoblastic leukemia/lymphoma with t(1;19)(q23;p13.3);*TCF3-PBX1*

T lymphoblastic leukemia/lymphoma

NOS, not otherwise specified.

Table 19.4 Immunophenotype of ALL

Lineage	Immunophenotype	Frequency (%)	
		Pediatric	Adult
B lineage ≈85%			
Pro B	HLA-DR+,TdT+,CD19+	5	11
Common	HLA-DR+,TdT+,CD19+,CD10+	65	51
Pre B	HLA-DR+,TdT+,CD19+,CD10±,cIgM	15	10
B cell	HLA-DR+,TdT+,CD19+,CD10±,sIgM	3	4
T lineage≈15%			
Pre T	TdT+,cCD3+,CD7+,	1	7
T cell	TdT+,cCD3+,CD1a/2/3+,CD5+	11	17

c, cytoplasmic; s, surface.

- t(9;22)—the Ph chromosome—results in constitutive tyrosine kinase activity which interferes with different signaling pathways such as RAS. Occurs in 20% of adult and only 5% of pediatric ALL and associates with poor prognosis.
- t(8;14) is associated with mature B cell (ALL-L3) phenotype and with dysregulation of c-myc proto-oncogene. 5% of ALL. Confers poor prognosis.
- T-ALL. Activating mutation in NOTCH1 is present in 60% of T-ALL and is associated with improved outcome.

Numerical changes in chromosomes are also very common. Hypodiploid (<46 chromosomes), pseudodiploid (46 chromosomes with other structural abnormalities) and hyperdiploid (>50 chromosomes). Hyperdiploidy confers favorable prognosis while hypodiploidy and pseudodiploidy have a poor prognosis.

D. Clinical features

- Bone marrow failure:
  - Anemia: weakness, lethargy, shortness of breath and palpitations.
  - Neutropenia: fever, infection (usually with Gram-negative organisms or *Staphylococcus* species).
  - Thrombocytopenia: purpura, menorrhagia, mucosal bleeding (epistaxis, gingival), retinal hemorrhage.
- Hyperleukocytosis with leukostasis: hypoxemia, retinal hemorrhage, confusion. Leukostasis is much less common than in AML.
- Bone pain: More common in children.
- Mediastinal mass with cough and superior vena cava syndrome in T-ALL.
- CNS involvement: headache, confusion, cranial nerve palsy. Occurs in 6% of patients at presentation.
- Lymphadenopathy (in 55%).
- Splenomegaly and hepatomegaly (in 45%).

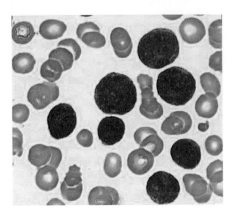

Figure 19.4 Lymphoid blasts in peripheral blasts.

E. Leukemia workup
As in AML. Immunohistochemistry positive for the terminal transferase lymphoid enzyme, TdT (Figure 19.4; Atlas Figure 41).

F. Differential diagnosis
- AML.
- Lymphoma with leukemic phase.
- Infectious mononucleosis.

G. Adverse prognostic factors
- Age >35 years.
- Elevated WBC at diagnosis (>30,000/µL for B lineage, >100,000/µL for T lineage).
- Presence of adverse cytogenetics: Philadelphia chromosome (t(9;22), t(4;11), t(8;14), complex karyotype (≥5 cytogenetic abnormalities), low hypodiploidy, near triploidy.
- Time to achieve CR (>4 weeks) has been found to correlate with a worse disease prognosis.
- Presence of minimal residual disease after induction and intensification.

H. Treatment

1. Supportive treatment
As in AML, except for greater likelihood of tumor lysis in ALL, especially with corticosteroids, necessitating optimal hydration and close observation.

2. Definitive treatment
Initial aim of chemotherapy is to achieve rapid and complete remission (CR), defined as for AML.

(a) Treatment for patients not intended for allogeneic HCT includes four phases
- **Remission induction.** Most induction regimens were designed based on pediatric models, which include two phases of induction, with multi-agent chemotherapy containing vincristine, dexamethasone, daunorubicin and L-asparaginase, cyclophosphamide and cytarabine in various combinations and time frames (usually lasting 2–4 weeks each). Treatment with the hyperfractionated "hyper-CVAD" regimen is used by some centers with a shorter duration of therapy.
- **Consolidation.** Four cycles of chemotherapy often using the same agents as given in induction with an aim to further decrease tumor burden and prevent relapse.
- **CNS prophylaxis.** Unlike AML, sanctuary site relapse is a common problem in ALL. Hence, periodic intrathecal chemotherapy, coupled with cycles of high dose methotrexate and cranial irradiation, is administered starting from induction and continuing throughout consolidation and maintenance. The latter is given to adults not planned for HCT (in a dose of 18–24 Gy over 12 fractions). Children are precluded from radiation due to cognitive impairment. CNS prophylaxis continues through all stages of treatment. With this approach the risk of CNS relapse decreases from 30% to 5%.
- **Maintenance therapy.** Maintenance therapy is given to complete 2.5-year treatment. It consists of daily 6-mercaptopurine (6-MP) and weekly methotrexate and vincristine plus prednisone ever 3 months. In contrast to AML, maintenance therapy using prolonged low-dose chemotherapy has demonstrated a significantly improved overall survival in ALL patients.
- **Novel agents in the treatment of ALL.** Clofarabine is a nucleoside analog that is approved for the treatment of patients with refractory or relapsed acute lymphoblastic leukemia (ALL). Clofarabine inhibits DNA synthesis at both DNA polymerase I and at RNA reductase. Overall response rates average 25%. Nelarabine (Arranon) is a novel purine nucleoside that is a prodrug of ara-G, the deoxyguanosine nucleoside analog 9-β-D-arabinofuranosylguanine. Complete responses are reported in 31% of patients with T-cell ALL. The dose-limiting toxicity of this drug is neurotoxicity. Monoclonal antibodies such as rituximab (anti CD20), epratuzumab (a humanized anti CD22), alemtuzumab (anti CD52) and blinatumomab (BiTE—anti CD19 and CD3) are currently being explored as additional non-myelosuppressive treatment in ALL.

(b) Allogeneic hematopoietic cell transplantation
Allogeneic HCT is recommended for adults or high-risk pediatric patients in CR1 following remission induction and for all patients in ≥CR2. Data from large cooperative trials and meta-analyses have demonstrated the beneficial impact of allogeneic HCT from a matched sibling donor on overall survival, implying potent graft-versus-leukemia effect. In the largest study to date, by the Eastern Cooperative Oncology Group (ECOG) in the United States and

Medical Research Council (MRC) in the United Kingdom, this effect was most prominent in the standard risk group, while in other studies it was more beneficial in the high risk category. Improved supportive care and use of RIC (explained earlier) HCT in the elderly population are likely to reduce transplant-related mortality, while preserving the beneficial effect of transplant. Alternative donors such as matched unrelated, umbilical cord and haploidentical donors are increasingly used for patients lacking a matched sibling, with encouraging results (see Chapter 26).

I. Treatment of Ph + ALL

Presence of Ph chromosome with the t(9;22)/BCR-ABL is associated with poor prognosis across all age groups. Its frequency increases with age (~50% of patients >60 years old). Introduction of the tyrosine kinase inhibitors (TKIs), imatinib and dasatinib (specifically inhibiting the fusion protein of bcr-abl and thus preventing its proliferative action) in combination with chemotherapy has led to a marked improvement in the outcome of ALL therapy, with a CR rate of 94%. This fact enables more patients to proceed to allogeneic HCT. In the elderly population it offers the option of using a less toxic RIC, although the role of transplantation has to be reassessed since there are long-term survivors even without transplantation.

J. Conclusions

The cure rate in pediatric ALL is between 80 and 90%. In adults, however, although ~90% attain CR, post-remission relapse rates are high and the long-term disease free survival is only ~30–40%. Allogeneic HCT increases the long-term overall survival to about 60% in standard risk patients. Innovative approaches both in transplantation and in targeted therapy (new TKIs, anti-CD22 antibody, anti-NOTCH) are being increasingly developed and used with an anticipation of improved survival.

Further reading

Döhner H, Estey EH, Amadori S, et al. Diagnosis and management of acute myeloid leukemia in adults: recommendations from an international expert panel, on behalf of the European Leukemia Net. Blood 2010;115:453–74.

Rowe JM, Tallman MS. How I treat acute myeloid leukemia. Blood 2010;116:3147–56.

Rowe JM. Optimal induction and post-remission therapy for AML in first remission. Am Soc Hematol Educ Program 2009:396–405.

Rowe JM. Optimal management of adults with ALL. Br J Haematol 2009;144:468–83.

Swerdlow SH, Campo E, Harris NL, et al., eds. WHO Classification of Tumours of Haematopoietic and Lymphoid Tissues, 4th edn. Lyon, France: IARC Press, 2008.

Vardiman JW, Thiele J, Arber DA, et al. The 2008 revision of the World Health Organization (WHO) classification of myeloid neoplasms and acute leukemia: rationale and important changes. Blood 2009;114:937–51.

20 Classification of Lymphoma

Yi-Hua Chen and Amy Chadburn

Northwestern University, Feinberg School of Medicine, Chicago, IL, USA

I. Introduction

A. Overview of lymphoma classification

Lymphoma is a neoplasm derived from lymphocytes at various stages of maturation and presents primarily as a solid tumor in the lymphoid or non-lymphoid tissues. Various classification systems have been used over the years including Rappaport classification, Kiel classification, Lukes–Collins classification, Working Formulation, Revised European–American classification (REAL) and World Health Organization (WHO) classification. The earliest classification systems were mainly based on the architecture and cytomorphology of the neoplastic cells. More recent classifications use a combination of morphology, immunophenotype, genetic characteristics and clinical features to define specific subtypes of lymphoma. This chapter will discuss the lymphoma classification based on the latest WHO classification updated in 2008.

Lymphoid neoplasms are classified into five major categories according to the WHO classification: precursor lymphoid neoplasms, mature B-cell neoplasms, mature T- and NK-cell neoplasms, Hodgkin lymphoma and immunodeficiency-associated lymphoproliferative disorders. Each category is further classified into various subtypes based on their clinical, morphologic, biological, phenotypic and genetic features. Hodgkin lymphoma is derived from mature B cells in the vast majority of cases, but is classified as a separate entity from the other B-cell lymphomas due to its unique clinicopathologic features. Many cases of immunodeficiency-associated lymphoproliferative disorders are similar to those occurring in immunocompetent individuals except for a few entities.

This chapter will impart basic information on the common subtypes of lymphoma (Box 20.1). Lymphoid neoplasms that primarily involve peripheral

Concise Guide to Hematology, First Edition. Edited by Alvin H. Schmaier, Hillard M. Lazarus.
© 2012 Blackwell Publishing Ltd. Published 2012 by Blackwell Publishing Ltd.

> # Box 20.1 Classification of lymphoma*
>
> **Precursor lymphoid leukemia/lymphoma**
> > B-lymphoblastic leukemia/lymphoma
> > T-lymphoblastic leukemia/lymphoma
>
> **Mature B-cell lymphoma**
> > Chronic lymphocytic leukemia/small lymphocytic lymphoma
> > Follicular lymphoma
> > Mantle cell lymphoma
> > Extranodal marginal zone lymphoma of mucosa-associated lymphoid tissue (MALT)
> > Nodal marginal zone lymphoma
> > Splenic B-cell marginal zone lymphoma
> > Lymphoplasmacytic lymphoma
> > Burkitt lymphoma
> > Diffuse large B-cell lymphoma, not otherwise specified (NOS)
> > > T cell/histiocyte-rich large B-cell lymphoma
> > Primary mediastinal large B-cell lymphoma
> > Plasmablastic lymphoma
> > Primary effusion lymphoma
>
> **Mature T- and NK-cell lymphoma**
> > Peripheral T-cell lymphoma, NOS
> > Specific subtype of peripheral T-cell lymphoma
> > > Anaplastic large cell lymphoma
> > > Angioimmunoblastic T-cell lymphoma
> > > Hepatosplenic T-cell lymphoma
> > > Adult T-cell leukemia/lymphoma
> > > Extranodal NK/T-cell lymphoma, nasal type
> > > Mycosis fungoides and Sézary syndrome
>
> **Hodgkin lymphoma (HL)**
> > Nodular lymphocyte predominant HL
> > Classical HL
> > > Nodular sclerosis
> > > Mixed cellularity
> > > Lymphocyte-rich
> > > Lymphocyte-depleted
>
> *Lymphoid neoplasms that primarily involve peripheral blood and/or bone marrow and some rare entities are not listed.

blood and/or bone marrow (such as hairy cell leukemia and plasma cell myeloma), and the relatively rare immunodeficiency-associated lymphoproliferative disorders will not be discussed. For a more comprehensive review of lymphoma subtypes, refer to the suggested readings at the end of the chapter.

B. Role of ancillary studies in diagnosis and classification of lymphoma

Morphologic examination of the tissue biopsy is an important initial step in the evaluation of lymphoma. However, ancillary studies are now widely used and play an important role in diagnosis and subclassification of lymphoma as well as in predicting prognosis and directing therapy.

1. Flow cytometry (FC) immunophenotyping

(a) FC analyzes the expression of various antigens, most frequently the clusters of differentiation (CD) antigens (e.g., CD20, a B-cell antigen; CD3, a T-cell antigen), using specific antibodies. Single-cell suspensions prepared from fresh tissue biopsies, peripheral blood, bone marrow aspirate or body fluid can be used for analysis.

(b) FC not only determines the "clonality" of B cells based on monotypic immunoglobulin (Ig) light chain (κ or λ) expression, but also aids in the subclassification based on the expression of various other markers (Table 20.1).

(c) The assessment of T-cell "clonality" by FC is much more complicated and less commonly performed. However, detection of an aberrant T cell immunophenotype, most commonly abnormal expression of pan T-cell antigens (CD2, CD3, CD5 and CD7), may support a diagnosis of T-cell lymphoma.

2. Immunohistochemistry (IHC)

IHC is the localization of antigens (e.g., CD20, CD3) in tissue sections by enzyme-labeled specific antibodies. The final reaction products are visible under the microscope. Most markers analyzed by FC can also be examined by IHC in formalin-fixed tissue sections. In addition, some of the protein products derived from chromosomal translocation, e.g., cyclin D1 from t(11;14) in mantle cell lymphoma, can be readily detected by IHC.

3. Genetics

(a) Increasing numbers of chromosomal abnormalities have been identified and associated with specific subtypes of lymphoma. Some of these

Table 20.1 Common immunophenotype of mature B-cell lymphoma by flow cytometric analysis

Lymphoma	CD19	CD20	CD5	CD10	CD23	FMC7	CD79b
Chronic lymphocytic leukemia/ small lymphocytic lymphoma	+	Dim+	+	−	+	−	−
Follicular lymphoma	+	+	−	+	−	+	+
Mantle cell lymphoma	+	+	+	−	−	+	+
Marginal zone lymphoma	+	+	−	−	−	+	+
Lymphoplasmacytic lymphoma	+	+	−	−	−	+	+

Table 20.2 Common genetic aberrations associated with subtypes of lymphoma and the detection techniques in the clinical laboratories

Lymphoma	Chromosomal abnormality	Involved genes	CG/iFISH/PCR*	Dysregulated protein	IHC**
FL	t(14;18)(q32;q21)	IgH-BCL-2	Yes/Yes/Yes	BCL-2	Yes
MCL	t(11;14)(q13;q32)	CCND1-IgH	Yes/Yes/Yes	BCL-1 (Cyclin D1)	Yes
BL	t(8;14)(q24;q32)	MYC-IgH	Yes/Yes/Yes	MYC	No
MALT lymphoma	t(11;18)(q21;q21)	API2-MLT1	Yes/Yes/Yes	API2-MALT1	No
ALCL	t(2;5)(p23;q35)	ALK-NPM	Yes/Yes/Yes	ALK	Yes
HSTCL	Isochromosome 7q	Unknown	Yes/Yes/No	Unknown	No

*CG/iFISH/PCR: Cytogenetics/interphase fluorescence in-situ hybridization/polymerase chain reaction.
** IHC: Immunohistochemistry. ALCL, anaplastic large cell lymphoma; BL, Burkitt lymphoma; FL, follicular lymphoma; HSTCL, hepatosplenic T-cell lymphoma; MALT, mucosa associated lymphoid tissue; MCL, mantle cell lymphoma.

abnormalities have important diagnostic and/or prognostic value (Table 20.2).

(b) Molecular analysis, most commonly polymerase chain reaction (PCR) using DNA extracted from fresh or fixed tissues, is frequently used to detect monoclonal immunoglobulin heavy chain (IgH) gene and T-cell receptor (TCR) gene rearrangement in B- and T-cell lymphomas, respectively. Molecular studies can also be used to detect various specific genetic abnormalities (Table 20.2).

(c) Interphase FISH analysis identifies specific genetic abnormalities using fluorescent probe(s) (synthetic small fragments of DNA or RNA) with a specific sequence complimentary to the target sequence (Table 20.2).

(d) Conventional cytogenetic studies analyze metaphase chromosomes prepared from cultured cells from fresh biopsy tissue by the G-banding technique to identify numerical and/or structural abnormalities in chromosomes.

II. Classification of lymphoma

A. Precursor lymphoid neoplasms

Precursor lymphoid neoplasms are derived from lymphocyte progenitors (lymphoblasts), and include B lymphoblastic leukemia/lymphoma (B-ALL/LBL) and T lymphoblastic leukemia/lymphoma (T-ALL/LBL).

1. Clinical features

ALL/LBL is primarily a disease of children, but also occurs in adults. LBL is the solid tissue counterpart of ALL, and is defined as a mass lesion with <25%

blasts in the bone marrow. T-ALL/LBL more commonly presents as a solid tumor (lymphoma), usually as a rapid growing mediastinal mass, whereas B-ALL/LBL more frequently involves peripheral blood and bone marrow (leukemia). CNS involvement may occur in both B- and T-ALL/LBL.

2. Morphology
B-lymphoblasts and T-lymphoblasts are morphologically indistinguishable. The blasts vary from small cells with indistinct nucleoli to larger cells with variably prominent nucleoli.

3. Immunophenotype
(a) Terminal deoxynucleotidyl transferase (TdT), the most important marker for identifying lymphoblasts, is positive in nearly all B- and T-ALL/LBL.
(b) B-ALL/LBL often expresses B-cell antigens (CD19, cytoplasmic CD79a, cytoplasmic CD22, PAX-5) and is usually CD10+.
(c) T-ALL/LBL is often cytoplasmic CD3+, but variably expresses other T-cell-associated antigens (CD2, CD5, CD7, CD4 and CD8). A subset of cases is CD34+ and/or CD10+.

4. Molecular and cytogenetic features
(a) Specific subtypes of B-ALL/LBL are recognized and characterized by recurrent genetic abnormalities which have prognostic implication (Table 20.3).
(b) Approximately 50–70% of T-ALL/LBLs have an abnormal karyotype. The most common genetic abnormality involves 14q11 (TCR α and δ loci) and 7q35 (TCR β locus) with a variety of partner genes, leading to the dysregulation of transcription of the partner genes. Currently no genetic markers in T-ALL/LBL reliably predict treatment response or outcome.

Table 20.3 Recurrent genetic abnormalities in B-lymphoblastic leukemia/lymphoma

Genetic subgroups	Genes involved	Prognosis
Hyperdiploidy	–	Favorable
t(12;21)(p13;q22)	TEL-AML1	Favorable
Hypodiploidy	–	Unfavorable
t(v;11)(v;q23)	MLL	Unfavorable
t(9;22)(q34;q11)	BCL-ABL	Worst
t(1;19)(q23;p13.3)	E2A-PBX1	No value*
t(5;14)(q31;q32)	IL3-IgH	Uncertain**

*In early studies, it was associated with poor prognosis, but now it has no prognostic significance with modern intensive therapy.
**There are too few cases to be certain.

B. Mature B-cell lymphomas

Mature B-cell neoplasms are monoclonal proliferations of mature (TdT-negative) B cells at various stages of differentiation, ranging from naïve B cells to mature plasma cells. The B cell neoplasms appear to recapitulate stages of normal B-cell differentiation, and this resemblance is a major basis for their classification and nomenclature (e.g., follicular lymphoma morphologically and immunophenotypically mimics normal germinal center cells of lymphoid follicles). Mature B-cell neoplasms comprise over 90% of lymphoid malignancies; diffuse large B-cell lymphoma (Atlas Figure 47) and follicular lymphoma (Atlas Figure 46) account for more than 60% of all B-cell lymphomas.

1. Chronic lymphocytic leukemia/small lymphocytic lymphoma (CLL/SLL)

CLL is the leukemic manifestation whereas SLL is the tissue counterpart of the same disease.

(a) **Clinical features:**

  (i) Most patients are asymptomatic; the diagnosis is often made following an incidental finding of peripheral blood lymphocytosis. The majority of patients also present with peripheral lymphadenopathy.

  (ii) The clinical course is generally indolent. Transformation to large B-cell lymphoma (Richter's transformation) occurs in 2–8% of patients.

(b) **Morphology:** The neoplastic lymphocytes in the peripheral blood are predominantly small with round to slightly irregular nuclei, clumped chromatin and scant cytoplasm (Figure 20.1a). The lymph node architecture is diffusely replaced by small lymphocytes with scattered "proliferation centers" consisting of collections of prolymphocytes (larger transformed lymphoid cells with a single prominent nucleolus) (Figure 20.1b & c; Atlas Figures 34 and 35).

(c) **Immunophenotype:**

  (i) The neoplastic lymphocytes are monotypic (i.e., positive for either Igκ or Igλ), expressing pan B-cell antigens (e.g., CD19, CD20, CD22), and are CD5+, CD23+ and CD10– (Table 20.1).

  (ii) CD38 and/or ZAP-70 are expressed in a subset of cases, and may be associated with an adverse prognosis.

(d) **Molecular and cytogenetic features:**

  (i) CLL with somatic hypermutation of the variable region of the immunoglobulin heavy chain (*IgVH*) genes (an indication that the cells giving rise to CLL have undergone germinal center maturation) is found in 50–60% of CLL/SLL, and is associated with a good prognosis. CLL with unmutated *IgVH* genes (indicative of pre-germinal center origin) is associated with a poor prognosis.

  (ii) FISH analysis is commonly used to detect genetic abnormalities in CLL/SLL. Deletion of 11q22-23 (*ATM* gene) and deletion of 17p13 (*P53*, a tumor suppressor gene) are associated with a poor prognosis, whereas isolated deletion of 13q14 is associated with a favorable prognosis.

(a)

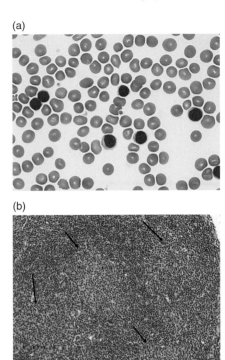

(b)

Figure 20.1 Chronic lymphocytic leukemia/
small lymphocytic lymphoma (CLL/SLL).
(a) CLL/SLL in the peripheral blood smear
showing lymphocytosis composed
predominantly of small lymphocytes with
clumped chromatin (1000×). (b) Low-power
view of CLL/SLL in lymph node showing
"proliferation centers" (arrows to lighter area)
that are composed of prolymphocytes, the
characteristic feature of CLL/SLL in lymph
node sections (200×). (c) At higher
magnification, the neoplastic lymphocytes are
small with clumped chromatin and scant
cytoplasm. (1000×).

(c)

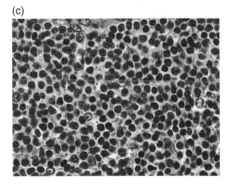

2. Follicular lymphoma (FL)

FL is the second most common non-Hodgkin lymphoma (NHL) in the United
States and Western Europe. It affects predominantly elderly individuals with
a slight female predominance.

(a) **Clinical features:** Most patients present with widespread disease involving lymph nodes and bone marrow. Extranodal sites may also be involved.

(b) **Morphology:**
  (i) FL shows nodular (follicular) and/or diffuse growth patterns
       (Figure 20.2a). The neoplastic follicles are composed of centrocytes
       and centroblasts in various proportions (Figure 20.2b).

(a) (b) (c) (d)

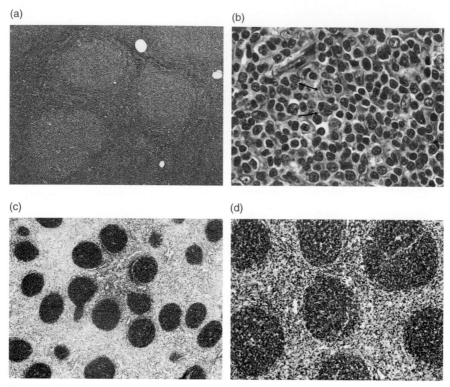

Figure 20.2 Follicular lymphoma (FL). (a) Lymph node biopsy showing an abnormal nodular (follicular) proliferation of lymphocytes (100×). (b) The neoplastic follicles contain variable numbers of centrocytes and centroblasts (arrows) (1000×). (c) The neoplastic cells are CD10+ by immunostaining (brown; 100×). (d) In contrast to normal lymphoid follicles, the neoplastic follicles in FL are positive for BCL-2 by immunostaining (brown; 200×).

> (ii) FL is graded by the average number of centroblasts per 40× high power field (HPF) in 10 neoplastic follicles: grade 1 = 0–5 centroblasts/ HPF; grade 2 = 6–15 centroblasts/HPF; grade 3 = >15 centroblasts/ HPF. Distinction between grade 1 and 2 is not encouraged since both are clinically indolent according to the current WHO classification.

(c) Immunophenotype: The neoplastic cells are monotypic, expressing pan B-cell antigens and are often CD5−, CD10+, BCL-6+ and BCL-2+ (normal germinal center cells are negative for BCL-2) (Table 20.1) (Figure 20.2c & d).

(d) Molecular and cytogenetic features: The majority of cases have t(14;18) (q32;q21) involving *BCL-2* and *IgH* genes, resulting in the overexpression of BCL-2, an anti-apoptotic protein.

3. Mantle cell lymphoma (MCL)

MCL comprises 3–10% of NHL and occurs in middle-aged to older individuals with a male predominance. It is genetically characterized by t(11;14)

(a)   (b)

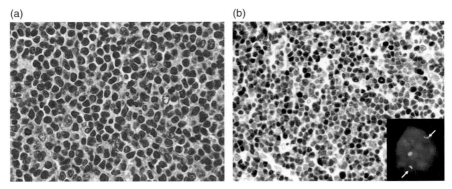

Figure 20.3 Mantle cell lymphoma (MCL). (a) Lymph node biopsy showing a proliferation of small to medium-sized lymphocytes with slightly irregular nuclei (1000×). (b) The neoplastic cells show nuclear positivity for cyclin D1 by immunostaining (brown; 1000×). FISH showed the presence of t(11;14) translocation (inset). Red signal: *CCND1* gene at chromosome 11; green signal: *IgH* gene at chromosome 14; yellow signals (arrows): fusion of *CCND1* and *IgH*.

(q13;q32) involving the *CCND1* gene encoding for a cell cycle protein, cyclin D1 (BCL-1).

(a) **Clinical features:** Most patients present with advanced stage disease. Transformation to large B-cell lymphoma is exceedingly rare, but aggressive variants (blastoid or pleomorphic MCL) may occur.

(b) **Morphology:** MCL may show nodular, diffuse or mantle zone growth patterns. The neoplastic cells are usually composed of monomorphic (uniform) small to medium-sized lymphocytes with irregular nuclear contours and inconspicuous nucleoli (Figure 20.3a). The blastoid variant may resemble lymphoblastic lymphoma while the pleomorphic variant may be indistinguishable from large cell lymphoma.

(c) **Immunophenotype:** The neoplastic cells are monotypic, expressing pan B-cell antigens and are CD5+, CD23−, CD10− and cyclin D1+ (Table 20.1) (Figure 20.3b).

(d) **Molecular and cytogenetic features:** Most cases have t(11;14)(q13;q32) involving *CCND1* and *IgH* genes, leading to the overexpression of cyclin D1, a positive cell cycle regulator (Figure 20.3b).

4. Marginal zone lymphoma (MZL)

MZL arises from post-germinal center B cells and consists of three distinct diseases: extranodal marginal zone B-cell lymphoma of mucosa associated lymphoid tissue (MALT lymphoma), splenic B-cell MZL and nodal MZL.

(a) **Clinical features:**

(i) MALT lymphoma comprises 7–8% of B-cell lymphomas. The gastrointestinal tract is most commonly involved. Gastric MALT lymphoma is associated with *Helicobacter pylori* infection.

(ii) Nodal MZL and splenic B-cell MZL are rare. Both primarily affect adults with an equal gender incidence. Nodal MZL often presents as asymptomatic lymphadenopathy. Splenic B-cell MZL presents with splenomegaly; peripheral lymphadenopathy is extremely uncommon.

(b) **Morphology:** MZL is usually composed of small lymphocytes; some may show plasmacytic differentiation. Transformation of MZL to large B-cell lymphoma may occur.

(c) **Immunophenotype:** The neoplastic cells are monotypic, expressing pan B-cell antigens and are CD5–, CD10– and CD23– (Table 20.1).

(d) **Molecular and cytogenetic features:** Chromosomal translocations associated with MALT lymphomas include t(11;18)(q21;q21) (*API2/MALT1*), t(14;18)(q32;q21) (*IgH/MALT1*), t(1;14)(p22;q32) (*BCL-10/IgH*) and t(3;14) (p14;q32) (*FOXP1/IgH*). Gastric MALT lymphoma with t(11;18) is resistant to *H. pylori* eradication therapy.

5. Lymphoplasmacytic lymphoma (LPL)

LPL represents 2–3% of NHL, and primarily occurs in adults with a slight male predominance.

(a) **Clinical features:** Most cases involve the bone marrow, but lymph nodes and extranodal sites may also be involved. The majority of patients have a serum IgM paraprotein, and serum hyperviscosity is seen in 30% of patients. Bone marrow involvement with a serum IgM monoclonal protein of any concentration constitutes Waldenström macroglobulinemia according to the current WHO classification.

(b) **Morphology:** The involved lymph nodes or bone marrow show infiltration by small lymphocytes, plasmacytoid lymphocytes and plasma cells in variable proportions.

(c) **Immunophenotype:** The neoplastic cells are monotypic, expressing pan B-cell antigens and are CD5–, CD10– and CD23– (Table 20.1).

(d) **Molecular and cytogenetic feature:** No specific molecular or cytogenetic abnormalities are recognized in LPL.

6. Burkitt lymphoma (BL)

BL is a highly aggressive B-cell lymphoma characterized by a chromosomal translocation involving the *MYC* gene at chromosome 8q24 and one of the three immunoglobulin genes, most commonly IgH gene (14q32) and less commonly Igκ (2p12) or Igλ (22q11) genes. These translocations lead to the overexpression of c-MYC protein, a pleiotropic transcriptional regulator involving in cell proliferation, differentiation and apoptosis. BL accounts for 30% of non-endemic pediatric lymphomas and less than 1% of adult B-cell lymphomas.

(a) **Clinical features:**
  (i) Patients present with rapidly growing tumor masses, often with evidence of tumor lysis. CNS involvement is seen in 15% of patients at diagnosis and frequently at relapse.

(a)   (b)

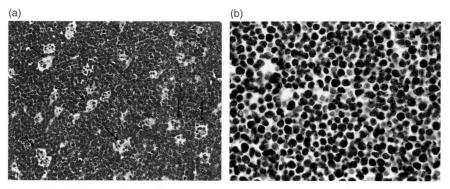

Figure 20.4 Burkitt lymphoma (BL). (a) Lymph node biopsy showing a "starry sky" pattern, which is the presence of scattered macrophages (arrows) with ingested apoptotic tumor cells in a diffuse proliferation of neoplastic lymphocytes (400×). (b) Immunostaining for Ki-67 (a proliferation marker) showing virtually 100% of the neoplastic lymphocytes are positive (brown; 1000×).

    (ii) Three distinct variants are recognized: endemic, sporadic and immunodeficiency-associated. The endemic form occurs most frequently in children in equatorial Africa and commonly presents as jaw and other facial bone lesions. The sporadic form occurs worldwide and often presents as an abdominal mass. The immunodeficiency-associated form primarily affects HIV+ individuals, and nodal involvement is common.

(b) Morphology: BL consists of a diffuse proliferation of uniform, medium-sized lymphocytes with frequent mitoses and apoptotic bodies. Frequent macrophages containing ingested cellular debris (tingible body macrophages) are present, reflecting the high cell turn-over and creating a "starry sky" pattern in tissue sections (Figure 20.4a).

(c) Immunophenotype: The neoplastic cells are monotypic, expressing pan B-cell antigens and are CD10+, BCL6+ and BCL-2−. Virtually 100% of the neoplastic cells are positive for Ki-67, a cell proliferation marker (Figure 20.4b). Epstein–Barr virus (EBV) is present in almost all endemic forms, but is less frequently seen in sporadic or immunodeficiency-associated forms.

(d) Molecular and cytogenetic features: Virtually all BL have a translocation involving the *MYC* gene at 8q24. t(8;14)(q24;q32) (*MYC/IgH*) is the most common translocation; t(2;8)(p12;q24)(*Igκ/MYC*) and t(8;22)(q24;q11) (*MYC/Igλ*) are less common.

7. Diffuse large B-cell lymphoma (DLBCL)

DLBCL is the most common subtype of B-cell lymphoma. It is more common in the elderly and slightly more common in males. DLBCL may arise de novo or represent progression or transformation from a less aggressive lymphoma.

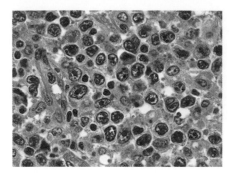

Figure 20.5 Diffuse large B-cell lymphoma showing diffuse proliferation of large lymphoid cells; some have prominent nucleoli (1000×).

A number of clinicopathologic distinct subtypes of DLBCL have been recognized (Box 20.1).

(a) **DLBCL, not otherwise specified (NOS):**
   (i) DLBCL, NOS, typically presents as a rapidly enlarging nodal or extranodal tumor mass.
   (ii) There is a diffuse proliferation of large lymphoid cells with centroblastic (centroblastic variant), immunoblastic (immunoblastic variant), or highly pleomorphic (anaplastic variant) cytomorphology (Figure 20.5).
   (iii) Based on the expression of CD10, BCL-6 and MUM-1, DLBCL, NOS, is subdivided into germinal center B-cell-like (GCB; better prognosis) and non-germinal center B-cell-like/activated B-cell-like (non-GCB/ABC; poorer prognosis).
   (iv) *BCL-6* and *BCL-2* gene rearrangements are relatively common. Rearrangements involving *MYC* gene occur less commonly and are associated with a poor prognosis.

(b) **T cell/histiocyte-rich large B-cell lymphoma (THRLBCL):**
   (i) Patients often present with hepatosplenomegaly and B symptoms, and are refractory to chemotherapy.
   (ii) Morphologically, there is a limited number of large neoplastic B lymphocytes associated with many reactive T lymphocytes and histiocytes.

(c) **Primary mediastinal (thymic) large B-cell lymphoma (PMBL):**
   (i) PMBL occurs predominantly in young adults with female predominance, and frequently presents with superior vena cava syndrome due to a large mediastinal mass.
   (ii) PMBL shows frequent gains of 9p24 and 2p15, but *BCL-6*, *BCL-2* and *MYC* gene rearrangements are rare.

(d) **Plasmablastic lymphoma (PBL) and primary effusion lymphoma (PEL):**
   (i) Both lymphomas preferentially affect HIV+ individuals. PBL often occurs in the oral cavity while PEL usually presents as a pleural, peritoneal or pericardial effusion.

(ii) Both lymphomas are usually positive for plasma cell markers (CD138, CD38 and MUM-1), but negative for B-cell markers. PBL is often EBV+ and PEL is HHV-8+.

C. Mature T-cell lymphomas

Mature T-cell lymphomas are derived from mature (post-thymic, TdT-negative) T cells, and are clinically and morphologically diverse and generally exhibit aggressive clinical behavior. They are relatively uncommon and occur more frequently in Asia. Mature T-cell lymphomas are difficult to subclassify, thus, the majority of cases are categorized as peripheral T-cell lymphoma, NOS. However, some T-cell lymphomas with distinct clinicopathologic features are recognized and classified as specific subtypes (Box 20.1).

1. Peripheral T-cell lymphoma (PTCL), NOS

(a) PTCL, NOS usually arises in lymph nodes, and consists of T-cell lymphomas that do not fit into any specific subtype of mature T-cell lymphoma. PTCL, NOS, comprises approximately 25–30% of all peripheral T-cell lymphomas in Western countries.

(b) **Clinical features:** Most patients present with generalized lymphadenopathy and B symptoms (fever, night sweats and unintentional weight loss). These tumors are aggressive and respond poorly to therapy.

(c) **Morphology:** The number of malignant cells in a lesion is variable and often associated with a background of non-neoplastic inflammatory cells. The neoplastic cells may range from small cells indistinguishable from the normal lymphocytes to large and highly pleomorphic cells (Figure 20.6).

(d) **Immunophenotype:** PTCL may show aberrant T-cell antigen expression, most commonly diminished or absent expression of one or more of the pan T-cell antigens (CD2, CD3, CD5, CD7).

(e) **Molecular and cytogenetic features:** These lymphomas often show clonal rearrangement of TCR genes and a complex karyotype.

2. Specific subtypes of mature T-cell lymphoma
(a) **Anaplastic large cell lymphoma (ALCL):**

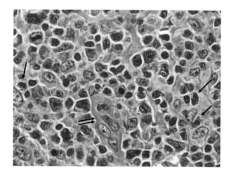

Figure 20.6 Peripheral T-cell lymphoma, NOS. Lymph node biopsy showing diffuse proliferation of lymphocytes varying from small to large, accompanied by vascular proliferation (double arrows) and a reactive cellular infiltrate including eosinophils (single arrows) (600×).

(i) Most ALCLs express anaplastic lymphoma kinase (ALK) as a result of t(2;5)(p23;q35) translocation involving the *ALK* gene. ALCL-ALK+ accounts for 10–20% of childhood lymphomas and 3% of adult NHL. Most patients present with advanced stage disease with involvement of lymph nodes and extranodal sites. ALCL-ALK+ has a better prognosis than its ALK– counterpart.

(ii) Morphologically, most cases consist of a diffuse proliferation of large cells with large nuclei, prominent nucleoli and abundant cytoplasm. "Hallmark" cells, the large cells with horseshoe- or kidney-shaped nuclei, are present in all cases (Figure 20.7a).

(a)

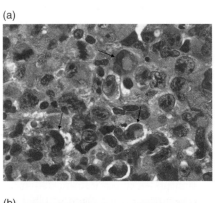

(b)

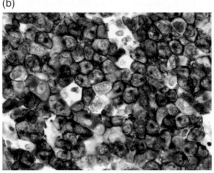

(c)

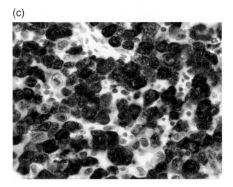

Figure 20.7 Anaplastic large cell lymphoma (ALCL). (a) Lymph node biopsy showing proliferation of large cells and the presence of the "hallmark" cells with horseshoe-like nuclei (arrows) (1000×). (b & c) The neoplastic cells are positive for CD30 (b) and ALK-1 (c) by immunostaining (brown; 1000×).

    (iii) All ALCL are CD30+ and the majority of cases are ALK+ (Figures 20.7b & c). T cell-associated antigens are variably expressed.

    (iv) The most frequent genetic alteration is t(2;5)(p23;q35) (*ALK/NPM*). Variant translocations involving *ALK* gene and other partner genes also occur.

(b) Angioimmunoblastic T-cell lymphoma (AITL)

    (i) AITL is a more common subtype of PTCL and accounts for approximately 15–20% of all PTCL. AITL is derived from a unique T-cell subset in the germinal center, the CD4+ follicular helper T cells.

    (ii) Patients often present with generalized lymphadenopathy, hepatosplenomegaly, pruritic rash and systemic symptoms. Clinical features associated with dysregulated immune responses are frequently present such as polyclonal hypergammaglobulinemia, circulating immune complexes, cold agglutinins with hemolytic anemia, positive rheumatoid factor and anti-smooth muscle antibodies. The clinical course of the disease is generally aggressive.

    (iii) Morphologically, the involved lymph nodes often show a diffuse polymorphic infiltrate composed of small to medium-sized neoplastic lymphocytes admixed with reactive lymphocytes, eosinophils and plasma cells. Vascular proliferation is prominent.

    (iv) AITL, similar to normal follicular helper T cells, expresses CD4, CD10 and BCL-6. Many cases contain EBV+ B cells.

    (v) Clonal TCR gene rearrangements are present in most cases. The most common cytogenetic abnormalities are trisomy 3, trisomy 5 and an additional X chromosome.

(c) Hepatosplenic T-cell lymphoma (HSTCL):

    (i) HSTCL is rare and predominantly affect young males. Patients often present with marked splenomegaly with no lymphadenopathy. The clinical course is aggressive.

    (ii) HSTCL is derived from CD4–, CD8– and TCRγδ+ T cells in contrast to the majority of other T cell lymphomas that are predominantly from TCR αβ T cells. Isochromosome 7q is present in most cases, and can be readily detected by FISH or conventional cytogenetics.

(d) Adult T-cell leukemia/lymphoma (ATLL):

    (i) ATLL is associated with T-cell leukemia virus type 1 (HTLV-1) infection, and most commonly seen in Japan and the Caribbean. The disease affects adults and often present with widespread lymph node, peripheral blood and bone marrow involvement.

    (ii) The neoplastic cells in the peripheral blood are described as "flower cells" because of the multiple nuclear convolutions.

(e) Extranodal NK/T-cell lymphoma, nasal type

    (i) This lymphoma is more prevalent in Asia and is strongly associated with EBV infection. The nasal cavity is most commonly involved.

    (ii) The neoplastic cells are mostly NK cells; some cases are derived from cytotoxic T cells. The tumor often shows necrosis and high mitotic activity. No specific genetic abnormalities have been identified.

(f) Mycosis fungoides (MF) and Sézary syndrome
   (i)   MF is a peripheral T-cell lymphoma involving skin. It is associated with an indolent clinical course. The disease may progress to Sézary syndrome where the patient has erythroderma, generalized lymphadenopathy, and peripheral blood involvement by neoplastic cells with convoluted nuclei (Sézary cells).
   (ii) A skin biopsy of MF shows abnormal lymphocytes with highly indented (cerebriform) nuclei in the upper dermis and epidermis. Small epidermal collections of neoplastic cells called "Pautrier microabscesses" are often seen. Complex karyotypes are present in many cases.

D. Hodgkin lymphoma (HL)
HL accounts for approximately 30% of all lymphomas. It is classified into two major categories: nodular lymphocyte predominant HL (NLPHL) (5%) and classical HL (CHL) (95%). CHLs are further subclassified into four subtypes: nodular sclerosis, mixed cellularity, lymphocyte-rich and lymphocyte-depleted. NLPHL is a B-cell neoplasm, as are the vast majority of CHL.

1. Clinical features
(a) **NLPHL** predominantly affects young males and usually presents as localized peripheral lymphadenopathy. NLPHL has very good prognosis, but multiple relapses and transformation to DLBCL may occur.
(b) **CHL** has a bimodal age distribution with a peak at 15–35 years of age and a second peak in late life (>50 years of age). CHL often involves cervical lymph nodes and the mediastinum. B symptoms are present in up to 40% of patients.

2. Morphology
(a) **NLPHL** is characterized by a nodular or nodular/diffuse proliferation of lymphocytes with scattered large neoplastic cells known as "popcorn cells" or lymphocyte predominant cells (LP cells).
(b) **The four subtypes of CHL** differ in composition of cellular background and growth pattern. In general, all types of CHL show a proliferation of large neoplastic cells composed of mononucleated Hodgkin cells or multinucleated Reed-Sternberg cells in a reactive inflammatory background containing variable numbers of eosinophils (Figure 20.8a & b; Atlas Figure 48).

3. Immunophenotype
(a) **The large neoplastic cells in NLPHL** are typically CD45+, CD20+, CD30– and CD15–.
(b) **The large neoplastic cells in all types of CHL** are typically CD45–, CD20–, CD30+ and CD15+ (Figure 20.8c & d). EBV is present in a subset of CHL.

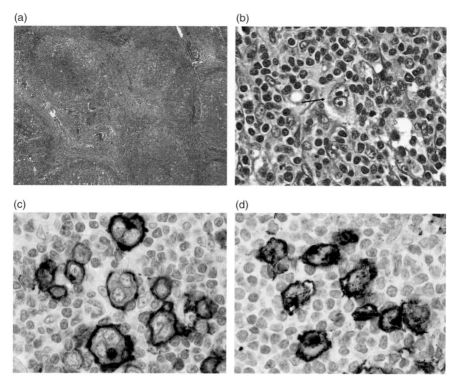

Figure 20.8 Nodular sclerosis classical Hodgkin lymphoma (NSHL). (a) Lymph node biopsy showing fibrous collagen bands dividing the lymph node into nodules (40×). (b) A typical binucleated Reed–Sternberg cell (arrow) in a background of reactive inflammatory cells including eosinophils (1000×) (c & d). The large neoplastic cells are positive for CD30 (c) and CD15 (d) by immunostaining (brown; 1000×).

4. Molecular and cytogenetic features

No specific molecular or cytogenetic abnormalities have been identified in HL.

Further reading

Armitage JO, Weisenburger DD. New approach to classifying non-Hodgkin's lymphomas: clinical features of the major histologic subtypes. Non-Hodgkin's Lymphoma Classification Project. J Clin Oncol 1998;16(8):2780–95.

Aster JC. Diseases of white blood cells, lymph nodes, spleen, and thymus. In: Kumar V, Abbas AK, Fausto N, eds. Robbins and Cotran Pathologic Basis of Disease, 7th edn. Philadelphia: Elsevier Saunders, 2004:661–709.

Rizvi MA, Evens AM, Tallman MS, Nelson BP, Rosen ST. T-cell non-Hodgkin lymphoma. Blood 2006;107(4):1255–64.

Swerdlow SH, Campo E, Harrie NL, Jaffe ES, Pileri SA, Stein H, Thiele J, Vardiman JW. WHO Classification of Tumours of Haematopoietic and Lymphoid Tissues. Lyon, France: IARC, 2008.

21 Clinical Evaluation and Management of Lymphoma

Makiko Ban-Hoefen, Jonathan W. Friedberg and Richard I. Fisher

James P. Wilmot Cancer Center, University of Rochester Medical Center, Rochester, NY, USA

I. Introduction

Hodgkin and non-Hodgkin lymphoma are two distinct malignant disorders arising from cells that populate the lymph nodes. Establishing the histopathologic diagnosis of either Hodgkin or non-Hodgkin lymphoma is crucial because the prognosis and treatment regimen for each disease is different.

II. Distinctions between Hodgkin and non-Hodgkin lymphoma

A. Epidemiologic factors

1. Hodgkin lymphoma is about one-third as common as non-Hodgkin lymphoma. In the United States, there were about 66,000 new cases of non-Hodgkin lymphoma in 2008, and non-Hodgkin lymphoma is associated with an estimated 19,500 deaths per year with a prevalence of approximately 250,000.
2. The incidence of non-Hodgkin lymphoma is rising rapidly due to known factors such as HIV and unknown factors, while the incidence of Hodgkin lymphoma is not rising. Non-Hodgkin lymphoma now ranks fifth among cancers in incidence and cause of death from cancer.
3. Hodgkin lymphoma has a bimodal age distribution; it peaks at 20–29 years of age and again at 60 years of age and older. The incidence of non-Hodgkin lymphoma increases with age, especially above age 50 years.
4. Both Hodgkin and non-Hodgkin lymphoma have a moderate male predominance.

B. Clinical presentation

1. Causes of lymphadenopathy include:

Concise Guide to Hematology, First Edition. Edited by Alvin H. Schmaier, Hillard M. Lazarus.
© 2012 Blackwell Publishing Ltd. Published 2012 by Blackwell Publishing Ltd.

Table 21.1 Distinctions between palpable lymph nodes		
Normal	*Reactive*	*Malignant*
Small (0.5–1.0 cm)	Moderately large (<2 cm)	Large (>1 cm, especially >2 cm)
Soft, flat, ellipsoid, fixed	Firm, spherical, movable	Firm, spherical, especially matted
Nontender	Tender or nontender	Usually nontender
Usually multiple	Single to multiple (depends on disease)	Single or multiple (depends on type of cancer)
Usually high neck, submandibular, submental areas; occasionally inguinal	Usually cervical	Any anatomic nodal area
Usually stable	Should resolve 1–2 months after acute process stops	Progressive growth

(a) Infections, such as common cold, local acute or chronic infection, infectious mononucleosis (Atlas Figure 32), tuberculosis, syphilis, toxoplasmosis, cytomegalovirus, HIV, cat-scratch fever.
(b) Drugs (e.g., phenytoin).
(c) Connective tissue disorders (e.g., systemic lupus erythematosus, dermatomyositis, scleroderma).
(d) Metastatic cancer.
(e) Primary lymphoid malignancies (e.g., Hodgkin lymphoma, NHL).

2. Malignant vs. non-malignant causes of lymphadenopathy. Enlarged lymph nodes as a result of infection tend to be tender, smaller and transiently enlarged as opposed to those arising from malignancy (Table 21.1).

3. Differences in clinical presentation arise, in part, from distinct differences in the pattern of spread of disease. Hodgkin lymphoma generally spreads in a contiguous fashion from one anatomic lymph node group to another. Non-Hodgkin lymphoma is less predictable in its spreading pattern. It can have characteristics of both hematogenous dissemination as well as lymphatic contiguity.

4. Hodgkin lymphoma rarely involves the mesenteric nodes, central nervous system, skin, gastrointestinal tract, or Waldeyer's ring (adenoids, palatine and lingual tonsil). These sites are much more likely to be affected by non-Hodgkin lymphoma.

5. While mild to moderate enlargement of the spleen can be observed in any form of lymphoma, gross splenomegaly is rare in Hodgkin lymphoma; it is more common in non-Hodgkin lymphoma.

6. B symptoms, or systemic constitutional symptoms such as fever (in the absence of infection), drenching night sweats, and weight loss (unexplained and greater than 10% body weight within 6 months), can accompany both disorders. However, generalized pruritus and pain soon after drinking alcohol are much more likely to be associated with Hodgkin lymphoma.

Table 21.2 The Ann Arbor Staging Classification	
*Stage**	*Description*
I	Involvement of a single lymph node region (I) or a single extralymphatic organ or site (IE)
II	Involvement of two or more lymph node regions on same side of diaphragm (II) or local involvement of an extralymphatic organ or site and one or more lymph node regions on same side of diaphragm (IIE)
III	Involvement of lymph node regions on both sides of diaphragm (III), which may also be accompanied by involvement of the spleen (III$_S$) or by local involvement of an extralymphatic organ or site (IIIE) or both (III$_S$E)
IV	Diffuse or disseminated involvement of one or more extralymphatic organs or tissues, with or without lymph node involvement

*Letters following the roman numerals are used to subclassify the stage. Fevers, night sweats, or unexplained loss of 10% or more of body weight in the 6 months preceding diagnosis is denoted by B. A indicates absence of these symptoms. E indicates involvement of an extralymphatic site; S indicates splenic involvement.
(Reproduced with permission from Hoffman R, et al. Hematology: Basic Principles and Practice. New York: Churchill-Livingstone, 1991.)

C. Staging

1. The TNM Classification of Malignant Tumours (TNM), developed and maintained by the International Union Against Cancer (UICC), is a cancer staging system that describes the extent of cancer in a patient's body. T describes the size of the tumor and whether it has invaded nearby tissue, N describes regional lymph nodes that are involved, and M describes distant metastasis (spread of cancer from one body part to another). This system is generally reserved for use in solid tumors and is not applicable to lymphoma, since it is based upon the concept of a primary tumor and metastasis.

2. The prognosis and treatment of Hodgkin and non-Hodgkin lymphoma are greatly influenced by the stage (degree of known spread) of the disease at time of diagnosis.

3. The *Ann Arbor staging system* (Table 21.2) is used for both Hodgkin and non-Hodgkin lymphoma.

4. Cases are subclassified to indicate the absence (A) or presence (B) of constitutional symptoms.

5. The tools used to stage Hodgkin and non-Hodgkin lymphoma are similar. These tools are used to determine the overall stage and identify prognostic factors that may influence the outcome within stages of the disease.

   (a) **History:**
      (i) Unexplained fever.
      (ii) Weight loss.
      (iii) Night sweats.
      (iv) Pruritus.
      (v) Alcohol intolerance.

      (vi)   Fatigue.

      (vii) Pain.

      (viii) Overall performance status:
- is an attempt to quantify cancer patients' general well-being that impacts upon tolerance to therapy and prognosis.
- assessed using a simple scale such as the Eastern Cooperative Oncology Group (ECOG) scale of:

          0 = asymptomatic, fully active.

          1 = symptomatic but completely ambulatory.

          2 = symptomatic but in bed <50% of the time.

          3 = symptomatic and in bed >50% of the time.

          4 = bed-bound, completely disabled.

          5 = death.

      (ix)   Overall tempo of the disease, e.g., indolent growth or more rapid enlargement of nodes and other organs.

(b) Physical examination:
- (i)   Areas of palpable lymphadenopathy.
- (ii)   Size of liver and spleen.
- (iii)   Bony tenderness.
- (iv)   Neurologic abnormalities.

(c) Laboratory studies:
- (i)   Complete blood count, differential and platelet count, erythrocyte sedimentation rate (especially for Hodgkin lymphoma).
- (ii)   Peripheral blood smear.
- (iii)   Serum electrophoresis.
- (iv)   Serum alkaline phosphatase, lactic dehydrogenase, albumin, uric acid, calcium.
- (v)   Renal function (creatinine, blood urea nitrogen [BUN]).
- (vi)   Liver function tests.

(d) Radiologic studies:
- (i)   Chest radiograph.
- (ii)   Computed tomography scan of the chest, abdomen, and pelvis.
- (iii)   Bone scan or bone radiograph if symptoms of bone involvement are present.
- (iv)   Positron emission tomography (PET) scan.

(e) Biopsies
- (i)   Diagnostic biopsy of affected lymph node.
- (ii)   Bone marrow biopsy, especially when treatment may be modified.
- (iii)   Biopsy of suspicious disseminated extranodal sites (e.g., pulmonary or liver lesions) if clinically indicated.

D. Pathology

1. **Classical Hodgkin lymphoma:** Presence of Reed–Sternberg cells with the following variants:

(a) Nodular sclerosing.

(b) Mixed cellularity.

(c) Lymphocyte rich.

(d) Lymphocyte depleted.

2. **Nodular lymphocyte-predominant Hodgkin lymphoma:**

(a) Very uncommon.

(b) Represents a more indolent disease than classical Hodgkin lymphomas, and is therefore managed uniquely (see Section IV-E).

3. **Non-Hodgkin lymphoma:**

(a) B-cell (i.e., diffuse large B-cell, follicular, marginal zone, Burkitt's, B-cell chronic lymphocytic leukemia):

(i) Gene expression profiling studies, or studies measuring the activity of genes, have revealed at least two distinct subtypes of diffuse large B cell lymphoma (germinal center B-cell subtype and activated B-cell subtype). Gene expression profiling studies are important for understanding the malignant microenvironment and how it affects the outcome following therapy.

(b) T-cell (i.e., mycosis fungoides, T-cell chronic lymphocytic leukemia).

III. Treatment of Hodgkin lymphoma

A. Early stages (I–II)

1. **Radiation or chemotherapy alone.** Historically, the mainstay of treatment for early-stage Hodgkin lymphoma was radiation therapy. Because of the contiguity of spread of Hodgkin lymphoma to adjacent lymph node groups, radiation was given to the clinically involved areas and the next contiguous clinically uninvolved nodal groups. This approach resulted in the development of standard radiation fields (i.e., mantle, para-aortic, pelvic) to fit the individual situation (Table 21.3). Studies now have shown that either chemotherapy or radiation therapy alone is associated with a higher risk of recurrence than combined chemotherapy and radiation therapy. Long-term toxic effects may befall an organ that is within the radiation field, including premature coronary artery disease with irradiation to the heart, or secondary malignancies such as breast cancer if chest radiation therapy includes the breast.

2. **Chemotherapy followed by radiation.** The use of chemotherapy before radiation is designed to eradicate disease in the next contiguous clinically uninvolved nodal groups. Beginning therapy first with chemotherapy treatment potentially allows the fields of radiation to be smaller and limited to clinically involved areas, thereby lessening the exposure of the patient to radiation. A standard approach is administration of two to four cycles of chemotherapy (ABVD or Adriamycin, bleomycin, vinblastine, and dacarbazine) followed by involved-field radiation.

3. **Overall results.** The combined chemotherapy and radiation has the lowest rate of relapse (10% to 15%) compared to either modality alone. Regardless of the approach used, a 5-year freedom from relapse rate of at

Table 21.3 Radiation field designs used in lymphoma

Radiation field	Involved lymph nodes
Mantle	Submental, cervical, supra- and infraclavicular, axillary, hilar and mediastinal lymph nodes.
Mantle and para-aortic ± splenic	Para-aortic lymph nodes in addition to the mantle field. The spleen is included in the treatment field in patients who do not undergo surgical staging and splenectomy. Also known as subtotal nodal or lymphoid irradiation.
Total nodal irradiation	Most of the lymphoid tissue, with the addition of a pelvic field to the mantle and para-aortic field. Does not include other nodal groups such as the brachial, epitrochlear, popliteal, sacral, and mesenteric nodes.
Inverted-Y	Para-aortic and pelvic lymph nodes.
Involved-field	Includes at least the entire contiguous lymph node group, but may also contain the next echelon of nodes (i.e., in a patient presenting with an enlarged cervical lymph node, radiation would include the entire ipsilateral cervical chain and the supraclavicular region, as these nodes are considered one region).

Table 21.4 International Prognostic Score for Hodgkin Lymphoma

One point is given for each of the characteristics below present in the patient

Serum albumin <4 g/dL
Hemoglobin <10.5 g/dL
Male gender
Age >45 years
Stage IV disease
White blood cell count ≥15,000/microL
Absolute lymphocyte count <600/microL and/or <8% of the total white blood cell count

Score	5-year freedom from progression	5-year overall survival
0	84%	89%
1	77%	90%
2	67%	81%
3	60%	78%
4	51%	61%
5 or more	42%	56%

Abstracted from Hasenclever DH, Diehl V, et al. A prognostic score for advanced Hodgkin's disease. N Engl J Med 1998; 339:1506–14. Copyright © 1998 Massachusetts Medical Society. All rights reserved.

least 80% is expected for patients with early-stage disease with no unfavorable factors (Table 21.4). However, the longer patients are followed, the more treatment-related mortality increases; thus, death from Hodgkin lymphoma is becoming less of a concern than the late consequences of treatment (see Section III-D).

Table 21.5 Initial chemotherapy for advanced (stage III–IV) Hodgkin lymphoma		
ABVD	Doxorubicin, bleomycin, vinblastine, and dacarbazine	Preferred modality. 80% with complete response.
BEACOPP	Bleomycin, etoposide, doxorubicin, cyclophosphamide, vincristine, procarazine, and prednisone	Given in standard or escalated doses Compared with ABVD, escalated BEACOPP has superior progression-free survival rates, but has increased toxicity and no difference in overall survival rates.
Stanford V	Doxorubicin, vinblastine, mechlorethamine, vincristine, bleomycin, etoposide, and prednisone	Uses a brief intensive chemotherapy regimen combined with radiation to bulky lymph node sites. The cumulative doses of doxorubicin, mechlorethamine, and bleomycin are reduced compared with ABVD and MOPP.
MOPP	Mechlorethamine, vincristine, procarbazine, and prednisone	Less efficacy and greater toxicity compared to ABVD.

B. Later stages (III–IV)

1. **Chemotherapy alone.** Chemotherapy with ABVD is the primary form of treatment in advanced cases of Hodgkin lymphoma. Other regimens include complex schedules of combination chemotherapy such as BEACOPP and Stanford V (see Table 21.5 for other regimens as well). The role of radiation therapy after completion of chemotherapy, referred to as consolidation, is controversial in certain situations.

2. **Overall results.** As with early-stage disease, a number of adverse prognostic factors affect the outcome of late-stage disease. The prognosis according to the number of unfavorable factors is shown in Table 21.4.

C. Salvaging treatment failures

1. Chemotherapy, usually ABVD, is used at the time relapse for patients treated with radiation therapy alone. These patients do as well or better with salvage combination chemotherapy as patients with advanced disease who have never received radiation, with a 10-year survival of nearly 90%. Whether or not adjunctive radiotherapy is associated with improved response in patients previously treated with radiation alone is not yet known.

2. For patients who relapse after receiving chemotherapy as part of the initial treatment, salvage with standard-dose chemotherapy is far less successful. These patients are generally treated with either conventional chemotherapy combined with radiation therapy or high dose chemotherapy and autologous hematopoietic cell transplantation given with or without radiation therapy (Section V).

D. Complications of treatment

1. Despite the high rate of success in the treatment of Hodgkin lymphoma, long-term follow-up indicates a continuous pattern of mortality related

to the agents used in therapy. Death from complications of treatment now approximates, if not exceeds, death from Hodgkin lymphoma in certain stages.

2. Secondary leukemias were the first major concern to emerge. Previously, the risk of developing leukemia was approximately 5% at 5–7 years after exposure to chemotherapy. This risk appears to have decreased with the broad use of ABVD rather than the previously used alkylating agent-containing regimen nitrogen mustard, vincristine, procarbazine, and prednisone (MOPP).

3. Solid tumors (e.g., breast, lung, sarcoma) have now emerged as the principal problem. There appears to be no plateau to the incidence over time.

4. Lung fibrosis and early coronary artery disease are among late problems.

5. It is hoped that reducing the fields of radiation and the radiation dose will curb the incidence of these late events. Alterations in chemotherapeutic regimens may also help.

E. Lymphocyte predominant Hodgkin lymphoma

This disease is often categorized with the other histologic types of Hodgkin lymphoma. However, there is considerable doubt that this entity should be classified as Hodgkin lymphoma. Its clinical behavior (high response rate but late relapses) and immunophenotype are more akin to low-grade or follicular B-cell non-Hodgkin lymphoma. Unlike treatment in classical Hodgkin lymphoma, treatment of patients in the early stage (stage I/II) of lymphocyte predominant Hodgkin lymphoma should be with local-regional radiation therapy alone. Patients with advanced stage disease (i.e., stage III/IV) respond to treatment in a similar fashion to patients with classical Hodgkin lymphoma.

IV. Treatment of non-Hodgkin lymphoma

A. Overview

Treatment recommendations are highly dependent on the histologic type of disease. Therefore, it is imperative that a thorough and expert review of pathologic specimens be performed before initiation of treatment and in some cases before staging.

1. Multiple classification schemes have been employed for these diseases (e.g., Working Formulation, Revised European-American [REAL] Classification, and the World Health Classification).

2. In order to classify the non-Hodgkin lymphomas within the context of the clinical behavior of the disease, the following three terms are routinely used: **indolent**, **aggressive**, and **highly aggressive**.

B. Indolent, usually incurable non-Hodgkin lymphomas

These lymphomas account for approximately 35–40% of lymphomas. The median age of presentation is 50–60 years. The most common types are the follicular lymphomas, followed by the small lymphocytic lymphomas. Chronic lymphocytic leukemia (CLL) (see Section IV.C) can be regarded as a type of small lymphocytic lymphoma whose features also include a large number (at least 5000 cells/mcL) of circulating lymphoma cells in the blood. More than 80% of these lymphomas are diagnosed in an advanced stage. Despite the advanced stage of the disease, most patients are not symptomatic, and the disease often behaves in an indolent manner (i.e., stays stable in size for long periods, slowly increase in size, or decreases in size). The natural history of the disease typically is long, with median survivals of 7–10 years.

1. **Initial observation.** Given that treatment may lessen the quality of life and that the disease appears incurable, can be slow growing, may not produce symptoms for some time, and may spontaneously regress, patients can be observed without treatment until intervention is clinically necessary (i.e., when symptoms emerge, the pace of the disease increases, blood counts are compromised, or a vital organ such as the lung, liver or kidney is infiltrated and not properly functioning).

    (a) Approximately 20% of patients have spontaneous remissions lasting longer than one year, making treatment unnecessary for this sub-group. The death of malignant cells may occur by necrosis or by apoptosis. *Apoptosis* is the body's genetic program that induces the programmed death of cells that lose normal growth regulation. When cancer cells are unable to subvert apoptosis pathways that would otherwise permit cancer cells to survive, spontaneous remissions of malignancies are possible.

    (b) Studies have indicated that there is no difference in the survival of patients who receive immediate treatment compared to those who are just observed (Fig. 21.1).

    (c) The median time from diagnosis to treatment using this observational approach is approximately 2–3 years.

    (d) Although some have questioned the observation approach in the modern therapeutic era, it remains a standard option in most centers for appropriate patients.

2. **Monoclonal antibodies.**

    (a) Rituximab is a chimeric monoclonal antibody (human-mouse hybrid) directed against the CD20 antigen expressed by nearly all lymphomas of B-cell origin (approximately 85% of lymphomas).

    (b) Rituximab binds to the CD20 antigen on the cell surface, activating B-cell depletion via one or more of several antibody-dependent mechanisms, including:

        (i)   B-cell apoptosis.
        (ii)   Complement-mediated cell lysis.
        (iii) Antibody-dependent cytotoxicity.
        (iv)   Growth arrest.

    (c) Rituximab is detectable in the serum 3–6 months after completion of treatment. B-cell recovery begins approximately 6 months and

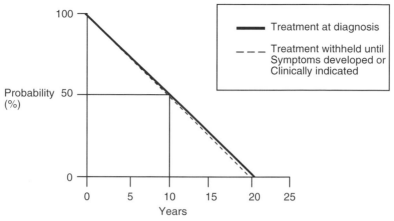

Figure 21.1 Survival of patients with indolent lymphoma with or without initial treatment.

returning to normal by 12 months following completion of treatment. Absorption by intravenous therapy is immediate and results in a rapid and sustained depletion of circulating and tissue-based B cells. Half-life elimination is proportional to the dosage used.

(d) Use of rituximab alone or in combination with chemotherapy has been effective in a number of clinical settings in patients with indolent non-Hodgkin lymphoma. When it is given by intravenous infusion weekly for 4 weeks, the response rate in patients with indolent lymphomas that have relapsed after chemotherapy is approximately 50% (mostly partial remission). The median response duration is approximately 9–12 months.

3. **Chemotherapy.** Although indolent lymphomas are responsive to initial treatment with chemotherapy, relapse of disease is inevitable (median of 2–4 years after initial treatment) regardless of the intensity of treatment. Chemotherapy with immunotherapy (i.e., rituximab) rather than chemotherapy alone is recommended. Commonly used regimens include cyclophosphamide, vincristine, and prednisone plus rituximab (R-CVP), R-CHOP (rituximab, cyclophosphamide, doxorubicin, vincristine, and prednisone), fludarabine plus rituximab (FR), and fludarabine, mitoxantrone, dexamethasone plus rituximab (R-FMD), and bendamustine plus rituximab (BR). The addition of rituximab improves response rates, progression-free survival, and may impact overall survival. Unfortunately, each successive remission after relapse is of decreasing duration.

4. **Radiation therapy.** At times, only one site of disease may cause symptoms. In these instances, local radiation may be appropriate to palliate symptoms. In the uncommon setting of stage I disease, long-term local disease control is frequently possible with this approach, with patients enjoying long disease-free intervals (median of close to 10 years) and long

overall survival (median of approximately 17 years). However, in most instances the disease is widespread, and there is no curative treatment. In these cases, survival curves continue on a downward slope without clear evidence of a plateau. In addition, the indolent lymphoma may transform to an aggressive form of disease, which portends a poorer prognosis. The progression of an indolent lymphoma such as follicular lymphoma to the more aggressive variant of diffuse large B-cell lymphoma occurs regardless of whether follicular lymphoma is treated aggressively or conservatively, at a rate of about 3% per year.

5. **Hematopoietic cell transplantation.** The use of either autologous or allogeneic hematopoietic cell transplantation in the indolent lymphomas is still a matter of some debate (see Section V).

6. **Radiolabeled monoclonal antibodies.** CD20 antibodies bound to radioisotopes to target CD20 may improve efficacy over antibody therapy alone. Anti-CD20 antibodies tagged with radionuclides, such as iodine-131 (Bexxar) and yttrium-90 (Zevalin), have been shown to produce higher overall response rates (60–80%) and higher complete response rates (20–40%) in patients with chemotherapy-relapsed or refractory indolent lymphomas than their unlabeled counterparts. The main side effect of radiolabeled monoclonal antibodies is reversible bone marrow suppression. Therefore, it is not recommended in patients with inadequate marrow reserves (i.e., platelet count <100,000), or significant bone marrow involvement with lymphoma. These agents are generally reserved for relapsed or refractory disease.

7. **Interferon.** This biologic has activity in indolent lymphoma and has historically been used in combination with chemotherapy or as a single agent after chemotherapy in an effort to maintain remission. The use of interferon in front line therapy has been largely abandoned since monoclonal antibodies offer a similar benefit in survival with a more favorable toxicity profile.

8. **Vaccines.** The clonal immunoglobulin idiotype displayed on the surface of most malignant B cells is a patient- and tumor-specific antigen that can be used for therapeutic vaccination. However, vaccinations for patients with lymphoma remain a non-approved, experimental therapeutic option for patients. Various strategies are being developed to optimize these vaccines, such as enhancing T-cell function to induce a better killing of the tumor cells, especially given that many patients are immunosuppressed. Also, lymphoma vaccines will need to define optimal integration with standard therapies, in particular with rituximab.

9. **Mucosa associated lymphoid tissue (MALT).** MALT lymphoma of the stomach is the only indolent lymphoma that may be curable with antibiotics. If MALT lymphoma is associated with a *Helicobacter pylori* infection of the stomach, antibiotic eradication of the infection results in frequent and complete remission. 50–80% of patients with localized gastric MALT achieve histologic complete remission, which will be maintained

long-term for the majority of patients. If irradiation is not successful, local radiation therapy is generally utilized. For marginal zone/MALT lymphomas involving other disease sites, management is similar to other indolent histologies as detailed above.

10. **Cutaneous T-cell lymphomas.** Although most lymphomas in the United States are of B-cell lineage, a form of T-cell lymphoma involving the skin (i.e., mycosis fungoides) can also be included in the indolent lymphoma category. T-cell lymphomas typically present with plaque-like lesions and can be treated with *ultraviolet light, radiation therapy,* and *various topicals* (i.e., nitrogen mustard, retinoids, corticosteroids). In some cases, the disease can progress to invade lymph nodes or to produce tumors on the skin, in which case the prognosis becomes poorer. Treatment in these stages can include *chemotherapy, interferon,* and *interleukin-2 conjugated to diphtheria toxin (Ontak).* Ontak is a recombinant interleukin-2 (IL-2)-diphtheria toxin fusion protein that targets lymphoma cells expressing the CD25 component of the IL-2 receptor

C. Chronic lymphocytic leukemia (CLL)

CLL can be considered part of the spectrum of small lymphocytic lymphomas. It is the most common leukemia in the western Hemisphere, affecting 20 in 100,000 persons older than 60 years of age. The diagnosis is often incidental on routine blood screening, and patients frequently have no symptoms. There is a monoclonal lymphocytosis in the blood (i.e., absolute lymphocyte count of at least 10,000/μL). More than 95% of cases of CLL are derived from B-cell lineage.

1. **Staging and prognosis:** The prognosis depends on the stage of disease (Table 21.6). Median survival ranges from 12 or more years for stage 0 to

Table 21.6 Rai and Modified Rai Clinical Staging System

Modified Rai stage	Rai stage	Description	Median survival from the time of diagnosis
Low risk	0	Lymphocytosis only (in blood and marrow)	150 months
Intermediate risk	1	Lymphocytosis plus enlarged nodes	101 months
	2	Lymphocytosis plus enlarged spleen and/or liver with or without enlargement of nodes	71 months
High risk	3	Lymphocytosis plus anemia (hemoglobin <11.0 g/dL), with or without enlarged nodes, spleen, or liver	19 months
	4	Lymphocytosis plus thrombocytopenia (platelets <100 × 10^9/μL), with or without anemia and/or enlarged spleen, or liver	

From Blood by Kanti Rai. Copyright 1975 by American Society of Hematology (ASH). (Reproduced with permission of American Society of Hematology.)

1.5 years for stage 4. Two staging systems exist for CLL, the Rai and the Binet systems.

    (a) **Rai system:** This system is based upon the concept that in CLL there is a gradual and progressive increase in the body burden of leukemic lymphocytes, starting in the blood and bone marrow (lymphocytosis), progressively involving lymph nodes (lymphadenopathy), spleen and liver (organomegaly), with eventual compromise of bone marrow function (anemia and thrombocytopenia). The *Modified Rai system* was developed as a more practical method to stratify patients for prospective trials, consisting of three groups (low, intermediate, and high).

    (b) **Binet system:** In this staging system, patients are classified according to the number of involved sites (cervical, axillary, and inguinal lymph nodes, spleen, and liver) plus the presence of anemia and/or thrombocytopenia.

    (c) **Although an integrated system** using both the Rai and the Binet staging systems is recommended, it has not been widely accepted and most clinicians today use either the Rai or Binet method for patient management and therapeutic investigation.

2. As with other indolent lymphomas, some patients with CLL can be observed without initial treatment.

3. There are several initial treatment options for patients with symptomatic CLL, including fludarabine (a purine analog), alkylating agents (e.g., chlorambucil, bendamustine), monoclonal antibodies (e.g., rituximab) or combination of these agents. Most have not been directly compared. Similar to indolent lymphoma, response rates improve when rituximab is combined with initial chemotherapy. A choice between these therapies is made based upon patient characteristics and goals of therapy. Median overall survival with each of these regimens is approximately five years. For most patients, fludarabine-based therapies are used. Combination therapy with fludarabine, cyclophosphamide, and rituximab results in overall response rate of 95%. Alemtuzumab has demonstrated superior response rates compared to chlorambucil, but has not been compared directly with fludarabine-based therapy.

4. **Alemtuzumab** is a monoclonal antibody that binds to CD52, a nonmodulating antigen present on the surface of B and T lymphocytes, a majority of monocytes, macrophages, NK cells, and a subpopulation of granulocytes. After binding to CD52+ cells, an antibody-dependent lysis of leukemic cells occurs. Clearance of Alemtuzumab decreases with repeated dosing due to loss of CD52 receptor-mediated clearance. Therefore, half-life elimination is only 11 hours after the first dose, but 6 days following the last dose.

5. **For refractory disease**, non-myeloablative allogeneic hematopoietic cell transplants achieve complete remissions in select cases.

6. **Complications of CLL.** Since CLL is characterized by the progressive accumulation of monoclonal, functionally incompetent lymphocytes,

common complications of CLL are associated with the intrinsic immune dysfunction that results in immunodeficiency and the development of autoimmune disorders (i.e., autoimmune hemolytic anemia, autoimmune thrombocytopenia, hypogammaglobulinemia and increased infection rate).

D. Aggressive, potentially curable non-Hodgkin lymphomas

These are the most common lymphomas. By far the most common type is diffuse large B-cell lymphoma. It is more common to diagnose these lymphomas in a lower stage than indolent lymphomas, e.g., stage I–II versus III–IV. Because of their rapid growth and propensity to invade vital organs, staging and treatment of these lymphomas should be initiated soon after diagnosis. Certain sites of involvement (i.e., bone marrow, sinuses, testes) pose a higher risk of CNS involvement. The International Prognostic Index (Table 21.7) identifies risk factors for prognosis, including age, stage, serum lactate dehydrogenase, number of extralymphatic sites, and performance status

1. Chemotherapy, the primary treatment for aggressive non-Hodgkin lymphomas, can be curative. CHOP combination chemotherapy plus rituximab (CHOP-R) is used for CD20+ disease.
    (a) The addition of rituximab to chemotherapy results in an approximately 10% overall increase in survival beginning at one year from initiation of therapy in patients with diffuse large B-cell lymphoma, with almost no increase in toxicity.
    (b) Patients with low-stage disease and no other adverse factors have a good prognosis. The usual recommended treatment for patients with localized disease is CHOP for three cycles plus rituximab followed by locoregional radiation therapy.
    (c) For patients with bulky stage II [tumorous masses greater than 5 cm in diameter] or stage III or IV disease, 6–8 cycles of CHOP plus rituximab for CD20+ disease is used. Elderly patients have a poorer prognosis overall.

IPI	Expected complete remission rate	Predicted 2-year survival rate	Predicted 5-year survival rate
0-1	87%	84%	73%
2	67	66	51
3	55	54	43
4-5	44	34	26

Table 21.7 International Prognostic Index for Aggressive Non-Hodgkin Lymphoma

IPI, International Prognostic Index. Each risk factor [age>60, stage III or IV, LDH elevation, ≥2 extra-lymphatic sites, and performance status ≥2 (on a scale from 0–4)] is assigned a value of one. The number of IPI values (0–5) is indirectly correlated with prognosis.

(d) Less than 20% of patients who do not achieve a complete remission with initial therapy can be cured.

2. Autologous hematopoietic cell transplantation (HCT) is not currently used in the initial treatment of aggressive NHL. This is principally because HCT is associated with significant morbidity and survival is the same in patients administered chemotherapy with or without HCT.

E. Moderately aggressive incurable non-Hodgkin lymphomas

A prime example of such a lymphoma is mantle cell lymphoma (MCL). This B-cell lymphoma has a clear male predominance and a median survival of 4–5 years. It usually presents in an advanced stage, often with splenomegaly, circulating lymphoma cells, or intestinal involvement.

1. Combination chemotherapy is the main treatment modality. Surgery is usually not of benefit, but may be of value in certain circumstances such as bowel obstruction. Radiation therapy is usually reserved for palliative purposes.

2. Two most commonly used chemotherapy regimens are:
   (a) CHOP (Cyclophosphamide, doxorubicin, vincristine, and prednisone) or CVP (cyclophosphamide, vincristine, prednisone) either program with rituximab.
   (b) Hyper-CVAD (hyperfractionated cyclophosphamide, vincristine, doxorubicin, and dexamethasone, alternating with high-dose methotrexate and cytarabine) with rituximab.

3. For patients over 70 years of age or for those with comorbidities that exclude more aggressive treatment options, conventional chemotherapy such as R-CHOP or R-CVP without subsequent autologous HCT is used. This regimen is also used off protocol for patients younger than 70 years of age without comorbidities who do not fall into the high risk group under the International Prognostic Index (Table 21.7).

4. For patients less than 65 years old with the blastic variant of MCL or a high International Prognostic Index score, an aggressive treatment program such as R-Hyper-CVAD alone or R-CHOP followed by autologous HCT is considered.

F. Highly aggressive, potentially curable, non-Hodgkin lymphomas

These include Burkitt's lymphoma (BL) and lymphoblastic lymphoma.

1. Despite their tendency for rapid proliferation, these lymphomas are often responsive to chemotherapy, which are aggressive and of short duration. These regimens use intensive alkylating agents, delivered in a hyperfractionated way or as a continuous infusion. Since the different regimens have not been directly compared, the physician's experience with administration becomes very important when choosing among these regimens.

2. **Burkitt's lymphoma.** One treatment used is the CODOX-M/IVAC protocol (cyclophosphamide, doxorubicin, vincristine, methotrexate, leukovorin, colony-stimulating factor, ifosfamide, etoposide, cytarabine, and

intrathecal cytarabine/methotrexate). There is a significant risk of tumor lysis syndrome in patients treated for BL. Also, patients with BL are at high risk for developing CNS involvement and so CNS prophylaxis is a standard component of first line therapy.

3. **Lymphoblastic lymphoma.** Treatment resembles that of acute lymphocytic leukemia. Combination chemotherapy is the primary treatment modality. There is no role for surgery or total body radiation therapy in the induction phase. Multiple induction regimens have been developed, with none having been directly compared in a prospective randomized trial. These chemotherapy regimens contain vincristine, a corticosteroid (i.e., prednisone), and an anthracycline in addition to other agents. Some form of CNS prophylaxis is also incorporated. For patients with newly diagnosed Philadelphia chromosome positivity, induction chemotherapy plus imatinib (Gleevec) rather than chemotherapy alone is recommended.

V. Hematopoietic cell transplantation (HCT)

Both autologous and allogeneic HCT are important treatment modalities for patients with relapsed Hodgkin and non-Hodgkin lymphomas. Unlike *allogeneic* HCT, where donor cells are used, *autologous* HCT infuses the patient's own hematopoietic cells to reestablish bone marrow function after the administration of high-dose chemotherapy and/or radiation. These reinfused hematopoietic cells can come from the patient's bone marrow or peripheral blood, or both. Because a major limitation to the use of allogeneic HCT is that only a few patients have an HLA-matched sibling donor, the use of autologous hematopoietic cells greatly increases the number of patients eligible for transplantation. Autologous transplantation can also be used safely in older patients because of the absence of graft-vs.-host disease, which is a major concern with allogeneic HCT, especially in the elderly population. A disadvantage of autologous HCT is the risk of contaminating the graft with viable tumor cells. Although patients undergoing autologous transplantation have higher relapse rates than do patients undergoing allogeneic transplantation, the lower rate of other complications with autologous transplantation seems to translate into similar long-term outcomes. On the other hand, allogeneic HCT offers a potential for cure, due to the graft-vs.-tumor effects conferred by alloreactive donor cells. The goals and outcomes of hematopoietic transplantation are unique in each histology, as detailed below.

A. Hodgkin lymphoma

1. **Indications.** Due to the up to 5% early mortality and the appreciable risk of late myelodysplastic syndrome and/or acute myeloid leukemia, this approach should be considered as a treatment of choice only in patients with a poor prognosis who have one of the following features:

(a) Early relapse after initial chemotherapy (less than 12 months after treatment) or induction failure (i.e., resistant disease), suggesting cellular drug resistance to conventional doses.

(b) Second relapse after conventional treatment for first relapse.

(c) Generalized systemic relapse after initial chemotherapy even beyond 12 months, suggesting an aggressive biologic behavior.

2. **Autologous HCT.** Most centers perform autologous HCT with up to 5% early mortality and relapse rates of 40 to 50%, depending upon patient risk factors. Event-free survival is 35 to 60% at five years for patients transplanted after first relapse. Outcomes of relapse following autologous HCT are poor.

3. **Preparative regimens.** The most common preparative regimens prior to autologous transplantation in Hodgkin lymphoma are CBV (cyclophosphamide, BCNU [carmustine], etoposide) and BEAM (BCNU, etoposide, cytarabine, and melphalan). Total body radiation has often been given in conjunction with etoposide and cyclophosphamide, however may be associated with increased late toxicities, including leukemia. Adjuvant involved-field irradiation is widely used either before or after autologous HCT.

4. **Allogeneic HCT** are generally considered in young patients with Hodgkin lymphoma who recur after autologous HCT.

B. Indolent non-Hodgkin lymphoma

1. **The use of either autologous or allogeneic HCT** in the indolent lymphomas is still a matter of some debate because of:

   (a) the high frequency of bone marrow and peripheral blood infiltration in the indolent lymphomas, resulting in contamination of the reinfused marrow or peripheral blood stem cells with viable tumor cells.

   (b) the treatment-related complications including short-term (e.g., graft vs. host disease, infection) and long-term (e.g., myelodysplastic syndrome, acute myeloid leukemia, other secondary malignancies).

   (c) the belief that this is a disease with a very long natural history, in which excessive treatment-related toxicities associated with aggressive therapy would not be acceptable.

2. **Relapsed disease:** There have been mixed results from studies examining the role of autologous HCT in relapsed indolent NHL. One trial demonstrated that high-dose therapy followed by autologous HCT was more effective than combination chemotherapy in relapsed or progressive follicular lymphoma. However, that study was performed before rituximab was available for the treatment of follicular lymphoma. The tremendous responses seen with rituximab treatment have made some clinicians question whether the benefit of HCT still holds true in the rituximab era.

3. **Histologic transformation:** Studies indicate 4- to 5-year overall survivals in the range of 37 to 63% and suggest that aggressive therapy with autologous HCT is a reasonable treatment option for selected patients

(i.e., age <60 and chemosensitive disease) with transformed follicular lymphoma.

4. **Indications:** Young, otherwise fit patients with a poor response to initial therapy, or short remission duration should be considered for autologous HCT early in the disease.

5. **Allogeneic transplantation:** This may represent a curative modality for selected patients with relapsed indolent lymphoma. Treatment-associated mortality has ranged between 20 to 50%, usually due to complications of graft-versus-host disease, opportunistic infection, or pneumonitis. Other approaches to improve results of allogeneic HCT, such as non-myeloablative conditioning, donor lymphocyte infusions, and use of rituximab are ongoing. Generally these transplants are pursued in the context of a clinical trial.

C. Recurrent or refractory aggressive non-Hodgkin lymphoma

1. **Autologous hematopoietic HCT** is not currently used in the initial treatment because of its association with significant morbidity with no difference in survival between patients administered chemotherapy with or without HCT. Studies in selected high-risk subgroups of patients are ongoing.

2. **Indications** in recurrent or refractory aggressive NHL:
   (a) Patients with chemosensitive relapse (bone marrow negative). The quality of evidence for patients with positive bone marrows is not quite as high.
   (b) Front line therapy in selected patients with high-intermediate to high risk disease, according to the International Prognostic Index.

3. **Patients who receive high dose chemotherapy** followed by autologous HCT have been shown to have a superior event-free survival (46 vs. 12%) and overall survival (53 vs. 32%) compared to patients receiving chemotherapy alone. Several pilot trials lend support to the use of rituximab as an adjunct to autologous HCT in patients with relapsed or resistant aggressive NHL. The goal of these transplants is curative therapy.

VI. Summary

The curability of Hodgkin lymphoma is one of the great success stories of 20th century medicine. Most patients can now expect to be cured with chemotherapy with or without radiation therapy. However, this success has its price in that second malignancies and organ toxicity from treatment have emerged as serious problems developing several years after treatment. The emphasis of current research is the search for ways to decrease the late consequences of treatment while maintaining the high level of cure.

The non-Hodgkin lymphomas are a diverse collection of lymphoid malignancies ranging in clinical behavior from indolent to rapidly progressive and in prognosis from curable to incurable. New treatment modalities besides those of traditional chemotherapy and radiation therapy such as monoclonal antibodies have made a profound impact on the natural history of these diseases. Current studies are evaluating the use of targeted agents directed against specific proteins in the malignant cells.

Further reading

Abeloff M, ed. Clinical Oncology. New York: Churchill, Livingstone, 2008.

Dave SS, Wright G, Tan B, et al. Prediction of survival in follicular lymphoma based on molecular features of tumor-infiltrating immune cells. N Engl J Med 2004;351:2159–69.

Devita V, ed. Cancer: Principles and Practice of Oncology, 8th edn. New York: Lippincott, 2008.

Friedberg JW, Fisher RI. Diffuse large B cell lymphoma. Hematology/Oncology Clinics of North America 2008;22:941–52.

Hoffman R, ed. Hematology: Basic Principles and Practice, 5th edn. New York: Churchill Livingstone, 2008.

Mendler JH, Friedberg JW. Salvage therapy in Hodgkin lymphoma. Oncologist 2009;4:425–32.

Re D, Thomas RK, Behringer K, Diehl V. From Hodgkin disease to Hodgkin lymphoma: biologic insights and therapeutic potential. Blood 2005;105:4553–60.

Rosenwald A, Wright G, Chan WC, et al. The use of molecular profiling to predict survival after chemotherapy for diffuse large B-cell lymphoma. N Engl J Med 2002;346:1937–47.

CHAPTER 22

22 | Plasma Cell Disorders

Sumit Madan and Philip R. Greipp

Mayo Clinic, Rochester, MN, USA

I. Introduction

Monoclonal gammopathies comprise a group of disorders characterized by the clonal proliferation of Immunoglobulin (Ig) secreting plasma cells. The spectrum of plasma cell proliferative disorders range from the asymptomatic premalignant conditions of "monoclonal gammopathy of undetermined significance" (MGUS) and "smoldering multiple myeloma" (SMM) to incurable hematologic diseases such as multiple myeloma (MM) or plasma cell myeloma, light chain amyloidosis (AL) and Waldenström's macroglobulinemia (macroglobulinemia, WM) (Figure 22.1a). In addition, a small percent of lymphoproliferative disorders, solitary plasmacytomas or miscellaneous disorders make-up the remaining cases with plasma monoclonal gammopathies (Figure 22.1a).

II. Identification of the monoclonal (M) protein

- Malignant plasma cells produce a monoclonal M-protein which appears as a dense, localized band on agarose gel serum protein electrophoresis (SPEP) and as a tall, narrow spike in the gamma (γ), beta (β) or β-γ region when converted to a densitometer tracing (M-spike) (Figure 22.2a, b). This confirms the presence of a monoclonal gammopathy such as MGUS, MM, WM, AL amyloidosis or another plasma cell proliferative disorder. On the other hand, a polyclonal proliferation of Ig (polyclonal gammopathy) usually manifests as a broad peak in the γ region, and is often seen in non-hematologic diseases such as liver disease, connective tissue disorders (rheumatoid arthritis and systemic lupus erythematosus) and chronic infections (osteomyelitis).

Concise Guide to Hematology, First Edition. Edited by Alvin H. Schmaier, Hillard M. Lazarus.
© 2012 Blackwell Publishing Ltd. Published 2012 by Blackwell Publishing Ltd.

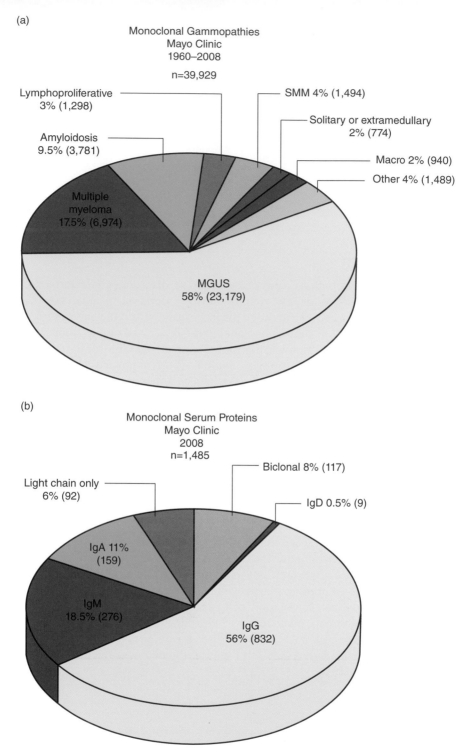

Figure 22.1 (a) Monoclonal gammopathies diagnosed at the Mayo Clinic between 1960 and 2008. MGUS: monoclonal gammopathy of undetermined significance; Macro: macroglobulinemia; SMM: smoldering multiple myeloma. (b) Type of monoclonal protein detected at the Mayo Clinic in 2008.

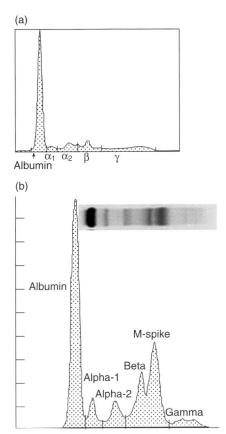

Figure 22.2 (a) Serum protein electrophoresis from a normal serum sample. (b) Serum protein electrophoresis from a patient with multiple myeloma. The monoclonal protein appears as an abnormal band on the agarose gel electrophoresis that is converted to an M-spike on the densitometric tracing.

- The size of the M-spike provides a measure of the number of bone marrow plasma cells (BMPCs). At least 5×10^9 BMPCs should be present in order to identify an M spike on SPEP.
- Upon the identification of a spike or a localized band on SPEP, an immunofixation (IF) with agarose gel should be performed to confirm the presence of an M protein, and to determine the heavy chain class (Figure 22.1b) [gamma (IgG), alpha (IgA), mu (IgM), or delta (IgD)]. Epsilon (IgE) is quite uncommon and light chain disease itself can be an isolated disease. Additionally, the light chain type [kappa (κ) or lambda (λ)] in the immunoglobulin needs to be identified. IF is more sensitive than SPEP, and is able to detect smaller amounts of M protein. Ig quantification should be performed which can yield higher results than predicted by the SPEP tracing.
- When suspecting MM or amyloidosis, a 24-hour urine protein electrophoresis (UPEP) is recommended. It may show an M-spike or heavy albuminuria.
- The serum free light chain (FLC) assay measures the κ and λ light chain that are not bound to the Ig heavy chain. The normal FLC ratio is 0.26 to

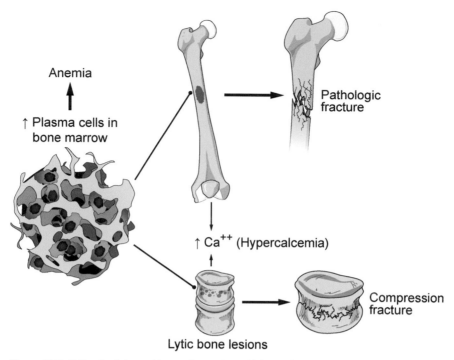

Anemia

↑ Plasma cells in bone marrow

Pathologic fracture

↑ Ca^{++} (Hypercalcemia)

Compression fracture

Lytic bone lesions

Figure 22.3 Pathophysiology of bone disease in multiple myeloma.

1.65 gm/dL. An abnormal ratio identifies clonality, with values <0.26 and >1.65 indicating an excess production of monoclonal λ and monoclonal κ light chains, respectively. The involved FLC and FLC ratio should be used in monitoring disease activity in non-secretory MM, and monoclonal light chain disorders such as light chain MM, AL amyloidosis, and light chain deposition disease (LCDD).

III. Multiple myeloma

Multiple myeloma, more recently termed plasma cell myeloma by the World Health Organization, is the prototype of monoclonal plasma cell dyscrasias.

A. Epidemiology
- MM affects more than 20,000 people each year in the United States. It is the second most prevalent hematologic malignancy with an annual incidence of approximately 4 to 5 per 100,000 individuals.
- It accounts for 10% of all hematologic cancers and approximately 1% of all newly diagnosed cancers in the US each year. Approximately 10,000 patients will die of MM each year.
- MM is usually diagnosed in the late middle-aged and elderly (median age at diagnosis = 72 years); only 2% patients are under the age of 40 at the time of diagnosis.

Table 22.1 Diagnostic criteria for monoclonal gammopathy of undetermined significance, smoldering multiple myeloma and multiple myeloma

Disease stage	Diagnostic criteria
Monoclonal gammopathy of undetermined significance	Serum M protein <3 g/dL BMPC <10% Very low or no amount of urine monoclonal light chains (Bence Jones proteins) Absence of CRAB features (hypercalcemia, renal failure, anemia, and lytic bone lesions)
Smoldering multiple myeloma	Serum M protein (IgG or IgA) ≥3 g/dL and/or BMPC ≥10% Absence of CRAB features
Multiple myeloma	Presence of a serum and/or urine M protein BMPC ≥10% Presence of CRAB features directly attributable to the monoclonal plasma cell disorder

BMPC, bone marrow plasma cells; CRAB, hypercalcemia, renal failure, anemia, and lytic bone lesions.

- The prevalence of MM varies by ethnicity. African-Americans (AA) are twice as likely to suffer from MM, and the mortality is twice as high as that of Caucasians. In contrast, the prevalence in Asians is lower than the Caucasians. However, within the different ethnic and geographical groups, MM is slightly more common in men than in women (approximately 1.4:1).

B. Clinical features

- MM is caused by the uncontrolled proliferation of abnormal, atypical or immature BMPCs that leads to an increased production of a monoclonal Ig (M protein). It is characterized by bone destruction, and marrow replacement by malignant BMPCs that leads to suppression of normal hematopoiesis (Table 22.1; Figure 22.3).
- Classically, the MM patient presents with pain in the lower back that is exacerbated by standing and relieved by lying down. Anemia resulting in weakness and fatigue are also common at initial presentation. Impaired humoral immunity predisposes some MM patients to recurrent infections, especially with encapsulated organisms such as *Streptococcus pneumoniae* and *Haemophilus influenzae*.
- The initial diagnosis of MM may also be made due to the clinical manifestations related to renal failure, spinal cord compression (most common with IgA MM), severe hypercalcemia or hyperviscosity syndrome (mucosal and gastrointestinal bleeding, nausea, vertigo, visual disturbances, and altered mental status).
- The common tetrad used to define the end organ damage in MM is *CRAB*: C = hypercalcemia, R = Renal failure, A = Anemia, B = Lytic bone lesions.

C. Bone disease

- Bone disease characterized by hypercalcemia, osteolytic bony lesions, pathologic fractures of the axial skeleton, compression fractures of the spine and osteoporosis cause significant morbidity and mortality.
- Bone pain in areas of active hematopoiesis such as the vertebrae, pelvis, ribs and proximal long bones is present at the time of diagnosis in approximately 60% patients.
- The bone lesions are purely lytic in nature, and are best seen on conventional radiograph as sharply defined and spheroid with smooth borders ("punched-out lesions").
- Myeloma bone disease occurs due to an excessive osteoclastic-mediated bone resorption and impaired osteoblastic bone formation. An increase in the ratio of receptor activator of nuclear factor kappa-B ligand (RANKL) and its decoy receptor osteoprotegerin (OPG) mediates osteoclast activation and excessive bone resorption. Additionally, cytokines such as macrophage inflammatory protein (MIP)-1alpha, interleukin (IL)-3, IL-1 beta and IL-6 produced by marrow stromal cells are also implicated as potential osteoclast activating factors. On the other hand, increased activity of IL-7, DKK1, and IL-3 inhibit osteoblast differentiation and decrease bone formation.

D. Hypercalcemia and renal failure/insufficiency

- Abnormal bone metabolism leads to hypercalcemia and its associated symptoms in approximately 25% of MM patients at initial diagnosis.
- Both acute and chronic renal failure occur in almost half of MM patients at diagnosis, and serum creatinine is >2 mg/dL in approximately 25%.
- Two major causes of renal insufficiency in MM are hypercalcemia and myeloma cast nephropathy (myeloma kidney). Myeloma kidney occurs due to tubular damage from the light chain portion of the Ig (Bence Jones proteins) (Figure 22.4).

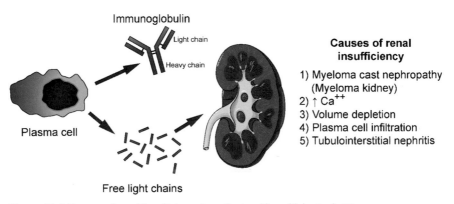

Immunoglobulin

Light chain

Heavy chain

Plasma cell

Free light chains

Causes of renal insufficiency

1) Myeloma cast nephropathy (Myeloma kidney)
2) ↑ Ca^{++}
3) Volume depletion
4) Plasma cell infiltration
5) Tubulointerstitial nephritis

Figure 22.4 Causes of renal insufficiency in patients with multiple myeloma.

- Other causes of renal failure in MM include concurrent AL amyloidosis and light chain deposition disease (LCDD).
- In 15% of MM patients, the Ig heavy chain (IgH) is undetectable but a light chain is found on UPEP or urine IF (Light chain MM). The serum creatinine is $\geq 2\,mg/dL$ in about one-third of these patients at diagnosis.
- Approximately 3% MM patients lack M-protein in the serum or urine on IF, and are considered to have nonsecretory MM. These patients may have low levels of monoclonal FLC and are at low risk for myeloma kidney.

E. Anemia
- Marrow replacement with myeloma cells and erythropoietin deficiency from renal insufficiency results in signs and symptoms of anemia (Figure 22.3).
- A normocytic, normochromic anemia is present in 73% at diagnosis and almost all patients at some time during the disease course.

F. Pathogenesis
- The etiology of MM is unknown.
- The first step in pathogenesis of MM is the development of MGUS clone.
- The pathogenetic event in almost all MGUS patients is believed to be the occurrence of either a primary chromosomal translocation or hyperdiploidy.
- Primary translocations usually occur due to errors in IgH (immunoglobulin heavy locus) switch recombination or somatic hypermutation. They are observed in approximately 60% MM patients and 45% MGUS patients. The most common IgH translocations is t(11;14) (q13;q32) identified in 25%, whereas t(4;14) (p16;q32) and t(14;16) (q32;q23) are recognized in a smaller subset of MGUS patients. These translocations dysregulate a variety of oncogenes present on the partner chromosome such as cyclin D1 (11q13) or D3 (6p21), fibroblast growth factor receptor 3 (FGFR3) and MMSET (4p16), and c-MAF (6p21).
- Most of the remaining cases of MGUS have evidence of hyperdiploidy (non-IgH translocated MGUS), usually of one or more of the odd numbered chromosomes (except chromosome 13).
- The precise mechanisms for the evolution of MGUS to MM are poorly understood; however, the constant lifelong risk of progression of MGUS (irrespective of the time period of the preceding MGUS phase) is strongly suggestive of a random 2-hit model resulting in the malignant transformation to MM or another malignant gammopathy.
- Changes in bone marrow microenvironment including induction of angiogenesis, and dysregulation of various cytokines (IL-6, IL-1) are implicated in the transition of MGUS to MM.
- RAS (N and K RAS) mutations, p16 methylation, p53 mutations, myc abnormalities, and secondary translocations are also associated with transition to symptomatic disease.

Table 22.2 Staging systems for multiple myeloma	
International staging system	
Stage I	Serum beta 2-microglobulin <3.5 mg/L
	Serum albumin > = 3.5 g/dL
Stage II	Neither stage I or III
Stage III	Serum beta 2-microglobulin > = 5.5 mg/L
Durie Salmon Staging	
Stage I	Requires all of the following:
	Hemoglobin >10 g/dL
	Normal serum calcium
	Skeletal survey: normal or single plasmacytoma or osteoporosis
	Serum paraprotein level <5 g/dL if IgG, <3 g/dL if IgA
	Urinary light chain excretion <4 g/24 h
Stage II	Fulfilling the criteria of neither I nor III
Stage III	Requires one or more of:
	Hemoglobin <8.5 g/dL
	Serum calcium >12 mg/dL
	Skeletal survey: > = 3 lytic bone lesions
	Serum paraprotein >7 g/dL if IgG, >5 g/dL if IgA
	Urinary light chain excretion >12 g/24 h
Subclass A	Serum creatinine <2 mg/dL
Subclass B	Serum creatinine ≥2 mg/dL

G. Staging systems for MM

- The International Staging System (ISS) was developed in 2005 utilizing database on 10,750 MM patients. It provides a prognostic index using simple variables (serum albumin and beta-2 microglobulin) in patients who meet the diagnostic criteria for MM. The median survival is 62, 44 and 29 months for stage I, II, and III disease, respectively. However, the ISS is not a reliable indicator of tumor burden.
- The Durie Salmon Staging (DSS) System is based on the total tumor burden but correlates less well with prognosis. Table 22.2 lists the staging and prognostic systems used in MM patients.

H. Laboratory findings

Patients suspected of having MM should initially undergo all of the following:

- A complete history and physical examination.
- Blood tests: CBC with differential, serum electrolytes, blood urea nitrogen (BUN), creatinine, calcium, magnesium, phosphorus, uric acid, albumin, β2M, lactate dehydrogenase (LDH), C-reactive protein, and peripheral blood smear (Atlas Figure 43).
- SPEP, IF, and quantitative Ig levels (The M spike usually increases with disease progression and relapse, and decreases with response to treatment).

- Serum FLC assay.
- UPEP and urine IF.
- Skeletal survey including X-rays of the skull, chest, axial skeleton and all long bones. A CT scan, PET/CT scan, or MRI can be used in patients with bone pain without an abnormality seen on the X-rays. A bone scan is less sensitive to detect osteolytic lesions, and is therefore not required in the initial diagnosis of MM.
- Bone marrow aspirate and biopsy with conventional cytogenetic studies, and FISH analysis for the identification of certain translocations which carry a poor prognostic significance (Atlas Figure 42).

It is not necessary to repeat a bone marrow biopsy to assess disease progression or response to treatment; an M protein level in the serum or urine and/or FLC level can be used to monitor disease activity.

I. Treatment

Important prognostic factors in multiple myeloma are listed in Table 22.3.

- The median survival for patients diagnosed with MM between 1996 and 2006 was approximately 45 months. However, the use of novel agents has resulted in significant improvement, with various studies demonstrating a median 3-year survival rate of approximately 90%. Despite the recent therapeutic advances, MM still remains an incurable disease.
- The treatment armamentarium of MM consists of conventional chemotherapy, corticosteroids, high-dose therapy (HDT) with chemotherapeutic agents including melphalan followed by autologous hematopoietic cell transplant (AHCT), allogeneic hematopoietic cell transplant, and the novel therapies such as thalidomide and lenalidomide, and the proteasome inhibitor bortezomib.
- Previous studies demonstrated no difference in the overall survival (OS) of MM patients treated with either melphalan and prednisone or a

Table 22.3 Prognostic factors in multiple myeloma	
1	Poor performance status
2	Elevated LDH
3	Plasmablastic morphology
4	Deletion 17p, t(4;14) or t(14;16) on FISH analysis
5	Deletion of chromosome13 or hypodiploidy on metaphase cytogenetic
7	Elevated plasma cell labeling index (PCLI)* ≥3%
8	Age ≥70 years
9	CRP
10	Serum calcium ≥11 mg/dL
11	Elevated creatinine ≥2 mg/dL
12	Platelet count <150,000/microL

*PCLI is a slide based immunofluorescence method that provides a measure of the proliferative rate of the malignant BMPC. It is a powerful and independent predictor of survival in patients with newly diagnosed MM.

combination of cytotoxic drugs. However, in the 1980s, the introduction of HDT and AHCT was shown to improve response rates and prolong OS when compared with conventional chemotherapeutic regimens.

- Therefore, in MM patients who are considered transplant eligible, HDT followed by AHCT is now routinely incorporated in the treatment paradigm, either upfront or at the time of initial relapse.
- Thalidomide, lenalidomide, and bortezomib (used either alone or in combination with steroids) are widely used as either induction therapy before transplant, in patients considered ineligible for transplant, and/or at disease relapse. Their use has led to improved outcomes both in disease relapse as well as from the time of diagnosis.
- Although patients with relapsed disease usually respond to further chemotherapy, the response rates and the response duration progressively decrease with each salvage regimen.
- The use of recombinant human erythropoietin for anemia, and better management of patients with renal failure have also contributed to improving the OS in MM.
- Additionally, bisphosphonate (zoledronic acid and pamidronate) therapy reduces the number of skeletal events by inhibiting osteoclastic bone resorption observed in MM.

IV. Monoclonal gammopathy of undetermined significance

A. Introduction

- Recent evidence suggests that almost all cases of MM evolve from an age-dependent, pre-malignant, asymptomatic disease stage termed MGUS.
- MGUS is characterized by the limited clonal proliferation of the BMPCs, small amount of a serum M protein, and absence of end organ damage (Table 22.1).
- The term MGUS indicates the uncertain nature of the malignant plasma cell clone that usually remains stable; however, substantial proliferation can occur to cause a plasma cell cancer.
- Although MGUS is clinically under-recognized due to the asymptomatic nature of this condition, it is still the most commonly diagnosed plasma cell dyscrasia (Figure 22.1a).
- It is usually diagnosed in an outpatient setting as an incidental finding of an M protein during the evaluation of an unrelated disease or in an apparently healthy individual undergoing routine health examination.

B. Epidemiology

- MGUS has been observed in 3.2% and 5.3% of Caucasians over the age of 50 and 70 years, respectively.
- African-Americans have two-threefold higher age-adjusted prevalence of MGUS compared with Caucasians. On the other hand, the age-

adjusted prevalence of MGUS in Asians is lower (2.4% in persons over 50 years).
* Within the different ethnic groups, the age-adjusted rates are higher in men than in women.

C. Natural history
* MGUS carries a lifelong risk of 1% per year progression to MM (most common), AL amyloidosis or WM (with IgM MGUS).
* Since the MGUS population is generally older with multiple comorbid conditions, the true probability of MGUS progression is much lower (11% at 25 years) when the competing causes of death are taken in account. Therefore, it is important to realize that the majority (approximately 75–90%) of MGUS patients will not progress to MM or a related disorder, and will usually die from a non-plasma cell disease.

D. Risk factors of progression
The important risk factors for MGUS progression are listed in Table 22.4.
* A model to stratify MGUS patients utilizes three important risk factors namely: non-IgG (IgA and IgM) MGUS, abnormal serum FLC ratio and serum M protein $\geq$1.5 g/dL (Figure 22.5).
* At 20 years of MGUS diagnosis, patients with all three risk factors (high risk) have a 58% risk of progression, compared with 37% with any two risk factors (high intermediate), 21% with one risk factor (low intermediate) and 5% when none of the risk factors are present (low risk, constitutes nearly 40% of MGUS patients).
* Identifying MGUS patients at high risk of progression is important for prognostication, and to help guide in the design of clinical trials aimed at preventing disease progression.

E. Clinical implications and disease associations of MGUS
* An increased risk of axial fractures and a slightly increased risk of venous thromboembolic disease (VTD) have been reported in MGUS patients compared with the general population.

Table 22.4 Major risk factors associated with progression of MGUS

1	Higher M protein at diagnosis
2	"Evolving" MGUS—progressively increasing M protein value
3	IgA or IgM MGUS
4	Abnormal free light chain ratio (<0.26 or >1.65 g/dL)
5	Percentage of bone marrow plasma cells (6–9% carries twice the risk compared with < = 5%)
6	Suppression of uninvolved immunoglobulins
7	Presence of peripheral blood circulating plasma cells or clonal B cells

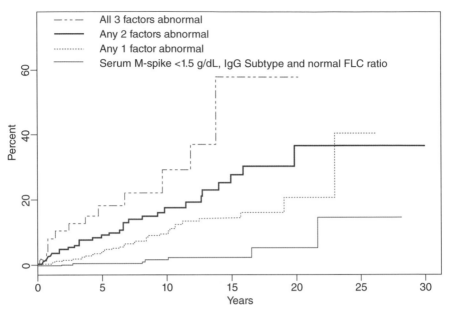

Figure 22.5 Risk of progression of MGUS to myeloma or related disorder using a risk-stratification model that incorporates the FLC ratio and the size and type of the serum monoclonal protein. The top curve illustrates risk of progression with time in patients with all three risk factors, namely an abnormal serum kappa–lambda FLC ratio (<0.26 or >1.65), a high serum monoclonal protein level (≥1.5 mg/dL), and non-IgG MGUS; the second gives the risk of progression in patients with any two of these risk factors; the third curve illustrates the risk of progression with one of these risk factors; the bottom curve is the risk of progression for patients with none of the risk factors. (Reproduced with permission from Rajkumar et al. © the American Society of Hematology.)

- Occasionally, an M protein may be found in association with skin diseases (scleromyxedema, pyoderma gangrenosum, discoid lupus erythematosus, erythema elevatum diutinum), hematologic disorders (malignant lymphoma, chronic lymphocytic leukemia), neurologic disorders (idiopathic peripheral neuropathy, motor neuron disease), connective tissue diseases (rheumatoid arthritis, polymyalgia rheumatica, systemic lupus erythematosus), and immune suppression (post-transplant in patients undergoing organ or bone marrow transplantation; acquired immune deficiency syndrome).

F. Management
- MGUS patients should undergo periodic lifelong follow-up; therapy is currently not indicated.
- A bone marrow biopsy and skeletal survey should be obtained when any of the risk factors of MGUS are identified.
- Low-risk MGUS can be followed at 6 months and every 2 years thereafter; all other subsets of MGUS patients should be reassessed in 6 months and

then yearly thereafter. A pattern of rising M protein ("evolving" MGUS) should be monitored more frequently.
- On return visits, a thorough history, physical exam, CBC, serum calcium and creatinine, and SPEP should be obtained. Further testing should be dictated by the clinical assessment and if suspicion is high, a complete workup including bone marrow examination, skeletal survey, and UPEP must be obtained.

V. Smoldering multiple myeloma

- Although clinically similar to MGUS, SMM is a far more advanced premalignant disease stage than MGUS (Table 22.1).
- In contrast to the fixed 1% risk of progression of MGUS, SMM progresses to symptomatic MM or AL amyloidosis at a rate of 10% per year for the first 5 years, approximately 3% per year for the next 5 years and 1% per year for the next 10 years, yielding a cumulative probability of progression of 73% at 15 years (Figure 22.6).
- The risk of progression is directly related to the proportion of BMPCs and the serum M protein level at diagnosis of SMM.

A. Management
- Although no treatment is required, SMM should be followed up more closely than MGUS, usually once every 3–4 months in the initial stages of diagnosis.

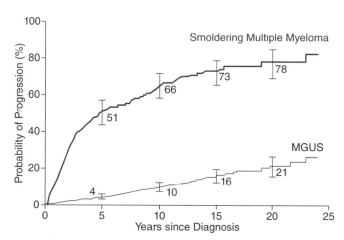

Figure 22.6 Probability of progression to active multiple myeloma or primary amyloidosis in patients with smoldering multiple myeloma or monoclonal gammopathy of undetermined significance (MGUS). I bars denote 95% confidence intervals. (Reproduced with permission from Kyle RA, Remstein ED, Therneau TM, et al. Clinical course and prognosis of smoldering (asymptomatic) multiple myeloma. N Engl J Med 2007;356(25):2582–90. Copyright © 2007 Massachusetts Medical Society. All rights reserved.)

- No benefit has been shown with early therapy compared with when progression to MM occurs.
- Ongoing clinical trials are testing thalidomide plus zoledronic acid versus zoledronic acid, interleukin-1β inhibitors, and thalidomide in an attempt to delay progression of SMM to active MM. However, outside of a clinical trial, no therapy is currently recommended.

VI. Amyloidosis

A. Introduction
- Amyloid is a fibrillar (7.5 to 10nm in width, aggregated in a β-pleated sheet conformation), proteinaceous material that can be detected by Congo red stain as a characteristic apple-green birefringence under polarized light.
- Amyloidosis represents a group of diseases in which progressive deposition of insoluble, aggregated fibrils occurs in various tissues that leads to organ dysfunction and death.
- It is a rare disorder occurring at an incidence of 9 per million per year, about 1/5 times as common as MM.
- In light chain (AL) amyloidosis, the fibrils are derived from Ig light chains secreted by clonal plasma cells.
- Fibrils composed of fragments of serum amyloid A (SAA) protein (a major acute-phase reactant protein produced predominantly by hepatocytes) are found in reactive systemic amyloidosis (AA). AA amyloidosis can occur in a variety of chronic inflammatory or infectious conditions, such as rheumatoid arthritis, inflammatory bowel diseases, and osteomyelitis.
- Hereditary systemic amyloidosis result from mutations in a specific protein, and comprise a group of extremely rare autosomal dominant disorders. Transthyretin (TTR) amyloidosis is the most common heritable form of amyloidosis and usually affects the nerves (familial amyloid polyneuropathy) and heart. Non-neuropathic amyloidosis (Ostertag type amyloidosis) results from mutations in the genes encoding lysozyme, fibrinogen A alpha-chain, apolipoprotein A1 and A2, cystatin C and gelsolin, and usually affects the kidney, liver and heart.
- Senile systemic amyloidosis occurs in up to 25% of the elderly population. It is characterized by the deposition of normal wild-type transthyretin (TTR) derived amyloid fibrils in the heart.
- AL amyloidosis represents the most common form of systemic amyloidosis and will be discussed below.

B. Clinical features of AL amyloidosis
Signs and symptoms
- The spectrum of presentation can be diverse, and a high index of suspicion is required for prompt diagnosis.
- AL amyloidosis should be suspected in patients presenting with nephrotic range proteinuria (mainly albuminuria, associated with amyloid deposition

(a)

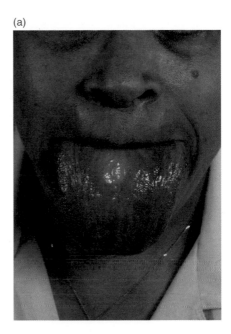

(b)

Figure 22.7 Clinical features of amyloidosis.
(a) Enlarged tongue (macroglossia);
(b) Periorbital purpura ("raccoon eyes").
© Mayo Foundation for Medical Education
and Research. All rights reserved.

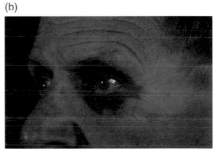

predominantly in the glomerulus), paresthesias, restrictive cardiomyopathy, hepatomegaly, peripheral edema, dyspnea, orthostatic hypotension, fatigue, weight loss, macroglossia and periorbital purpura (hallmark signs, Figure 22.7), in the presence of an M protein in serum or urine.
- The kidney, heart, nerves and liver are most commonly affected.
- Approximately 10% to 15% of MM patients can develop overt AL amyloidosis, either concurrent with the diagnosis of MM or during the course of their disease.
- MM patients with light chain MM and/or lambda light chain isotype may be at a higher risk of developing AL amyloidosis.

C. Laboratory findings
- The diagnosis of AL amyloidosis requires documentation of positive amyloid staining on a tissue biopsy (subcutaneous fat pad, bone marrow or organ) and evidence of a clonal plasma cell proliferative process.

- Further workup includes CBC, complete metabolic profile including liver function tests, and a 24-hour urine collection.
- Findings of septal or ventricular hypertrophy and diastolic dysfunction on the echocardiogram, a low voltage in limb leads and conduction abnormalities on electrocardiogram, and/or a high serum concentration of BNP, NT-proBNP and troponins (I and T) are frequently observed in patients with cardiac involvement from AL amyloidosis.

D. Treatment of AL amyloidosis

- The treatment of AL amyloidosis is aimed at the eradication of the underlying plasma cell clone to suppress the production of the amyloidogenic monoclonal light chain with the goal of improving organ function over time.
- The degree of cardiac involvement is the most important predictor of outcome in AL amyloidosis patients.
- HDT/AHCT is a commonly used and effective treatment that produces a high rate of hematologic and organ response. The transplant related mortality (TRM) with AHCT in AL amyloidosis is approximately 13%, significantly higher than seen in MM, and is often attributed to the presence of underlying cardiac involvement.
- The combination of dexamethasone with melphalan or thalidomide or lenalidomide or cyclophosphamide/thalidomide, and bortezomib can be used in patients who are considered ineligible for transplant.
- In rare circumstances, a heart transplantation or pacemaker insertion may be considered in AL patients with cardiac involvement.

VII. POEMS syndrome

A. Introduction

- POEMS syndrome (osteosclerotic myeloma) is a paraneoplastic syndrome associated with an underlying monoclonal gammopathy.
- Considerable elevation of pro-angiogenic and pro-inflammatory cytokines is seen. The production of VEGF (dominant driving cytokine in POEMS) is stimulated by both IL-1 beta and IL-6; and its levels in plasma and serum are found to correlate with disease activity.
- It is characterized by the constellation of **p**olyneuropathy, **o**rganomegaly, **e**ndocrinopathy, **M** protein and **s**kin changes.
- The diagnosis requires the presence of a monoclonal plasma cell disorder (usually lambda light chain type), peripheral neuropathy and at least one of the following seven features: osteosclerotic bone lesions, Castleman's disease, organomegaly, endocrinopathy (excluding diabetes mellitus or hypothyroidism), edema, typical skin changes and papilledema.

B. Clinical features

Signs and symptoms

- The peak incidence is seen in the 5th and 6th decades of life.

- Peripheral neuropathy often dominates the clinical picture, and muscle weakness is more marked than sensory loss. Clubbing, weight loss, pulmonary hypertension may also be seen.
- Unlike patients with MM, Bence Jones proteinuria, renal insufficiency, and hypercalcemia are uncommon.

C. Laboratory findings
- The size of the M-protein is small, and the bone marrow usually contains <5% BMPCs.
- Increased levels of proangiogenic and proinflammatory cytokines, especially VEGF are seen and correlate with disease activity.
- Solitary or multiple sclerotic bone lesions are observed on skeletal survey in approximately 95% patients.

D. Treatment
- Radiation therapy has been used effectively for localized lesions; alkylator based therapy or systemic therapy with HDT and AHCT can be used for widespread bone lesions.
- Novel therapies such as bevacizumab (monoclonal antibody against VEGF), bortezomib, thalidomide and lenalidomide have been used with variable efficacy.
- Typically, the disease runs a chronic course; median survival was 13.8 years in a series of 99 patients with POEMS syndrome (independent of the number of syndrome features, bone lesions, or plasma cells at diagnosis).
- Respiratory features such as the presence of cough and respiratory muscle weakness predict a poorer prognosis.

VIII. Waldenström macroglobulinemia

A. Introduction
- Waldenström macroglobulinemia (WM) is a rare malignant lymphoproliferative disorder characterized by the marrow accumulation of clonal lymphoplasmacytic cells that produce IgM M protein. WM is part of a category termed lymphoplasmacytic lymphoma, and includes the majority of patients with this disorder. The median age at diagnosis is 63 years; WM is more prevalent in the Caucasians.

B. Clinical features
Signs and symptoms
- Patients with WM present with fatigue, weight loss, clinical manifestations of hyperviscosity, fever or night sweats, and peripheral neuropathy.
- Physical examination can reveal lymphadenopathy and hepatosplenomegaly.

C. Laboratory findings

- Presence of IgM M spike in the γ or β region. The bone marrow biopsy demonstrates infiltration by lymphoplasmacytic cells.
- Anemia, and rouleau formation on peripheral blood smear is common. The mean corpuscular volume and reticulocyte count should be evaluated to assess autoimmune hemolysis.
- The serum viscosity is usually increased above normal.

D. Treatment

- Plasmapheresis is required when patients develop symptomatic hyperviscosity syndrome.
- Oral alkylator (chlorambucil), nucleoside analogs (fludarabine or cladribine), rituximab (monoclonal antibody against B lymphocytes), and bortezomib are used for treatment of WM. Asymptomatic patients should be observed.

IX. Plasma cell leukemia

A. Introduction

Plasma cell leukemia (PCL) is a rare but aggressive form of plasma cell dyscrasia characterized by the proliferation of plasma cells in peripheral blood and bone marrow, associated with rapid progression and a poor prognosis. It can either develop spontaneously (*de novo* or primary PCL; 60%) or evolve as a leukemic transformation in patients with MM (secondary PCL; 40%).

B. Clinical features

Signs and symptoms

PCL has a more aggressive clinical presentation than MM, and is associated with a higher frequency of extramedullary involvement, anemia, thrombocytopenia, hepatosplenomegaly, lymphadenopathy, and renal failure.

C. Laboratory findings

In addition to a bone marrow aspiration and SPEP and UPEP with immunofixation, a peripheral smear should be performed in order to establish a diagnosis of PCL. The diagnosis requires the presence of at least 2000/µL circulating plasma cells for a blood leukocyte count of >10,000/µL or 20% circulating plasma cells for <10,000 leukocytes/µL in the peripheral blood.

D. Treatment

Treatment with conventional chemotherapeutic agents yields a poor survival of a few months. However, emerging data suggest some improvement in survival with use of SCT and/or novel agents, especially with bortezomib therapy.

Further reading

Blade J, Kyle RA. Nonsecretory myeloma, immunoglobulin D myeloma, and plasma cell leukemia. Hematol Oncol Clin North Am 1999;13:1259–72.

Dispenzieri A, Kyle RA, Lacy MQ, et al. POEMS syndrome: definitions and long-term outcome. Blood 2003;101:2496–2506.

Durie BG, Salmon SE. A clinical staging system for multiple myeloma. Correlation of measured myeloma cell mass with presenting clinical features, response to treatment, and survival. Cancer 1975;36:842–54.

Finnegan DP, Kettle P, Drake M, et al. Bortezomib is effective in primary plasma cell leukemia. Leuk Lymphoma 2006;47:1670–73.

Fonseca R, Bailey RJ, Ahmann GJ, et al. Genomic abnormalities in monoclonal gammopathy of undetermined significance. Blood 2002;100:1417–24.

Gertz MA. Managing plasma cell leukemia. Leuk Lymphoma 2007;48:5–6.

Greipp PR, San Miguel J, Durie BG, et al. International staging system for multiple myeloma. J Clin Oncol 2005;23:3412–20.

Jemal A, Siegel R, Ward E, Hao Y, Xu J, Thun MJ. Cancer statistics, 2009. CA Cancer J Clin 2009;59:225–49.

Kristinsson SY, Fears TR, Gridley G, et al. Deep vein thrombosis after monoclonal gammopathy of undetermined significance and multiple myeloma. Blood 2008;112: 3582–6.

Kumar SK, Rajkumar SV, Dispenzieri A, et al. Improved survival in multiple myeloma and the impact of novel therapies. Blood 2008;111:2516–20.

Kumar SK, Therneau TM, Gertz MA, et al. Clinical course of patients with relapsed multiple myeloma. Mayo Clin Proc 2004;79:867–74.

Kyle RA, Gertz MA, Witzig TE, et al. Review of 1027 patients with newly diagnosed multiple myeloma. Mayo Clin Proc 2003;78:21–33.

Kyle RA, Remstein ED, Therneau TM, et al. Clinical course and prognosis of smoldering (asymptomatic) multiple myeloma. N Engl J Med 2007;356:2582–90.

Kyle RA, Therneau TM, Rajkumar SV, et al. A long-term study of prognosis in monoclonal gammopathy of undetermined significance. N Engl J Med 2002;346:564–9.

Kyle RA, Therneau TM, Rajkumar SV, et al. Prevalence of monoclonal gammopathy of undetermined significance. N Engl J Med 2006;354:1362–9.

Landgren O, Kyle RA, Pfeiffer RM, et al. Monoclonal gammopathy of undetermined significance (MGUS) precedes multiple myeloma: a prospective study. Blood 2009.

Madan S, Dispenzieri A, Lacy MQ, et al. Clinical features and treatment response of light chain (AL) amyloidosis diagnosed in patients with previous diagnosis of multiple myeloma. Mayo Clin Proc 2010;85:232–8.

Melton LJ 3rd, Rajkumar SV, Khosla S, Achenbach SJ, Oberg AL, Kyle RA. Fracture risk in monoclonal gammopathy of undetermined significance. J Bone Miner Res 2004;19: 25–30.

Musto P, Rossini F, Gay F, et al. Efficacy and safety of bortezomib in patients with plasma cell leukemia. Cancer 2007;109:2285–90.

Noel P, Kyle RA. Plasma cell leukemia: an evaluation of response to therapy. Am J Med 1987;83:1062–8.

Rajkumar SV, Kyle RA, Therneau TM, et al. Serum free light chain ratio is an independent risk factor for progression in monoclonal gammopathy of undetermined significance. Blood 2005;106:812–17.

Sallah S, Husain A, Wan J, Vos P, Nguyen NP. The risk of venous thromboembolic disease in patients with monoclonal gammopathy of undetermined significance. Ann Oncol 2004;15:1490–94.

Skinner M, Sanchorawala V, Seldin DC, et al. High-dose melphalan and autologous stem-cell transplantation in patients with AL amyloidosis: an 8-year study. Ann Intern Med 2004;140:85–93.

Srkalovic G, Cameron MG, Rybicki L, Deitcher SR, Kattke-Marchant K, Hussein MA. Monoclonal gammopathy of undetermined significance and multiple myeloma are associated with an increased incidence of venothromboembolic disease. Cancer 2004;101:558–66.

Turesson I, Velez R, Kristinsson SY, Landgren O. Patterns of multiple myeloma during the past 5 decades: stable incidence rates for all age groups in the population but rapidly changing age distribution in the clinic. Mayo Clin Proc 2010;85:225–30.

23 Pediatric Hematology

Sanjay P. Ahuja

Rainbow Babies and Children's Hospital, Case Western Reserve University, Cleveland, OH, USA

I. Introduction

Pediatric hematology has contributed much of the pioneering work in hematopoeisis, granulocyte, and platelet function.

II. Development of hematopoiesis

1. The erythrocytes produced by the human fetus are different from the erythrocytes of an older child. Fetal erythrocytes have different hemoglobins, different membrane properties and a significantly shorter lifespan. These differences are necessary for the fetus to adapt to intra- and extra-uterine life. In various pathologic states, erythrocytes bearing some of the properties of the fetal erythrocyte appear in the circulation.
2. Embryonic and fetal hematopoiesis can be divided in to three periods: mesoblastic, hepatic, and myeloid. The mesoblastic period is predominantly in the yolk sac during the first trimester. The hepatic period predominates during the second trimester. The myeloid period, where the bone marrow takes over hematopoiesis predominates during the third trimester.
   A. All blood cells are derived from the mesenchyme or the embryonic connective tissue. The earliest signs of blood formation can be detected by the 14th day of gestation. The first blood cells produced belong to the red cell series. They arise as a result of either the primitive megaloblastic erythropoiesis or the definitive normoblastic erythropoiesis. By the 10th week of gestation, normoblastic erythropoiesis is responsible for 90% of the erythrocytic cells. Hematopoiesis in the yolk sac or the mesoblastic period typically ceases by 10–12 weeks of gestation.

Concise Guide to Hematology, First Edition. Edited by Alvin H. Schmaier, Hillard M. Lazarus.
© 2012 Blackwell Publishing Ltd. Published 2012 by Blackwell Publishing Ltd.

B. Blood formation begins in the liver by 5th to 6th week of gestation. From 3rd to the 6th fetal month, liver becomes the chief organ of hematopoiesis. During this period, hematopoietic precursors can also be found in the spleen, thymus, and the lymph nodes.

C. Medullary hematopoiesis begins during the fourth to fifth fetal month. By 30th gestational week, marrow cavity is maximally cellular. The volume of the marrow cavity occupied by hematopoeitic activity, though continues to increase until term. During the last 3 months, bone marrow is the predominant site of blood formation whereas the hepatic site continues to decline.

D. At birth, marrow tissue continue to grow, though the cellularity does not. Any increase in cell production during times of stress then happens with an expansion of hematopoietic tissue outside of the marrow giving rise to "extramedullary hematopoiesis", as seen in severe erythroblastosis fetalis or hemolytic disease of the newborn in the form of hepatosplenomegaly, or in the form of "hemolytic facies", distortion of facial bones (frontal bossing, maxillary prominence), seen in β-thalassemia major.

E. Umbilical cord blood is rich in bone marrow progenitor cells and contains multipotential stem cells. The number of hematopoietic progenitors in cord blood are sufficient for a successful hematopoietic cell transplant. Human umbilical cord blood has been successfully used for hematopoietic reconstitution in patients with malignancies of the hematologic system, storage disorders, Fanconi's anemia or other bone marrow failure syndromes, as well as several immunodeficiencies (see Chapter 26).

III. Hemoglobin synthesis in the fetus and the newborn

1. The major form of adult hemoglobin (Hb) is Hb A1 ($\alpha_2\beta_2$), whereas in the embryonic and fetal stages, different forms of hemoglobins exist

A. Within 2 weeks of gestation, primitive erythroblasts in the yolk sac are already synthesizing the most primitive Hb, Gower 1 {ζ(zeta)$_2$, epsilon(ϵ)$_2$}.

B. Synthesis of the α and γ chains begins in the yolk sac by 4-8 weeks gestation. Synthesis of the ζ and ϵ chains decreases as that of the α and γ chains increases.

C. By 6 weeks gestation, Hb F ($\alpha_2\gamma_2$) has become the major Hb of fetal life. By the time the fetus has a crown-rump length of about 30 mm, Hb F represents 50% of the total Hb, and at a length of 50 mm it forms more than 90% of the hemoglobin.

D. At birth, term infants typically have 50–95% Hb F and the remainder Hb A.

E. By 6 months to a year of life, Hb F declines to 1–2% and then persist at those levels throughout life.

2. The switch from fetal to adult Hb is delayed in infants who are small for gestational age, have chronic intrauterine hypoxia, or have been born to diabetic mothers.

IV. Erythropoiesis after birth

1. At birth, tissue oxygen levels increase, resulting in a marked decrease in the level of erythropoietin in the plasma. Production of red blood cells and hemoglobin decreases during the first week of life. In healthy term infants, no measurable decrease in hemoglobin values occurs during the first week of life. Term infants develop physiologic anemia by 8–10 weeks of life with a nadir Hb of 11 g/dL, whereas preterm infants nadir at 4–6 weeks with a Hb of 9–10 g/dL (Table 23.1).

   The lifespan of RBCs in term infants is shorter than that of the red cells of an adult. The lifespan is 60–70 days in term infants, 35–50 days in premature infants, whereas it is 120 days in an adult. Neonatal red cells are typically macrocytic with a mean MCV of 100 fL. The neonatal RBC also has lower cell hemoglobin (MCHC) concentrations than do adult RBCs. The macrocytosis decreases as age progresses reaching adult levels by 1 year of age (Table 23.1). Premature infants have more prominent macrocytosis probably as a result of immature splenic function.

2. The neonatal red cell membrane is slightly more resistant to osmotic lysis than those of adults. About 14% of the red cells from neonates show morphologic distortions such as spherocytes and poikilocytes of various types, whereas this percentage is only 3% in an adult. The RBC membrane is also different from an immunologic perspective. In the ABO system, the A and B antigen sites are weakly expressed on the neonatal red cell membrane and in the Ii antigen system, the I antigen is either weak or absent. The Ii RBC system is a minor antigen in contrast to the major ABO and Rh.

3. Hemoglobin and hematocrit values in neonates can differ based on the site of sampling. Capillary samples obtained by a heel or toe stick generally have a higher hemoglobin concentration than do simultaneously obtained venous samples. The average Hb difference between the two methods is approximately 3.5 g/dL but could be as high as 10 g/dL. In virtually all infants, the capillary/venous hematocrit ratio is also greater than 1 and gradually decreases with increasing gestational age.

V. Myelopoeisis in infancy and childhood

1. The number of circulating leukocytes as well as neutrophils is elevated after birth in both full-term and premature infants. The mean WBC count at birth is $18.1 \times 10^3/\mu L$ with 61% neutrophils and less than 15% bands. By the first month of life, mean WBC count is $10.8 \times 10^3/\mu L$, with 35% neutrophils and 56% lymphocytes. The relative lymphocytosis persists until

Table 23.1 Normal hematologic values in children

Age	Hemoglobin (g/dL) Mean:	-2 SD	Hematocrit (%) Mean:	-2 SD	Red cell count (10 ^{12}/L) Mean:	-2 SD	MCV (fL) Mean:	-2 SD	MCH (pg) Mean:	-2 SD	MCHC (g/dL) Mean:	-2 SD
Birth (cord blood)	16.5	13.5	51	42	4.7	3.9	108	98	34	31	33	30
1 to 3 days (capillary)	18.5	14.5	56	45	5.3	4.0	108	95	34	31	33	29
1 week	17.5	13.5	54	42	5.1	3.9	107	88	34	28	33	28
2 weeks	16.5	12.5	51	39	4.9	3.6	105	86	34	28	33	28
1 month	14.0	10.0	43	31	4.2	3.0	104	85	34	28	33	29
2 months	11.5	9.0	35	28	3.8	2.7	96	77	30	26	33	29
3 to 6 months	11.5	9.5	35	29	3.8	3.1	91	74	30	25	33	30
0.5 to 2 years	12.0	10.5	36	33	4.5	3.7	78	70	27	23	33	30
2 to 6 years	12.5	11.5	37	34	4.6	3.9	81	75	27	24	34	31
6 to 12 years	13.5	11.5	40	35	4.6	4.0	86	77	29	25	34	31
12 to 18 years Female	14.0	12.0	41	36	4.6	4.1	90	78	30	25	34	31
Male	14.5	13.0	43	37	4.9	4.5	88	78	30	25	34	31
18 to 49 years Female	14.0	12.0	41	36	4.6	4.0	90	80	30	26	34	31
Male	15.5	13.5	47	41	5.2	4.5	90	80	30	26	34	31

These data have been compiled from several sources. Emphasis is given to studies employing electronic counters and to the selection of populations that are likely to exclude individuals with iron deficiency. The mean ± 2 SD can be expected to include 95% of the observation in a normal population.

(Reproduced with permission from Nathan and Oski's Hematology of Infancy and Childhood, 6th edn, Vol. 2 (2003) Appendix 11, Appendix 26, and Appendix 34, pages 1841–13, Saunders-Elsevier.)

4–6 years of age. By age 6 years, WBC count declines to a mean value of $8.5 \times 10^3/\mu L$, with 53% neutrophils and 39% lymphocytes—adult values (Table 23.2).

2. The lower limit for normal neutrophil counts (neutrophil and band cells) is 1000 cells/μL in Caucasian infants between 2 weeks and 1 year of age. After infancy, the corresponding value is 1500 cells/μL. In African-Americans, the neutrophil counts are about 200–600 cells/μL lower relative to counts in Caucasians.

Table 23.2 Reference ranges for leukocyte counts in children

Age	Total leukocytes Mean	Range	Neutrophils Mean	Range	%	Lymphocytes Mean	Range	%	Monocytes Mean	%	Eosinophils Mean	%
Birth	18.1	9.0–30.0	11.0	6.0–26.0	61	5.5	2.0–11.0	31	1.1	6	0.4	2
12 hours	22.8	13.0–38.0	15.5	6.0–28.0	68	5.5	2.0–11.0	24	1.2	5	0.5	2
24 hours	18.9	9.4–34.0	11.5	5.0–21.0	61	5.8	2.0–11.5	31	1.1	6	0.5	2
1 week	12.2	5.0–21.0	5.5	1.5–10.0	45	5.0	2.0–17.0	41	1.1	9	0.5	4
2 weeks	11.4	5.0–20.0	4.5	1.0–9.5	40	5.5	2.0–17.0	48	1.0	9	0.4	3
1 month	10.8	5.0–19.5	3.8	1.0–9.0	35	6.0	2.5–16.5	56	0.7	7	0.3	3
6 months	11.9	5.0–17.5	3.8	1.0–8.5	32	7.3	4.0–13.5	61	0.6	5	0.3	3
1 year	11.4	6.0–17.5	3.5	1.5–8.5	31	7.0	4.0–10.5	61	0.6	5	0.3	3
2 years	10.6	6.0–17.0	3.5	1.5–8.5	33	6.3	3.0–9.5	59	0.5	5	0.3	3
4 years	9.1	5.5–15.5	3.8	1.5–8.5	42	4.5	2.0–8.0	50	0.5	5	0.3	3
6 years	8.5	5.0–14.5	4.3	1.5–8.0	51	3.5	1.5–7.0	42	0.4	5	0.2	3
8 years	8.3	4.5–13.5	4.4	1.5–8.0	53	3.3	1.5–6.8	39	0.4	4	0.2	2
10 years	8.1	4.5–13.	4.4	1.8–8.0	54	3.1	1.5–6.5	38	0.4	4	0.2	2
16 years	7.8	4.5–13.0	4.4	1.8–8.0	57	2.8	1.2–5.2	35	0.4	5	0.2	3
21 years	7.4	4.5–11.0	4.4	1.8–7.7	59	2.5	1.0–4.8	34	0.3	4	0.2	3

Numbers of leukocytes are in thousands per mm^3, ranges are estimates of 95% confidence limits, and percentages refer to differential counts. Neutrophils include band cells at all ages and a small number of metamyelocytes and myelocytes in the first few day of life. (Reproduced with permission from Nathan and Oski's Hematology of Infancy and Childhood, 6th edition, Vol 2 (2003) Appendix 11, Appendix 26, and Appendix 34 Pages 1841–1853, Saunders-Elsevier.)

VI. Platelets in infancy and childhood

1. Platelet count at birth may vary between $100–300 \times 10^3/\mu L$. Any platelet count less than $100 \times 10^3/\mu L$ is considered abnormal for full term as well as preterm infants.
2. After infancy, the normal platelet count of $150–400 \times 10^3/\mu L$ is similar to that of adults.

VII. Coagulation system in infancy and childhood

1. The development of the hemostatic system is a dynamic process which is age dependent. The neonate manifests physiologic alterations of this developing hemostatic system. Therefore normal values of the coagulation protein factors are unique in this population by virtue of changes that occur from prenatal period to about 6 months of age.
2. A number of factors are responsible for the alterations of the hemostatic system seen at birth and for the few months after. There is decreased hepatic synthesis of coagulation factors, increased rates of clearance, and the synthesis of fetal forms of many factors. For this reason, age-appropriate reference ranges are necessary to adequately interpret coagulation results in preterm and term neonates (Table 23.3).

Table 23.3 Reference values for coagulation tests in healthy, full-term newborns compared with normal adults

Test	Newborns	Adults	P<
PT (sec)	13.1 ± 0.9	11.9 ± 0.6	0.0001
APTT (sec)	35 ± 4.5	28.8 ± 2.7	0.0001
Platelets (×10^9/L)	214 ± 55	258 ± 66	0.0001
Fibrinogen (mg/dL)	251 ± 51	262 ± 44	NS
Factor II (%)	73 ± 7	100 ± 15	0.0001
Factor V (%)	93 ± 13	98 ± 19	NS
Factor VII (%)	88 ± 12	95 ± 18	0.005
Factor VIII (%)	113 ± 38	92 ± 21	0.0001
Factor IX (%)	86 ± 18	94 ± 16	0.003
Factor X (%)	72 ± 10	97 ± 15	0.0001
Hematocrit (%)	59 ± 3.0	44 ± 2.5	0.0001

Data were obtained in 71 newborns and 100 adults and expressed as mean ± SD. Samples were collected with a constant anticoagulant-to-blood ratio, based on a previous determination of hematocrit.

(Reproduced with permission from Nathan and Oski's Hematology of Infancy and Childhood, 6th edn, Vol 2 (2003) Appendix 11, Appendix 26, and Appendix 34, pages 1841–53, Saunders-Elsevier.)

3. Despite striking differences in the levels of individual components of the hemostatic system, the neonatal coagulation is equal to or somewhat more robust than that observed in adults. The balance of the coagulation system is more weighted towards hypercoagulability and potential thrombosis in the sick infant.

4. Coagulation proteins are synthesized by the fetus and present in measurable quantities by approximately 10 weeks of gestational age. Values of vitamin K-dependent factors, prekallikrein, factor XII, high molecular weight kininogen, and fibrinolytic and anticoagulant factors typically normalize by 6 months of age.

   A. PT and APTT is usually prolonged in the neonatal period secondary to physiologic deficiency of vitamin K-dependent factors at birth. However, the thrombin time is normal.

   B. Concentrations of fibrinogen, FV, and FXIII are similar to adult values at birth. In contrast, levels of FVIII and von Willebrand factor (vWF) are increased in the neonatal period. The mean activity of several factors (II, VII, IX, X, XI, XII) is slightly lower throughout childhood (Table 23.3).

   C. Plasma concentrations of antithrombin and heparin cofactor II are decreased at birth, whereas plasma concentrations of α2 macroglobulin are increased at birth and throughout childhood. Plasma concentrations of protein C are decreased at birth, with levels usually less than those reported for heterozygote-deficient adults. Although total amounts of protein S are decreased at birth, the overall activity remains similar to adults. Levels of protein C do not reach adult range until puberty.

VIII. Disorders of fetomaternal unit causing hematologic manifestations in the neonate

1. **Placental insufficiency:** The most common causes of placental insufficiency resulting in interuterine growth retardation (IUGR) are pregnancy-induced hypertension, pre-eclampsia, eclampsia, and the HELLP syndrome (hemolysis, elevated liver enzymes, and low platelets). Disruption of placenta causes hematopoeitic dysfunction and its severity is proportional to the degree of placental insufficiency and fetal growth restriction.

   A. Mild placental dysfunction with tissue hypoxia is associated with increased erythropoietin levels and polycythemia. Severe placental vasculopathy seen in babies with severe IUGR. This vasculopathy causes decreased erythropoiesis due to abnormal erythroblast function leading to fetal anemia. RBC destruction from microangiopathic injury in the placenta is an additional mechanism of fetal anemia.

   B. The normal nucleated RBCs (nRBCs) count in healthy term neonates is variable but rarely exceeds 8 nRBCs/100 white blood cells. An elevated nRBC count is associated with placental insufficiency and fetal stress, though it is a non-specific marker and can be seen in other forms of fetal/neonatal stress such as Rh isoimmunization (clarify if you mean hemolytic disease of the newborn), fetal hemorrhage, maternal diabetes mellitus and respiratory distress syndrome (RDS).

   C. About 40–50% of neonates born to mothers with placental insufficiency are neutropenic; the cause is decreased neutrophil production due to a placental inhibitor present in cord blood. Even though neutrophil counts below 500/cubic mm are frequently seen, there does not appear to be a significant risk of infection. The neutropenia usually resolves in less than 72 hours, but can last up to 5 days.

   D. Growth-restricted neonates born to mothers with placental insufficiency can also have thrombocytopenia, especially if the mother has HELLP syndrome. This phenomenon is more common in preterm infants and is caused by decreased platelet production.

2. **Abnormal fetomaternal cell traffic:** The placental barrier though protective, is not completely effective. The barrier also changes during pregnancy. The maternal proteins do not traverse the barrier with the exception of IgG, which can cross over from the mother to the fetus. Certain microbes such as Rubella, cytomegalovirus, are able to cross the barrier as well.

   Clinically important fetomaternal transfusions occur in up to 50% of all pregnancies, where some fetal cells can be demonstrated in the maternal circulation. Fetal-to-maternal hemorrhage is most common after traumatic diagnostic amniocentesis or external cephalic version before delivery, but it can also be seen after maternal abdominal trauma, with placental tumors, or spontaneously. They can present as neonatal anemia when associated with chronic blood loss, or as fetal hypotension and intrauterine demise when associated with acute blood loss. Fetomaternal transfusions can also result in alloimmunization of the mother against paternal antigens present on fetal blood cells. The transplacental transfer of these maternal antibodies in to the fetus can cause destruction of the fetal blood cells carrying the cognate antigen. Hematologic consequences of this abnormal antibody traffic are several:

A. **Hemolytic disease of the newborn (HDN, erythroblastosis fetalis):**

  (a) Overview. HDN is classically seen in a setting of blood group incompatibility between the mother and her fetus for markers of the Rh system, which includes five antigens: C, D, E, c, and e. HDN is also seen with ABO or minor blood group incompatibilities between the mother and her fetus. Rh-mediated HDN affects about 1 in 1200 pregnancies. In approximately 97 % of cases, erythroblastosis fetalis is caused by anti-Rh(D) antibody, with the remaining 3% of cases caused by a variety of other antibodies to less common RBC groups.

  (b) Pathophysiology. Passage of fetal Rh(D) positive RBCs across the placental barrier to an Rh-negative mother is the primary method of maternal alloimmunization. Feto-maternal bleeding at the time of delivery is the major cause of sensitization in Rh-mediated HDN. About 10–15% of Rh negative women are sensitized while bearing children of Rh positive men. The disparity between the numbers of incompatible versus allo-immunized pairs are due to:

   (i) Threshold effect in fetomaternal transfusions, where a certain amount of the immunizing blood cell antigen is required to activate the immune system. In ABO incompatibility, transfer of 0.1 mL of blood leads to sensitization in 3% of women as compared to 60% of women with transfer of 5 mL of blood.

   (ii) Type of antibody response—IgG antibodies are more efficiently transferred across the placenta to the fetus. In Rh-mediated HDN, IgM antibodies are produced initially which are replaced by IgG antibodies. In future pregnancies, these IgG antibodies can cross the placenta easily causing more severe disease as the number of pregnancies rise. Rh-related HDN is therefore usually a disease of the second and subsequent pregnancies.

   (iii) Differential immunogenicity of blood group antigens: hemolysis due to anti-A is more common (1 in 150 births) than due to anti-B antibodies in ABO HDN.

   (iv) Differences in maternal immune response: even though 15–25% of all maternal/fetal pairs are ABO-incompatible, ABO HDN occurs in about 1% of these pairs that have preexisting high-titer IgG antibodies.

  (c) **Clinical features:**

   (i) Anemia, mild to severe resulting from destruction of antibody coated RBCs, mainly in the spleen. Severe anemia can lead to cardiac dilatation, hypertrophy, and subsequent high-output failure, and ultimately hydrops fetalis, a dead fetus due to severe intrauterine anemia.

(ii) Jaundice (indirect hyperbilirubinemia) presenting during the first 24 hours. It may cause kernicterus, resulting from bilirubin deposition in the developing brain leading to reduced intellectual development.

(iii) Hepatosplenomegaly, as a result of compensatory extramedullary hematopoeisis.

(iv) Hypoalbuminemia and hepatic dysfunction leading to generalized edema, hydrops, and ultimately intrauterine death. Depending upon severity, stillbirth or delivery of a macerated fetus is also possible.

(v) Petechiae in severely affected infants. Hyporegenerative thrombocytopenia and neutropenia may occur during the first week. This is probably as a result of marrow exhaustion from chronic overstimulation.

(d) Laboratory findings

(i) Anemia with increased reticulocyte count.

(ii) Direct Coomb's test positive on fetal RBCs.

(iii) Increased nucleated RBCs, marked polychromasia, and aniso cytosis on peripheral smear.

(iv) Raised indirect serum bilirubin concentration.

(e) Management and prevention

(i) Both planned, careful prenatal monitoring and therapeutic intervention are needed for prevention and successful treatment of HDN. Mothers should be screened at their first antenatal visit for Rh and non-Rh antibodies. Rh negative women have to undergo determination of anti-Rh antibody titers to determine the degree of sensitization. Any titers above 1:16 or 1:32 are considered high risk for development of hydrops fetalis. Father's blood is tested for Rh zygosity.

(ii) Examination of amniotic fluid for spectrophotometric analysis of bilirubin is done to determine the most suitable time for delivery or to determine the indication for intrauterine fetal transfusion. Amniocentesis is indicated if (1) there is history of previous Rh disease severe enough to require an exchange transfusion or has caused stillbirth and (2) maternal titers of antibodies are between 1:8 to 1:64 or greater by indirect Coomb's test. Intensive maternal plasmapheresis antenatally using a continuous-flow cell separator can significantly reduce Rh antibody levels, reduce fetal hemolysis, and improve fetal survival in those mothers carrying highly sensitized Rh-positive fetuses.

(iii) Determination of fetal biophysical profile score, a criteria standard to determine if intrauterine intravascular transfusion

(IUIVT) should be performed, is done with the help of optical density of the amniotic fluid, ultrasound to assess hydrops, and amniotic phospholipid determination done to assess lung maturity. The fetal biophysical profile is a test scoring five fetal vital sign variables: fetal heart rate, fetal breathing, fetal movement, fetal tone, and amniotic fluid volume. If the biophysical profile estimates a severely affected fetus and the phospholipid estimations indicate marked immaturity, IUIVT should be carried out. IUIVT is the procedure of choice as compared to intraperitoneal transfusions.

(iv) The IUIVT procedure involves high resolution ultrasound guided fine needle insertion directly in to the umbilical cord to gain access to the intravascular space. Compatible Rh-negative RBCs are used for IUIVT. The risk of fetal loss with an IUIVT is about 2%.

(v) Modern neonatal care with rigorous attention to metabolic, ventilatory, and nutritional needs, and use of artificial surfactant delivered via inhalation has made successful deliveries possible with severe HDNs. The need for IUIVT and intraperitoneal transfusion is rarely, if ever, indicated.

(vi) Postnatally, the most frequent problem is hyperbilirubinemia. The umbilical cord blood is examined for Coomb's test, bilirubin, and Hb levels. A rapid increase in the bilirubin level of greater than 1.0 mg/dL/h and/or a bilirubin level approaching 20 mg/dL at any time in a full-term infant and 15 mg/dL in a preterm infant is an indication for exchange transfusion to prevent development of kernicterus. An exchange transfusion is done using 10–20 mL aliquots of group O (or ABO compatible) Rh-negative blood to replace twice the infant's blood volume. This procedure removes 50% of the anti-Rh antibody and can be repeated to keep the bilirubin below 20 mg/dL. A partial exchange transfusion or a double-volume exchange transfusion may be necessary to correct severe anemia in a hydropic infant at birth.

(vii) To prevent Rh-mediated HDN, routine administration of 300 µg of Rh immunoglobulin to all unsensitized Rh-negative mothers is recommended at 28 weeks of gestation and within 72 hours of delivery. It is also indicated for all unimmunized Rh-negative mothers who have undergone spontaneous or induced abortion, or a ruptured tubal pregnancy, or any event during pregnancy that may lead to transplacental hemorrhage. Antibody to Rh is infused to block any Rh positive blood that may have gotten into the maternal circulation and thus rear antibodies to the Rh antigen.

B. **Alloimmune neonatal neutropenia:**

   (a) Alloimmune neonatal neutropenia (ANN) is the neutrophil counterpart of HDN. Mother makes antibodies against paternal antigens (also present in the fetus) which cross the placenta and cause neutropenia in the fetus. These antibodies can be detected in up to 20% of pregnant and post partum women, but ANN occurs in only 0.2–2% of newborns. In the US, almost half of all cases of ANN are mediated by antibodies to HNA-1a, HNA-1b, or HNA-2a antigens.

   (b) Common presentations of ANN include delayed separation of the umbilical cord, mild skin infections, fever or pneumonia within the first 2 weeks of life. ANN can last up to 6 months, though usually resolves by 4–6 weeks. Recombinant human granulocyte colony stimulating factor (G-CSF) may be indicated for prolonged, severe neutropenia ($<500/mm^3$) or a severe infection.

C. **Neonatal alloimmune thrombocytopenia:**

   (a) Neonatal alloimmune thrombocytopenia (NAIT) is the platelet counterpart of HDN. NAIT occurs in approximately 1 in 2000 live births. Maternal antibodies directed against fetal platelet antigens lead to increased platelet destruction. The commonest antigens causing fetomaternal incompatibility in almost 95% of the cases are HPA-1a, HPA-5b, and HPA-15b either singly, or in combination.

   (b) It is characterized by marked thrombocytopenia in the fetus and the neonate with platelet counts as low as $10 \times 10^3/\mu L$. Infants affected with NAIT are born to mothers with a normal platelet count as compared to infants born with ITP (NITP) to mothers with immune thrombocytopenia.

   (c) NAIT is associated with mortality of about 15%, mostly due to the occurrence of intracranial hemorrhage which can occur even *in utero*. Daily ultrasound of the newborn's brain should be carried out during the acute phase to detect intracranial hemorrhage. Bleeding from the umbilicus, or gastrointestinal or renal tract may also occur.

   (d) Treatment depends on the platelet count and symptoms, and can include transfusion of random donor platelets or HPA-1a negative platelets or maternal platelets. The antigen system HPA-1a accounts for approximately 75% of the cases of NAIT. As maternal antibodies against fetal HPA-1a antigen is causing platelet destruction, transfusion of HPA-1a negative platelets can help stop this destruction and increase platelet count. IVIG and/or corticosteroids can also be used to reduce platelet destruction. IVIG flood the reticuloendothelial cell system with immunoglobulin reducing clearance of antibody-coated RBCs. Weekly IVIG may also be used antenatally for the mother from midgestation until birth. Unfortunately, antiplatelet antibody titers in the mother during pregnancy cannot be used to predict whether an individual fetus will be affected.

5. **Transplacental transfer of maternal autoantibodies:** Transplacentally transmitted maternal autoantibodies against RBC, neutrophil, and platelet antigens can cause destruction of 1 or more of these cell lines in the fetus. Autoantibodies against hematopoietic lineages are frequently of the IgG1 subclass, which are transmitted to the fetus with high efficiency.

(a) **Neonatal autoimmune hemolytic anemia** is seen in infants born to mothers with autoimmune hemolytic anemia, SLE, rheumatoid arthritis, or other immune disorders. It is a self limited condition and resolves within a few weeks to months. It is diagnosed by a positive Coomb's test in the mother and the infant. Treatment with steroids may be needed to decrease the severity of the illness.

(b) **Neonatal autoimmune neutropenia** is caused by transplacental transmission of maternal antineutrophil autoantibodies. Both mom and the baby are neutropenic. It is an asymptomatic condition and treatment with IVIG and/or G-CSF may be needed only in severe cases or in infants with an active infection.

(c) **Neonatal autoimmune thrombocytopenia** (NITP) is milder than NAIT and carries a low risk (<1 %) of intracranial hemorrhage or bleeding at other sites. It is seen in 10 % of infants born to mothers with ITP, SLE, or other immune disorders. Symptomatic infants can be effectively treated with IVIG.

Further reading

Andrew A, et al. Maturation of the hemostatic system during childhood. Blood 1998;80(8).

Black LV, et al. Disorders of the fetomaternal unit: hematologic manifestations in the fetus and neonate. Semin Perinatol 2009;33;12–19.

Christensen RD. Hematologic Problems of the Neonate. Philadelphia, PA: Saunders, 2000.

Goodnight SH, et al. Disorders of Hemostasis and Thrombosis, 2nd edn. New York, NY: McGraw-Hill, 2001.

Nathan DG, et al. Nathan and Oski's Hematology of Infancy and Childhood, 6th edn. Philadelphia, PA: Saunders, 2003.

CHAPTER 24

24 Blood Banking

Lawrence Tim Goodnough

Stanford University Medical Center, Stanford, CA, USA

I. Introduction

Blood transfusion is the oldest and most frequently performed type of human tissue transplantation. Only relatively recently has transfusion become a standard therapy. Blood groups were first discovered in 1901 when Landsteiner showed, by cross-testing red cells and serum, that blood specimens from healthy people were not all the same. Anticoagulation of blood with citrate, first described in 1914, permitted storage of blood and so-called indirect transfusion. The first hospital blood bank in the United States was established in 1936. Systemic blood collection services developed during World War II. Subsequently, the most significant technologic advance occurred with the development of plastic bags, which allowed the evolution from transfusion of whole blood to component (red cells, plasma, and platelets) therapy, in which one blood unit from one donor can benefit many recipients.

II. Blood donation

A. Criteria for donation

Blood donations may be allogeneic (for another person), autologous (for later transfusion back to the patient), or directed (designated for a particular recipient). The Food and Drug Administration establishes criteria for acceptability of blood donors. These include measures to protect the donor's health (e.g., minimum hematocrit, minimum time between donations) and those to protect the recipient (e.g., donor history or risk factors for transmitting infectious diseases). Donors undergo a focused medical history, limited physical examination, and laboratory screening. For allogeneic (including directed) donation

---

Concise Guide to Hematology, First Edition. Edited by Alvin H. Schmaier, Hillard M. Lazarus.
© 2012 Blackwell Publishing Ltd. Published 2012 by Blackwell Publishing Ltd.

the hematocrit must exceed 38%, and donations may be no more frequent than every eight weeks. The exclusion of paid donors and the deferral of potential volunteer donors who have risk factors for infectious disease transmission along with laboratory testing of units donated, have been the most important factors in advancing blood safety.

Criteria for donation of autologous blood are less stringent, since autologous blood is used blood for the benefit of the donor (patient). Autologous blood may be donated every 3 days, up to 3 days prior to elective surgery. The patient's hematocrit must exceed 33% prior to each donation.

B. Components of the donation

A single blood donation is 450 ± 45 mL of whole blood. The anticoagulant is usually acid citrate dextrose and the ratio of anticoagulant to whole blood is 1 part to 6 parts. This is usually processed into components of red blood cells, plasma and platelets. Apheresis (the process of removing whole blood, separating out some portion and returning the rest to the donor) may also be used for blood component donation. Apheresis has less effect on blood volume, so a greater amount of the intended component can be collected from one donor. Red blood cells, platelets or plasma can be collected by apheresis. Leukocyte components that include granulocytes, mononuclear cells or hematopoietic progenitor cells are collected only by apheresis since a whole blood donation does not contain sufficient numbers of these cells to be therapeutically effective.

C. Donor testing

Blood donations are tested for markers of infectious diseases that may be transmitted by transfusion (Table 24.1).

These either are tests for antibodies, tests for viral antigens, or most recently tests for viral genetic material. Current estimates of the risk for virus transmission per unit of blood are 1 in 1.4 to 2.4 million for human immunodeficiency virus (HIV) and 1 in 872,000 to 1.7 million for hepatitis C.

Table 24.1 Infectious disease testing for blood donors

Hepatitis B surface antigen (HBsAg)
Hepatitis B core antibody
Hepatitis C virus (HCV) antibody
Human immunodeficiency virus (HIV-1 and HIV-2) antibody
HIV p24 antigen
Human T cell lymphotropic virus (HTLV-I and HTLV-II) antibody
Serologic test for syphilis
HIV and HCV genome (nucleic acid testing, NAT)
Cytomegalovirus (CMV) antibody
Bacterial culture testing

III. Blood storage

A. 2,3 DPG loss from stored RBCs

Blood components stored in the liquid state over 35–42 days undergo changes that affect the post-transfusion efficacy. Stored red cells lose 2,3-diphosphoglycerate (2,3 DPG) and also leak potassium. Although K^+ concentrations in the supernatant of stored red blood cells may reach 35 meq/dL, the total amount of extracellular K^+ in a unit is less than the daily requirement of an adult. It usually poses no problem except for transfusion of newborns. Loss of 2,3 DPG shifts the oxygen dissociation curve of the red cell to the left, so that after transfusion, stored red cells hold onto oxygen more tightly; levels of intracellular 2,3 DPG are restored in 6–12 hours, but until that time transfused red cells hold oxygen more tightly and therefore do little to increase oxygen delivery or affect oxygen consumption (VO_2) in peripheral tissues. Thus, any acute benefits perceived from red cell transfusion may be more related to changes in intravascular volume (and cardiac output) rather than oxygen delivery.

B. Irreversible storage lesion in red cells

This is the aging process similar to senescence *in vivo*. By the end of the storage period (35 or 42 days depending on the preservative solution) as much as 25% of transfused red cells are cleared post-transfusion from the circulation within 24 hours. The lack of deformability and presence of microaggregates in the microcirculation may explain, in part, some evidence that aged blood (>14 days of storage) may be associated with adverse outcomes in some patients such as those undergoing cardiac surgery.

C. Coagulation factors

Functional levels of the labile coagulation factors V and VIII gradually decrease during inventory of liquid plasma to about 50% of the initial value. If held at room temperature, factors V and VIII will begin to deteriorate after 4h. Other coagulation factors are less affected by storage. Although if plasma is stored at 4°C, C1 inhibitor becomes inactivated and factor XII autoactivates on the surface of the plastic bag leading to factor VII activation, *in vitro* thrombin formation, and bradykinin formation leading to hypotension upon infusion.

D. Platelets

Platelets must be stored at room temperature with constant gentle agitation to maintain hemostatic activity. During storage, platelets undergo a variety of changes including expression of activation markers, degranulation, and apoptosis-like events. These events result in lower post-transfusion survival of stored platelets and the release of soluble mediators that may cause transfusion reactions.

E. Leukocytes

Leukocytes in stored red cells and platelets also undergo activation during storage. These activities result in the release of cytokines and other biological response modifiers. These activation products can cause transfusion reactions and changes in the immune status of the recipient. Pyrogenic cytokines, such as interleukin-1 and tumor necrosis factor, also may cause febrile nonhemolytic reactions. Chemokines such as interleukin-8 may affect the function of circulating leukocyte populations and may cause impaired immune and inflammatory responses. Lipid mediators similar to platelet activating factor may prime neutrophils to respond briskly to secondary inflammatory stimuli, and may cause transfusion-related acute lung injury (TRALI, a transfusion-related acute lung injury due to pulmonary infiltrates from leukocyte antigen activation of complement) (see Chapter 25). Methods of blood component preparation that significantly reduce the number of leukocytes, such as leukoreduction by filtration (by up to three logs) can abrogate many transfusion reactions attributed to these mediators.

IV. Blood group serology and pretransfusion testing

A. Steps required to issue blood for transfusion
These are summarized in Table 24.2.

Table 24.2 Steps in setting up blood for transfusion	
Steps	*Location*
Blood order entry	Bedside
Type and screen specimen:	Bedside
• Identification of transfusion recipient and collection tube labeling	
Testing of transfusion recipient's blood specimen:	Laboratory
• Blood specimen acceptability	
• ABO group and Rh type	
• Antibody screen	
• Antibody identification	
• Comparison of current and previous test results	
Donor RBC unit testing:	Laboratory
• ABO group confirmation and RH type confirmation	
Donor red cell unit selection:	Laboratory
• Selection of components of ABO group and Rh types that are compatible with the transfusion recipient and with any unexpected allogeneic antibodies to minor red cell antigens	
Compatibility testing (crossmatch):	Laboratory
• Serologic	
• Computer or electronic	
Labeling of blood or blood components with the patient's identifying information, and issue	Laboratory
Identification of transfusion recipient with blood unit	Bedside
Reproduced with permission from Roback JD, ed. Technical Manual, 16th edn. Bethesda, MD: AABB, 2008.	

B. Preparation for blood transfusion

In preparation for blood transfusion, a diagnostic specimen for requesting blood type and screen ordered and drawn. Careful identification of the patient (with at least two identifiers including full name and date of birth or medical record number) and labeling of the collection tube (at the bedside, in the presence of the patient) is mandatory. Upon receipt in the Blood Bank, proper specimen labeling is verified again along with information on the laboratory requisition. Misidentification of samples is the most common cause of blood banking errors.

C. Antibody screening

(i)   **Routine pretransfusion testing** consists of ABO typing (testing for A and B antigens and the corresponding anti-B or anti-A in the serum) and Rh typing (testing for the Rh(D) antigen) (Table 24.3). The ABO and Rh RBC antigens systems are "major" blood typing systems.

(ii)   **An antibody screen** for other red cell antibodies against minor RBC antigens is also performed. This screen is an indirect antiglobulin test using commercial RBC from two or three group O selected individuals of known RBC phenotype that are positive for the most common clinically significant red cell antigens.

(iii)   If there are **problems with identifying the ABO type**, or if the antibody screen is positive, further testing is required before compatible blood can be provided. Red cell antibody evaluation is performed using commercial kits of panels of typed donor cells. When an antibody is identified, donor units are typed to find ones that are RBC antigen negative for that specificity.

(iv)   **Immune responses** in transfusion recipients via antibodies formed against red cell antigens are a concern and potential cause of substantial

---

Table 24.3 Routine ABO blood type grouping

Reaction of red cells with antisera (Red cell grouping)		Reaction of serum with reagent red cells (serum grouping)		Interpretation		Prevalence (%) in US population	
Anti-A	Anti-B	A_1 Cells	B Cells	O Cells	ABO Group	European Ethnicity	African Ethnicity
0	0	+	+	0	0	45	49
+	0	0	+	0	A	40	27
0	+	+	0	0	B	11	20
+	+	0	0	0	AB	4	4

+ = agglutination; 0 = no agglutination.
(Reproduced with permission from Roback JD, ed. Technical Manual, 16th edn. Bethesda, MD: AABB, 2008.)

morbidity or even mortality. Such antibodies may be either naturally occurring or made in response to previous exposure though transfusion or pregnancy.

(v)   **Antibodies in the ABO** system are naturally occurring and usually formed in the first months of life as a result of exposure to environmental bacterial antigens (Table 24.3). Anti-A and anti-B are typically IgM (and IgG), fix complement, and cause rapid intravascular hemolysis.

(vi)   In contrast, **antibodies to most other minor red cell antigens**, such as Rh, are not naturally occurring. Previous transfusion or pregnancy is required before a patient will make such antibodies. These antibodies are typically IgG, do not fix complement, and cause extravascular consumption or hemolysis, although there are exceptions. Even then, minor red cell antigens vary considerably in immunogenicity.

(vii)   **Many patients do not make red cell antibodies** (except for anti-D in the RH system) despite repeated transfusion. Thus, patients are routinely typed only for blood groups ABO and for Rh; and women are given prophylactic anti-D immunoglobulin during pregnancy and delivery to prevent sensitization against this Rh antigen. Briefly, the antibody in the anti-D immunoglobulin binds RBCs expressing Rh antigen and prevent sensitization of maternal blood.

(viii)   Antibodies to the patient's own red cells (**autoantibodies**), also occur. These may cause hemolysis as in autoimmune hemolytic anemia. Autoantibodies may be idiopathic or associated with certain diseases such as systemic lupus erythematosis or chronic lymphocytic leukemia. In some cases, red cell autoantibodies may be present serologically but without clinically detectable red cell destruction.

(ix)   **In order to ensure compatible blood**, it is necessary to detect any red cell antibodies before transfusion. Such tests are based on agglutination in which clumping for red cells are caused by cross-linking of cells by antibodies. Antibodies in the ABO system and some other IgM antibodies can directly agglutinate red cells. Most IgG antibodies require a second antibody, anti-IgG (also called antiglobulin or Coombs reagent) for detection by agglutination. Thus, crossmatching involves testing an aliquot of the donor's red cells against the recipient's serum plus Coombs reagent (see Chapter 8).

(x)   **To detect antibody bound to the red cells**, a specimen of red cells drawn from the patient is incubated with serum, excess unbound IgG is washed away, and the red cells are tested for bound antibody with antiglobulin serum (Coombs reagent); this is known as the direct Coombs test (see Chapter 8). Serologic reactions are temperature dependent. Anti-A and anti-B are readily detected at room temperature, but detection of most IgG red cell antibodies via the Coombs reagent requires testing at 37°C.

1. Pretransfusion testing

(i) Routine

Testing for red cell antibodies is also useful in diagnosis and evaluation of anemias that are due to hemolysis. Red cells that are coated with IgG in circulation, as in autoimmune hemolytic anemia or during a hemolytic transfusion reaction, are detected by the direct antiglobulin test (DAT). The DAT is used to detect IgG on the surface of red cells in warm autoimmune hemolytic anemia. A DAT performed with anticomplement serum can detect the presence of complement activation products such as C3b on the red cell surface. This test is typically positive in cold agglutinin disease. Some drug-induced hemolytic anemias will also have a positive DAT. Red cell autoantibodies may be found in autoimmune diseases such as systemic lupus erythematous.

(ii) RBC compatibility

The final check of red cell compatibility is the crossmatch. If the patient has a negative antibody screen, the most important purpose of the immediate spin crossmatch (no incubation period) is to detect ABO incompatibility. It is also possible to perform an "electronic crossmatch" using a computer to verify ABO compatibility. If the patient's antibody screen is positive, a full Coombs crossmatch (at 37°C) is necessary to insure the red cell units are not only ABO/Rh compatible, but also compatible for minor red cell antigens against which the patient has an alloantibody.

2. Emergency transfusion

In emergency situations if there is not time to perform blood type determination and pretransfusion testing, group O red cells can usually be given safely. Rh negative red cells are often selected to avoid sensitization to Rh(D). However, group O Rh-negative individuals constitute only 15% of all blood donors. Since this resource is limited, women of child-bearing age are the first priority for this emergency resource. In an emergency, Rh-positive red cells may be used for men and women >50 years of age. Type-specific, crossmatched blood is then provided when time permits. Good communication between the treating physician and the Blood Bank is essential. The decision to use unmatched blood in an emergent situation needs to be made by experienced physicians.

D. Blood transfusion

After issue, blood units must be carefully matched with the intended recipient by again using at least two patient identifiers (full name and date of birth or medical record number) on the blood unit and the patient wristband. Morbidity and mortality rates from errors in transfusion medicine now exceed estimated rates of complications from transmission of viral disease. Adverse events associated with transfusion and estimated risks per unit transfused are summarized in Table 24.4.

Table 24.4 Transfusion-associated adverse reactions	
	Risk per unit infused
ABO incompatible blood transfusions	1 in 30,000 to 60,000
Symptoms	40%
Fatalities	1 in 600,000
Delayed serologic reactions	1 in 1600
Delayed hemolytic reactions	1 in 6700
Transfusion-related acute lung injury	1 in 8000
Graft-vs.-host disease	Rare
Fluid overload	Underestimated
Febrile, nonhemolytic transfusion reactions	
Red blood cells	1 in 200
Platelets	1 in 5–20
Allergic reactions	1 in 30–100
Anaphylactic reactions	1 in 150,000
Iron overload	After 80–100 U
Post-transfusion purpura	Rare
Immunosuppressive effects	Unknown

E. Transfusion reactions

1. Acute hemolytic transfusion reaction

An acute hemolytic transfusion reaction is most commonly defined as hemolysis of donor red cells by preformed alloantibodies in the recipient's circulation. Life-threatening acute hemolytic transfusion reactions are most commonly due to ABO-incompatible blood being transfused to a recipient with naturally occurring ABO alloantibodies (anti-A, anti-B, anti-A, B). Clerical errors (mislabeling blood or misidentification of patients) account for 80% of such reactions. Hemolysis can also occur due to undetected (labile) antibodies present pre-transfusion to minor RBC antigens.

Signs and symptoms of an acute intravascular hemolytic transfusion reaction may develop when as little as 10 to 15 mL of ABO-incompatible blood has been infused. Fever, which is the most common initial manifestation, is frequently accompanied by chills. The patient may have complaints such as a general sense of anxiety or uneasiness or may complain of pain at the infusion site or in the back or chest (or both). The most serious sequela is acute renal failure due to microvascular thrombosis from intravascular coagulation initiated by lysing RBCs. Diffuse bleeding may be the first indication of intravascular hemolysis and may be accompanied by hemoglobinuria and hypotension. Treatment begins with immediate cessation of the transfusion. The risk for renal failure may be reduced by the administration of crystalloid fluids, including sodium bicarbonate to maintain urine pH at 7.0 and by diuresis with mannitol or furosemide.

Every institution has a nursing blood administration policy that specifies how to transfuse blood and to handle possible blood transfusion reactions. In all cases, if a reaction is suspected, the transfusion must be stopped and a medical evaluation must be undertaken. If evaluation determines a possible transfusion reaction, a transfusion reaction report is initiated and the blood unit is returned to the Blood Bank, along with a post-transfusion blood specimen. The Blood Bank *excludes* a hemolytic transfusion reaction by (1) rechecking the paperwork and unit labels to ensure that the correct unit was issued and that the blood was ABO/Rh compatible; and (2) performing a DAT on the patient's post-transfusion specimen to determine whether antibody bound to red cells is detected. If the DAT is positive, further workup is undertaken to identify the specific antibody responsible for the reaction.

2. Febrile nonhemolytic transfusion reactions

Febrile nonhemolytic transfusion reactions are common and estimated to occur in 0.5% of all red cell transfusions and up to 25% of platelet transfusions in frequently-transfused patients. A febrile transfusion reaction is defined as a rise in temperature of greater than 1°C, which may be accompanied by chills or rigor, or both.

These reactions are thought to be due to a reaction of HLA or leukocyte-specific antigens (or both) on transfused lymphocytes, granulocytes, or platelets in the donor unit with antibodies in previously alloimmunized recipients. Multiply transfused individuals and multiparous women are most likely to experience this type of transfusion reaction. Febrile nonhemolytic transfusion reactions, especially those associated with platelet transfusions, may be caused by the infusion of soluble biologic response modifiers, such as cytokines, that have accumulated in the blood component unit during storage.

Symptoms may occur during the transfusion or not be manifested until 1 to 2 hours after its completion. The diagnosis of a febrile nonhemolytic transfusion reaction is generally made by excluding other causes of fever (e.g., bacterial contamination of blood, acute hemolytic transfusion reaction). Prestorage leukocyte reduction by filtration has been utilized to reduce these kinds of reactions.

3. Allergic reactions

Allergic reactions can be mild, moderate, or life-threatening in severity and are usually associated with the amount of plasma transfused. Up to 15% of all blood transfusion recipients experience mild allergic reactions, particularly in frequently transfused patients receiving plasma or platelets.

Anaphylactic transfusion reactions are sometimes associated with antibodies to IgA, which are common in the population and have an incidence of approximately 1 in 700 individuals. However, the incidence of anaphylactic transfusion reactions is much lower, 1 in 20,000 to 50,000.

Urticarial reactions are believed to be an interaction between antibodies in the recipient's plasma and plasma proteins in donor blood. There is not usually a specific identifiable antigen to which the patient is reacting.

Symptoms are generally mild and include localized urticaria, erythema, rash, and itching. However, anaphylactic or anaphylactoid reactions, which can occur after the transfusion of only a few milliliters of blood or plasma, include skin flushing, nausea, abdominal cramps, vomiting, diarrhea, wheezing, dyspnea, laryngeal edema, hypotension, shock, cardiac arrhythmia, cardiac arrest, and loss of consciousness. Management begins with discontinuation of the transfusion. Treatment is diphenhydramine, but more severe episodes may require additional therapy.

4. Bacterial contamination

Bacterial contamination may be introduced into a unit of blood through skin contaminants during venipuncture or from donors with asymptomatic bacteremia. Multiplication of bacteria may occur in red cells stored at refrigerated temperatures but is more likely to occur in platelets stored at room temperature.

Bacterial contamination of red cells is most often due to *Yersinia enterocolitica*, followed by *Serratia liquefaciens*, whereas platelets are most often contaminated with *Staphylococcus* and Enterobacteriaceae. The incidence of bacterial contamination of red cells has been approximately 1 in 60,000 with an overall fatality rate of 1 in 1,000,000. The incidence of bacterial contamination of platelets was approximately 1 in 5000 before the initiation of bacterial detection systems in 2004, but is now estimated to be 50% lower (1 in 10,000).

Recipients of units with low bacterial counts may have relatively mild symptoms such as fever and chills, but transfusion of units with high bacterial counts may result in severe or fatal reactions. Clinically, the patient may experience high fever, shock, hemoglobinuria, renal failure, and DIC. The blood transfusion must be stopped immediately, the patient's and any untransfused blood must be cultured, and broad-spectrum antibiotics should be started.

5. Circulatory overload

Acute pulmonary edema, caused by the inability of the circulatory system to handle an increased fluid volume, can occur in any patient who is transfused too rapidly. The true frequency of this type of transfusion reaction is unknown, but under-recognized. Susceptible populations are primarily the very young, the elderly, and patients with a small total blood volume or cardiopulmonary disease. Treatment is the same as for heart failure.

6. Delayed reactions

A delayed hemolytic transfusion reaction generally occurs 3 to 7 days after transfusion of the implicated unit. Hemolysis is usually extravascular, where

RBCs are coated with antibodies or have abnormal shape of membrane or abnormal inclusion (such as Heinz bodies in G6PD deficiency) and so they are attacked prematurely by the liver and spleen phagocytes. (In intravascular hemolysis, the RBCs are lysed within the blood vessel such as by mechanical damage of a heart valve, or because of complement fixation as in paroxysmal nocturnal hemoglobinuria.) Red cells are destroyed in the recipient's circulation by antibody produced as a result of an immune response induced by the transfusion. These reactions are most commonly due to an anamnestic response (secondary exposure to a red cell antigen) in a patient who had a negative antibody screen despite a low level of antibody as a result of previous exposure, either through pregnancy or transfusion, to a foreign red cell antigen. Exposure to the same antigen a second time may cause IgG antibody to reappear within hours or days of the transfusion. This subsequent exposure to the antigen produces an anamnestic antibody response resulting in increased production of IgG antibodies that are capable of reacting with any transfused cells present.

In most cases, anamnestic production of antibody does not result in acute hemolysis, but red cell destruction does occur between 3 days and 2 weeks after the transfusion. Patients are generally asymptomatic, and hemolysis may be noted only by a more rapid decline than usual in the patient's Hgb or absence of the expected rise in Hgb. Fever, the most common initial symptom, may occasionally be noted, along with jaundice; renal failure is rare.

7. Transfusion-related acute lung injury

Transfusion-related acute lung injury (TRALI) is an acute respiratory distress syndrome that occurs within 6 hours after transfusion and is characterized by dyspnea and hypoxia secondary to noncardiogenic pulmonary edema. Although the actual incidence is almost certainly underreported, the estimated frequency is approximately 1 in 8000 transfusions. In approximately 50% of cases, blood donor antibodies with HLA or neutrophil antigenic specificity can be shown to react with the recipient's leukocytes, thereby leading to increased permeability of the pulmonary microcirculation.

Most recently, reactive lipid products from donor blood cell membranes that arise during the storage of blood products have been implicated in the pathophysiology of TRALI. Such substances are capable of neutrophil priming, with subsequent damage to the pulmonary–capillary endothelium of the recipient, particularly in patients who receive massive transfusions in defined clinical settings such as cardiac surgery or trauma or in patients receiving chemotherapy for malignancy. In each of these settings, the true incidence of TRALI may be underreported because the findings may be blamed on the underlying disease process or the surgical procedure. As in other causes of acute respiratory distress syndrome, therapy is supportive, and 90% of patients recover.

V. **Summary**

Medical management of the blood bank addresses issues related to blood inventory and safety, as well as oversight of laboratory policies and procedures (Figure 24.1). Management of the transfusion service includes the coordination of blood transfusion and blood conservation activities, in addition to serving as a consultant to clinicians managing patients undergoing massive transfusion, apheresis, or transplantation or having problems such as

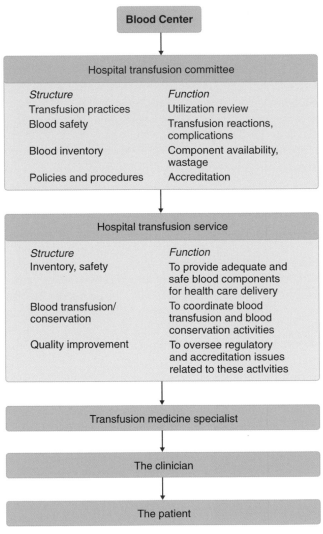

Figure 24.1 The flow of blood components.

difficulty finding compatible blood products. Finally, the transfusion medicine specialist supervises quality assurance to satisfy regulatory and accreditation requirements.

Further reading

Goodnough LT. What is a transfusion medicine specialist? Transfusion 1999;39:1031–3.

Goodnough LT, et al. Transfusion medicine. Blood transfusion and blood conservation (Parts I and II). N Engl J Med 1999;341:26–7.

King KE, ed. Blood Transfusion Therapy: A Physician's Handbook, 9th edn Bethesda, MD: AABB, 2008.

Mintz PD, ed. Transfusion Therapy: Clinical Principles and Practice. Bethesda, MD: AABB, 2010.

Roback JD, ed. Technical Manual, 17th edn. Bethesda, MD: AABB, 2011.

25 | Transfusion Therapy

Beth H. Shaz[1] and Christopher D. Hillyer[2]

[1]New York Blood Center, New York, NY, USA; Emory University School of
Medicine, Atlanta, GA, USA
[2]New York Blood Center; Weill Cornell Medical College, New York, NY, USA

I. Blood components

Blood components, including RBCs, plasma, platelets, and granulocytes, are prepared from either whole blood donation or by automated apheresis. Blood component manufacturing allows each component to be stored under optimal conditions, and component therapy has largely replaced the use of whole blood due to the ability to choose the appropriate component that target specific patient needs.

(a) **Whole blood:** Whole blood is the most common starting product for component preparation and manufacturing. In general, 500 mL of whole blood is collected into a bag with 70 mL of anticoagulant-preservative solution. The primary bag has up to three satellite bags attached for RBC, platelet, plasma, and/or cryoprecipitate component manufacturing. Due to the different specific gravities of RBCs (1.08–1.09), plasma (1.03–1.04), and platelets (1.023), differential centrifugation of the whole blood product is used to prepare blood components.

   (i)   Anticoagulant/preservative solutions allow blood components to be stored for extended periods of time generally without a significant detrimental effect on the quality of the RBCs. The commonly used anticoagulant/preservative solutions are acid-citrate-dextrose (ACD), citrate-phosphate-dextrose (CPD), citrate-phosphate-dextrose-dextrose (CP2D), and citrate-phosphate-dextrose-adenine (CPDA-1). The citrate (sodium citrate and citric acid) acts as an anticoagulant, and phosphate (monobasic sodium phosphate and trisodium phosphate), adenine and dextrose are substrates for cellular metabolism.

(b) **RBC products** are transfused to mitigate signs and symptoms of anemia and improve tissue oxygen delivery in situations where there is an

---

Concise Guide to Hematology, First Edition. Edited by Alvin H. Schmaier, Hillard M. Lazarus.
© 2012 Blackwell Publishing Ltd. Published 2012 by Blackwell Publishing Ltd.

inadequate circulating RBC mass. In the US ~15 million RBC units are transfused each year.

(i) The shelf life of RBC product depends on the anticoagulant-preservative solution, such that at a minimum 75% of the transfused RBCs remain viable 24 hours after transfusion. ACD, CPD and CP2D allow for RBC storage of 21 days, whereas RBCs stored in CPDA-1 have a self-life of 35 days. The majority of RBC products in the US contain additive solution (AS) in order to extend the RBC shelf life to 42 days. AS-1, AS-3 and AS-5 contain dextrose, adenine, sodium chloride; AS-1 and AS-5 contain mannitol, and AS-3 contains monobasic sodium phosphate, sodium citrate, and citric acid. Additive solutions products have a final volume of 350–400 mL and hematocrit of 55–65%, containing 100–110 mL of additive solution and 10–40 mL of plasma. RBC products are stored at 1–6°C.

(ii) In the US, ~85% of the RBC products are leukoreduced. Leukoreduction removes >99.9% of white blood cells (WBC) in the product. When transfused, WBCs have been associated with multiple adverse events including immunization to HLA antigens, febrile nonhemolytic transfusion reactions (FNTR), immunomodulation and cytomegalovirus (CMV) transmission (see below).

(iii) RBC products undergo changes during the storage period termed the RBC storage lesion, which may decrease their ability to oxygenate tissues.

(iv) RBCs are administered primarily based on laboratory values (hemoglobin/hematocrit) and clinical status (presence of symptomatic anemia or active bleeding). Multiple studies have demonstrated equivalent patient outcome using hemoglobin 7 g/dL vs. 9–10 g/dL transfusion trigger. Thus, hemoglobin of 7 g/dL is currently used in many patient populations, including critical ill patients without active coronary artery disease.

(v) RBC exchange, either manually or through automatic instruments, where patient RBCs are replaced with donor RBCs, may be indicated in patients with hemolytic disease of the fetus and newborn (Chapter 23), sickle cell disease, malaria, and babesiosis.

(vi) In an adult, a single RBC product increases the hemoglobin by 1 g/dL. Dosing in children is typically 10–15 mL/kg.

(c) **Plasma products** are transfused primarily to replace clotting factors. Multiple plasma products are available with similar efficacy: fresh frozen plasma (FFP), plasma frozen within 24 hours of collection (FP24), and thawed plasma.

(i) Each plasma product contains 200–300 mL and 0.7–1.0 IU/mL of coagulation factors. Plasma products are stored frozen at ≤–18°C for up to 1 year, then thawed at 30–37°C prior to transfusion. If the product is not transfused immediately it can be stored at 1–6°C for 24 hours (FFP, FP24) or 5 days (thawed plasma). During refrigeration storage coagulation factors decrease, particularly factor VIII (reduced by 35–41% by day 5), factor V (reduced by 9–16%, but reported as high as 50%), and factor VII (reduced by 4–20%). Thus, duration of storage is limited to coagulation factor activity loss.

(ii)   Plasma transfusion is indicated in the prevention or treatment of bleeding in patients with either congenital coagulation defects (when no factor concentrates are available) or acquired coagulation defect (disseminated intravascular coagulopathy, liver disease, massive transfusion, and rapid reversal of warfarin). Coagulation defects are most commonly determined by prothrombin time (PT)/ International Normalized Ratio (INR) and activated partial thromboplastin time (APTT).

(iii)   Plasma is used as the replacement fluid for therapeutic plasma exchange in patients with thrombotic thrombocytopenic purpura and other patients requiring coagulation factor replacement.

(iv)   The typical dose is 10–20 mL/kg which increases factor levels by >30% and should be adequate to control or prevent bleeding.

(v)   Outside the US, pathogen inactivated plasma products treated with pathogen reduction technologies including riboflavin with illumination, amotosalen with illumination, and solvent/detergent are available. These products have lower risks of transfusion-transmitted diseases.

(d) **Platelets products** are indicated in patients with thrombocytopenia or a qualitative platelet defect with active bleeding or at high risk of bleeding.

(i)   Platelets are stored at room temperature for up to 5 days.

(ii)   The platelet transfusion threshold is determined by the patient's clinical status and platelet count. For prophylactic platelet transfusions, a platelet count threshold of 10,000/μL is typically used in the absence of bleeding, fever, or sepsis. A threshold of 50,000/μL is used for minor surgical procedures (e.g., lumbar puncture and liver or transbronchial biopsies). A threshold of 100,000/μL is used for major procedures or procedures in critical areas (e.g., brain or eye). For therapeutic platelet transfusions, platelet transfusions typically are used on patients with platelet counts <50,000/μL.

(iii)   The use of platelets in patients with acquired or congenital dysfunctional platelets (Chapters 13 and 14) depends on the cause of the dysfunction. If the dysfunction is secondary to medication, the medication should be discontinued and platelets transfused if platelet defect requires immediate correction. In patients with uremia, treatment usually includes dialysis, desmopressin, hematocrit >30%, cryoprecipitate, and, perhaps, conjugated estrogens before platelet transfusions are given.

(iv)   Each adult platelet dose (1 apheresis or 5 pooled whole blood derived platelets) will increase the platelet count by 30,000–

60,000/μL. In children, the typical dose is 10mL/kg or 1 whole blood derived platelet concentrate per 10kg with an expected increase of 50,000–100,000/μL.

(v) Multiple factors can result in decrease response to platelet transfusions secondary to increased platelet consumption, such as fever, sepsis, active bleeding, disseminated intravascular coagulopathy platelet and HLA antibodies, and increased platelet splenic sequestration, (e.g. splenomegaly). A low response to platelet transfusions, <10,000/μL one-hour post transfusion, is termed platelet transfusion refractoriness.

(vi) The majority of platelet products are leukoreduced in order to mitigate transfusion reactions and HLA alloimmunization (discussed above).

(vii) Outside of the US, pathogen inactivated platelet products are available decreasing the risk of transfusion transmitted diseases.

(e) **Cryoprecipitated antihemophilic factor,** typically termed cryoprecipitate, contains fibrinogen, fibronectin, factor VIII, von Willebrand factor and factor XIII. Cryoprecipitate is stored at ≤–18°C for up to 1 year, must be thawed to 30–37°C, and 10 units are usually pooled prior to transfusion. Once the unit is thawed the shelf life is 6 hours, due to loss of factor VIII activity, or 4 hours, if pooled, due risk of bacterial contamination.

(i) Cryoprecipitate is indicated for fibrinogen replacement (secondary to disseminated intravascular coagulopathy, massive transfusion, and congenital hypofibrinogenemia), fibrin sealant, reversal of thrombolytic therapy and uremic bleeding. In an actively bleeding patient or prior to surgery, cryoprecipitate should be given when fibrinogen levels fall below 100mg/dL. Fibrin sealant is the combination of thrombin and fibrinogen mixed with calcium to form fibrin, which is used as a topical hemostatic agent. Products may contain antifibrinolytics (aprotinin) to reduce fibrinolysis or factor XIII to increase strength of the clot. Commercially FDA-approved fibrin sealant products consisting of human fibrinogen, human thrombin, calcium chloride, and aprotinin (bovine) are available in the US.

(ii) The typical adult dose is 10 units which raises the fibrinogen approximately 75mg/dL. The typical pediatric dose is 1 unit per 10kg which increases the fibrinogen by 60–100mg/dL. For patients with congenital deficiency, fibrinogen is administered daily or every other day depending on the presence of increased consumption; the half-life of fibrinogen is typically 4 days.

(iii) Cryoprecipitate should not be used in patients with hemophilia A (factor VIII deficiency), factor XIII deficiency or von Willebrand's disease because recombinant or pathogen-inactivated factor concentrates are available. Also, commercially available pathogen inactivated fibrin glues are available. Lastly, pathogen inactivated fibrinogen concentrate is available for patients with congenital fibrinogen defects.

(f) **Granulocytes products** are indicated for neonatal sepsis, neutrophil function defect and neutropenic patients with severe infection despite appropriate antibiotics.

(g) **Rh immune globulin (RhIg)** is a human-plasma derived product consisting of IgG antibodies to the D antigen. RhIg is used to prevent immunization to the D antigen in D-negative individuals and the treatment of idiopathic thrombocytopenic purpura (ITP).

   (i)   During pregnancy women have their blood type and antibody identification performed. If a woman is D-negative and does not have anti-D, she should receive RhIg during pregnancy (28 weeks' gestational age, at delivery (if neonate is D-positive), and following perinatal events (e.g., trauma, amniocentesis). Each dose of RhIg suppresses the immune response (masks the D-antigen) for up to a certain amount whole blood or D-positive RBCs: typical dose of 300 µg prevents immunization for up to 15 mL D-positive RBCs. Higher doses may be necessary if there is a large fetal maternal hemorrhage.

   (ii) Women who have clinically significant RBC alloantibodies (i.e., antibodies that can cause hemolytic disease of the fetus and newborn) should be closely followed during pregnancy and treated as appropriate.

   (iii) Hemolytic disease of the fetus and newborn is when maternal RBC antibodies (Chapter 23), that can be alloantibodies formed in response to a previous transfusion or pregnancy or more rarely autoantibodies, cross the placenta and result in hemolysis of the fetal/neonatal RBCs leading to anemia and, if severe, high-output cardiac failure (hydrops fetalis) and potentially death. After birth hemolysis also results in hyperbilirubinemia, which left untreated can result in kernicterus.

   (iv) RhIg is used in higher doses for the treatment ITP in individuals who are D-positive with an intact spleen.

II. Transfusion associated adverse events

Transfusion associated adverse events have been classified as acute (within 6 hours) versus delayed (days to years) reactions, infectious (termed transfusion transmitted diseases) versus non-infectious (termed non-infectious serious hazards of transfusion). The major causes of transfusion related mortality are mistransfusion, TRALI, and septic reactions.

(a) **Febrile nonhemolytic transfusion reactions (FNTR)** are defined as a temperature increase of $\geq 1°C$ and/or chills/rigors associated with transfusion that cannot be attributed to other etiologies.

   (i)   FNTRs occur in approximately 1% of platelet transfusions and 0.2% of RBC transfusions. This rate has significantly decreased with universal leukoreduction.

(ii)   In platelet products, these reactions are due to leukocyte-derived cytokines which accumulate in the product during storage.

(iii)   In RBC products, these reactions are due to donor leukocytes interacting with patient WBC antibodies.

(iv)   If a febrile reaction is suspected the transfused must be stopped and symptomatic care should be given.

(b) **Allergic reactions** are the result of an allergen interacting with a preformed antibody, resulting in a wide range of symptoms from mild, local urticarial reactions to life-threatening, systemic anaphylactic reactions.

(i)   Allergic reactions occur in ~0.5% of RBC transfusions and 1% of platelet and plasma transfusions. The majority of reactions are mild. Anaphylactic reactions occur in ~1:20,000 transfusions.

(ii)   Mild reactions consist of urticaria with or without generalized pruritus or flushing. More severe symptoms include hoarseness, stridor, wheezing, dyspnea, hypotension, gastrointestinal symptoms and shock.

(iii)   Mild reactions can be treated with antihistamine while more severe reactions can be treated with epinephrine, H1-receptor antagonist, and steroids.

(iv)   Premedication with antihistamine decreases the incidence of allergic reactions in patients with a history of allergic reactions. Premedication should not be used in patients without a history of allergic reactions.

(v)   Anaphylactic reactions may be secondary to anti-IgA which is usually formed in response to environmental factors, in patients with IgA deficiency. Not all patients with IgA deficiency who have anti-IgA will develop anaphylactic reactions. Patients who have severe allergic reactions should be tested for IgA deficiency and anti-IgA. If the patient has anti-IgA then the patient should receive IgA negative products, i.e., washed RBC and platelet products or plasma products collected from IgA deficient donors.

(c) **Acute hemolytic transfusion reactions (AHTR)** are a result of antigen–antibody complexes binding in the recipient and activating the complement cascade resulting in intravascular hemolysis. Most often severe reactions are a result of ABO incompatibility when the RBC antigens are incompatible with the recipient's plasma or, less often, when the plasma in the transfused unit contains antibodies against the recipient's RBC antigens.

(i)   The incidence of ABO incompatible RBC transfusion is ~1:50,000 transfusions and the risk of death is ~1:1,000,000. About 50% of ABO incompatible RBC transfusions have no adverse effect while 5% result in death.

(ii)   ABO incompatible RBC transfusions are most often associated with a mistransfusion event, blood transfused to the incorrect patient. Mistransfusion, a term generally used to describe an episode where "the wrong patient receives the wrong blood" is usually due to human error(s), and occurs for a variety of reasons including improper identification of the intended recipient during initial sample collection for blood typing, improper typing or pretransfusion testing of the blood component or recipient in the blood bank, or misidentification of the patient recipient and/or the blood product at the time of initiation of the blood transfusion.

(iii) The signs and symptoms of a hemolytic reaction are fever, chills/rigors, anxiety, chest and abdominal pain, flank and back pain, nausea and vomiting, dyspnea, hemoglobinuria, diffuse bleeding, and oliguria/anuria.

(iv) Diagnosis is based on the evidence of hemolysis (plasma free hemoglobin, decreased hematocrit, hemoglobinuria) as well as evidence of incompatible blood transfusion.

(v) AHTRs can occur secondary to RBC antigen–alloantibody complexes outside the ABO system or in patients with ongoing hemolytic disease. In addition, AHTRs can result from non-immune causes.

(d) **Delayed hemolytic transfusion reactions (DHTR)** are when transfused RBCs have decreased survival secondary to recipient RBC alloantibody formation. Delayed serologic transfusions are defined as a newly identified RBC alloantibody in the absence of evidence of increased RBC destruction. These reactions are secondary to an amnesic response to RBC antigens in individuals who had previously formed antibodies.

(i) The incidence of delayed hemolytic and serologic transfusion reactions is ~1:1500 RBC transfusions; serologic reactions occur four times more often than hemolytic reactions. Clinical signs of hemolysis usually appear 3–10 days post-transfusion.

(ii) DHTRs are characterized by unexpected decrease in hemoglobin or less than expected increase in hemoglobin post-transfusion. Other signs and symptoms include fever, chills, jaundice, malaise, back pain, and rarely renal failure.

(iii) To prevent future reactions, the patient should receive antigen negative RBCs for future transfusions.

(iv) A rare but severe form of DHTRs is termed hyperhemolytic transfusion reactions. These reactions are characterized by severe anemia (both the transfused and the recipient RBCs are destroyed) and reticulocytopenia. Most commonly these reactions occur in sickle cell patients.

(e) **Transfusion-associated circulatory overload (TACO)** results from circulatory overload following the transfusion of blood products.

(i) TACO occurs in ~1% of transfusion. Patients at increased risk are the young, elderly, female, those with cardiac dysfunction or positive fluid balance.

(ii) Symptoms include dyspnea, orthopnea, cough, chest tightness, cyanosis, hypertension, and headache. Symptoms usually present at the end of transfusion but may occur up to 6 hours post-transfusion.

(iii) Diagnosis is based on the presence of cardiogenic pulmonary edema.

(iv) Management includes discontinuing transfusion, diuretic therapy, oxygen supplementation, and sitting the patient upright.

(f) Transfusion related acute lung injury (TRALI) is defined as a new episode of acute lung injury which is not related to a competing etiology for acute lung injury. Competing etiologies include aspiration, pneumonia, toxic inhalation, severe sepsis, shock, trauma, burn injury, cardiopulmonary bypass, and drug overdose.

(i) TRALI results from neutrophil and pulmonary endothelial activation. The majority of cases (75%) are associated with WBC antibodies (human leukocyte antigen [HLA] and human neutrophil antigen [HNA] antibodies) in the donor reacting with the recipient's WBCs causing leukoagglutination, activation of the complement cascade and cytokine release, leading to fluid accumulation in the alveoli. Few cases (5%) are due to recipient WBC antibodies against donor WBCs. Non-immune mechanisms include bioactive lipids and CD40 ligand in the blood product, which prime neutrophils that are sequestered in the pulmonary vasculature resulting in TRALI.

(ii) The incidence of TRALI is ~1:250,000 transfusions. Products containing large volumes of plasma have a higher risk of TRALI (fatal TRALI 1:250,000 plasma products). TRALI has a 5–10% fatality rate.

(iii) Signs and symptoms include sudden onset of respiratory distress with dyspnea, tachypnea, hypoxia, fever, tachycardia, and hypotension after a transfusion. TRALI is secondary to noncardiogenic pulmonary edema.

(iv) The Canadian Consensus Conference criteria for TRALI is most commonly used: acute lung injury occurring during or within 6 hours of transfusion with bilateral infiltrates on chest X-ray, and no evidence of left atrial hypertension (i.e., circulatory overload), no pre-existing acute lung injury, and no temporal relationship to an alternative risk factor for acute lung injury. Possible TRALI is defined as the above except there is a clear temporal relationship to an alternative risk factor for acute lung injury. Acute lung injury is defined as acute onset and hypoxia ($PaO_2/FiO_2 \leq 300$, $SpO_2 < 90\%$, or other clinical evidence of hypoxemia).

(v) In cases of suspected TRALI, the transfusion should be discontinued. Medical management is primary supportive. The majority of patients improve within 2–4 days.

(vi) Blood banking practices in the US and worldwide are changing to decrease the risk of TRALI. High-risk donors (i.e., those with WBC antibodies) cannot donate high plasma volume containing products, such as platelets and plasma.

(g) **Septic reactions** are a result of bacterial contamination of the blood product. The highest risk component is platelets because they are stored at room temperature in a protein and oxygen rich environment. Bacteria can enter the blood product either through skin contamination or through asymptomatic donor sepsis. Methods to reduce the incidence of bacterial contamination include skin preparation with iodine scrub, diversion pouch to collect skin and hair from puncture site, culturing products and other assays to detect bacteria (outside the US pathogen inactivation technologies are available).

(i) The incidence of septic reactions for RBC products is ~1:250,000 products and ~1:75,000 for plateletpheresis products. ~5% of septic reactions are fatal.

(ii) Bacterial contamination of the product may result in no symptoms, mild symptoms (fever, chills), septic shock (high fever, rigors, hypotension, tachycardia, disseminated intravascular coagulopathy, renal failure), or death.

(iii) Diagnosis is by detection of bacteria in the patient and blood product.

(iv) Treatment includes discontinuing the transfusion, patient management as needed, and broad-spectrum antibodies.

(v) The most frequent bacterium implicated in RBC septic reactions is *Yersinia enterocolitica*. Platelet product contamination is most frequently due to skin flora, particularly *Staphylococcus* spp. The majority of fatalities from platelet products are due to Gram-negative organisms (e.g., Enterobacteriacea).

(vi) Prevention of septic reactions occurs through limiting and detecting of bacterial contamination particularly of platelet products. This is done through improved skin disinfection, diversion of the initial aliquot of blood, culturing products, and alternate testing for bacterial detection, which decrease contamination rate by about 50%. Outside the US, pathogen reduction and inactivation technologies are available which nearly eliminate bacterial contamination.

(h) **Post-transfusion purpura (PTP)** results in acute, profound thrombocytopenia (<10,000/μL). Patients present with unexplained purpuric rash, bruising, or mucosal bleeding 2–14 days post-transfusion. 10% of patients die secondary to hemorrhage and 30% have major hemorrhage.

(i) PTP is an immune thrombocytopenia resulting from antiplatelet alloantibodies, most often anti-HPA-1a. The transfused product contains the antigen, which triggers an amnesic response.

(ii) The incidence is ~1:330,000 transfusions.

(iii) Diagnosis is based on the clinical presentation and detection of platelet-specific alloantibodies.

(iv) The primary treatment is intravenous immunoglobulin resulting in a platelet count > 100,000/μL in 4–5 days.

(i) **Transfusion associated graft versus host disease (TA-GVHD)** results from engraftment of the transfused lymphocytes into the recipient resulting in pancyotpenia, erythemia, liver dysfunction, and gastrointestinal symptoms. The pancytopenia differentiates GVHD from transfusion versus from hematopoietic stem cell transplantation. There is a nearly a 100% fatality rate secondary to the profound pancytopenia resulting in infection, multiorgan failure and subsequent death.

    (i)   TA-GVHD results from viable lymphocytes in the product engraft into the recipient and mount an immune response that the recipient is unable to stop. An immunosuppressed individual is unable to mount a response against the transfused lymphocytes. In an immunocompetent individual the transfused lymphocytes are usually homozygous for HLA antigens while the recipient is heterozygous, thus the recipient does not see the donor lymphocytes as foreign but the donor lymphocytes see the recipient as foreign and subsequently mount an immune response against them.

    (ii)   The incidence is ~1:1,000,000 transfusions.

    (iii)   Patients at increased risk include those with congenital immunodeficiency, hematopoietic progenitor cell transplantation (current or potentially in the near future), Hodgkin's disease, acute leukemia and other hematologic malignancies, low birth weight infants, undergoing treatment with purine analog drugs (fludarabine, cladribine, deoxycoformycin), and undergoing intensive chemotherapy. Also at increase risk are those receiving HLA-match products, blood from relatives, granulocyte transfusions, intrauterine transfusions, and neonatal RBC exchange.

    (iv)   Patients at increased risk for TA-GVHD should receive irradiated cellular (red blood cells, platelets, and granulocytes) blood products. The US requires 2500 cGy at the center of the product with a minimum of 1500 cGy and maximum of 5000 cGy at any point. Irradiation results in the inability of leukocytes to replicate, and hence prevents TA-GVHD.

    (v)   Some institutions and countries irradiate all their cellular blood products. Countries with a more genetic homogenous population, such as Japan, have chosen to irradiate all cellular blood components.

(j) **Transfusion related immunomodulation (TRIM)** is when blood transfusion alters the recipients' immune system. Some effects of TRIM include RBC and HLA alloimmmunization, decreased renal allograft rejection, improvements in Crohn's disease, decreased repetitive spontaneous abortions, increased tumor recurrence, and increase post-operative infections.

    (i)   Proposed causes of TRIM include WBCs, soluble WBC-derived mediators accumulating, and soluble HLA peptides in the product. Therefore, leukoreduction may decrease its incidence.

    (ii)   Leukoreduction decreases the rate of HLA alloimmunization, which may result in platelet transfusion refractoriness (see above) and decreased ability to find compatible solid organ transplants (e.g., heart and kidney).

(k) Iron overload can occur in patients who are chronically transfused, particularly those with congenital anemia (thalassemia and sickle cell disease). Consideration for institution of iron chelation therapy should be made in any patient who will need chronic RBC replacement and who has received greater than 10 RBC transfusions. Patients are unable to actively excrete the excess iron.

    (i)   Each RBC product contains 200–250 mg of iron. Signs and symptoms of iron overload occur when the body iron reaches 10–25 g (50–100 RBC transfusions).

    (ii)   Clinical signs and symptoms include hepatomegaly, cirrhosis, congestive heart failure, cardiomyopathy, and endocrine dysfunction.

    (iii)   Iron chelating medications are available to treat iron overload.

(l) Transfusion transmitted diseases can be caused by viruses, protozoa and prions. The risk of transfusion-transmitted diseases continues to decrease to due to donor selection, improved testing and technologies to eliminate infectious agents (e.g., pathogen inactivation).

    (i)   **HIV:** The current risk of human immunodeficiency virus (HIV) in the US and other developed countries is <1:2,000,000 transfusions. Lowering the risk is secondary to donor screening and testing using both antibody serology and nucleic acid testing for HIV RNA, which reduces the window period (where the donor is infectious yet testing is negative) to 12 days.

    (ii)   **Hepatitis C:** The current risk of hepatitis C virus in the US and other developed countries is 1:1,400,000 transfusions.

    (iii)   **Hepatitis B:** The current risk of hepatitis B virus in the US is 1:300,000 transfusions.

    (iv)   **Human T-cell lymphotropic virus (HTLV):** The current risk in the US and other developed countries is 1:3,000,000 transfusions.

    (v)   **CMV:** CMV is transmitted through WBCs in the product. Recipients who are seronegative for CMV have 4% risk of transfusion transmission. CMV transmission is mitigated through leukoreduction and the use of CMV seronegative (CMV-safe) products. Patients who may benefit from CMV-safe products include low birth weight infants, solid organ recipients, hematopoietic progenitor cell transplant recipients, pregnant women, undergoing chemotherapy which results in neutropenia, and HIV-infected individuals. ~50% of the US population has previously been exposed to CMV.

    (vi)   **West Nile virus (WNV):** The current risk from transfusion transmission is low; two cases from a single donor of transfusion transmission were reported in 2008.

(vii) **Babesiosis:** Babesia is transmitted through RBCs in the component, thus most cases are associated with RBC products. More than 70 cases of transfusion transmission have been documented in the US resulting in 12 deaths.

(viii) **variant Creutzfeldt–Jakob disease (vCJD):** At least four cases of transfusion transmission of vCJD have occurred in the UK (no cases have been reported outside of the UK). It is estimated that transfusion transmission by donors who develop vCJD within several years of donation is about 14% for recipients who survive longer than 5 years post-transfusion. Prevention includes deferral for donors who have resided in the UK or Europe for over 6 months and through the use of prion removal by filters, which remove approximately half of the infectivity.

Further reading

Hillyer C, Shaz BH, Zimring JC, Abshire TC. Transfusion Medicine and Hemostasis: Clinical and Laboratory Aspects. San Diego: Elsevier, 2009.

Roback RD, Combs MR, Grossman B, Hillyer CD. Technical Manual, 16th edn. Bethesda: AABB, 2008.

The National Healthcare Safety Network (NHSN) Manual: biovigilance component: Protocol hemovigilance module. Division of Healthcare Quality Promotion, National Center for Preparedness, Detection, and Control of Infectious Diseases, Centers for Disease Control and Prevention. Atlanta, 2009.

26 Hematopoietic Cell Transplantation

Hillard M. Lazarus

Case Western Reserve University, University Hospitals Case Medical Center, Cleveland, OH, USA

I. Introduction

A. Hematopoietic cell transplantation (HCT)

HCT is a life-saving art applied as a curative treatment modality for patients with selected malignant and non-malignant diseases. The treatment and possible cure of certain malignant diseases depends on delivering doses of chemotherapy or chemotherapy plus radiation therapy that exceed the tolerance of bone marrow. Without restoring hematopoietic cell function, these patients would experience irreversible marrow toxicity leading to potentially fatal marrow aplasia (no cellular production). Formerly referred to as bone marrow transplantation, high-dose chemotherapy or chemoradiotherapy followed by infusion of hematopoietic progenitor cells allows full lympho-hematopoietic reconstitution. Further, in the case of infusion of cells that are obtained from another person, these cells exert an "allogeneic cellular effect" and eliminate residual malignant cells. HCT also may be used to correct immune deficiency disorders such as combined immune deficiency syndrome (SCIDS), bone marrow failure states such as severe aplastic anemia, congenital enzyme deficiency and autoimmune diseases, hemoglobinopathies and other conditions such as multiple sclerosis.

B. Definitions for graft sources

Terminally differentiated blood cells have a relatively short lifespan and must be replenished by the bone marrow. Decades ago investigators determined that bone marrow cells transplanted from one animal to another would restore blood production. Subsequently, others demonstrated that these long-term repopulating cells could be obtained from blood (known as blood progenitor cells) after recovery from chemotherapy or after exposure to certain drugs known as hematopoietic growth factors (G-CSF or filgrastim, GM-CSF or sargramostim) or more recently after plerixafor. Finally, umbilical cord blood

Table 26.1 Commonly used abbreviations in hematopoietic cell transplantation	
Abbreviation	*Definition*
auto	Autologous ("self")
allo	Allogeneic (another person)
HCT	Hematopoietic cell transplant
HSCT	Hematopoietic stem cell transplant
PBSC	Peripheral blood stem cell
DMSO	Dimethyl sulfoxide (cryoprotectant)
HLA	Human leukocyte antigen
GVHD	Graft-versus-host disease
GVL or GVT	Graft-versus-leukemia or graft-versus-tumor
UCB	Umbilical cord blood
RIC	Reduced-intensity conditioning
NMA or NST	Non-myeloablative or non-myeloablative stem cell transplant
t-MDS or t-AML	Therapy-related myelodysplastic syndrome or therapy-related acute myeloid leukemia
DLI	Donor lymphocyte infusion
G-CSF	Granulocyte colony-stimulating factor
TCR	T cell receptor
SCIDS	Severe combined immuno deficiency syndrome
CFU-GM	Colony-forming units granulocyte-macrophage
BFU-E	Burst-forming units-erythroid

(UCB) contains a high percentage of such cells and this product can be collected after a live birth from the placenta.

1. Autologous ("self"). The patient's own blood progenitor cells or bone marrow are collected, cryopreserved, and re-infused after high-dose chemotherapy.
2. Allogeneic (same species but "different genes"). Blood progenitor cells or bone marrow are obtained from another individual, such as a human leukocyte antigen (HLA) matched sibling donor, an HLA-mismatched family donor, or an HLA-matched unrelated donor. UCB cells are an increasingly used graft source even though usually not fully HLA-matched.
3. Syngeneic (identical twin, "same genes"). Marrow or stem cells are obtained from an identical twin.

C. Frequently used abbreviations in hematopoietic cell transplantation

Many abbreviations that often are used in this field are listed in Table 26.1.

II. Autologous hematopoietic cell transplantation

A. Overview

1. Using *in vitro* and *in vivo* preclinical models, many tumors show a steep dose–response curve. In other words, a small increment in the dose

Table 26.2 Diseases treated with autologous HCT	
Malignant disorders	*Non-malignant disorders*
Hodgkin lymphoma	Scleroderma
Non-Hodgkin lymphoma	Systemic lupus erythematosis
Acute myeloid leukemia	Multiple sclerosis
Multiple myeloma	
Germ cell tumors	
Pediatric solid tumors, e.g.,	
neuroblastoma, rhabdomyosarcoma	

of drug or radiation increase the number of cancer cells killed by many logs, especially for hematologic malignancies. This principle has been shown to be effective in a number of tumor types. As the dose of chemoradiotherapy is increased, organ toxicities also develop. The dose of the drug and radiation frequently is limited by marrow injury. Blood progenitor cells or marrow cells can be obtained from these patients before the high-dose therapy is given. These cells are frozen using sophisticated cryopreservation techniques that utilize cryoprotectant agents such as dimethyl sulfoxide and instruments such as controlled-rate liquid nitrogen freezing chambers. Cellular injury is minimized during freezing process and viability maintained upon thawing. Previously collected cells are frozen, the patient is given high-dose cytotoxic therapy and then the collected cells are infused after thawing and will reconstitute marrow function.

2. Autologous HCT depends almost entirely upon the administration of high-dose chemotherapy or chemo-radiation therapy to eliminate the malignancy. In contrast, allogeneic HCT can provide effective anti-tumor effect by virtue of both high-dose cytotoxic therapy as well as by the infused donor allogeneic cells that can exert an "allogeneic effect" against the tumor, i.e., graft-versus-tumor (GVT) effect (see Section III on Allogeneic HCT). In both autologous HCT and allogeneic HCT, the "transplanted" hematopoietic cells are a sophisticated support device that allows the high-dose therapy to be administered "safely" by repopulating chemotherapy-injured bone marrow. Without this cellular support or "rescue", the patient would succumb to the consequences of marrow aplasia, including infection, bleeding, and profound anemia.

3. Autologous HCT also are used as therapy in some severe autoimmune diseases because this treatment can be very immunosuppressive. Table 26.2 lists diseases treated with autologous HCT.

B. Phases of autologous HCT

1. Harvesting. During harvesting, blood progenitor cells or bone marrow are collected from the patient who has not been exposed to cytotoxic agents (chemotherapy or radiation) in a number of weeks. These cells represent a multilineage progenitor cell that gives rise to the entire lympho-hematopoietic system. Approximately 1 in 2000 nucleated marrow cells has the unique property of self-renewal; the daughter cells produced during cell division give rise to an undifferentiated cell as well as to a more differentiated progenitor cell, the later beginning the process toward further differentiation and ultimately production of the mature circulating cells. These early progenitor cells are identified as CD34+ by immunophenotyping. Some centers also continue to determine hematopoietic restoring potential by growing cells in *in vitro*, termed the colony-forming unit assay. This assay is reported as granulocyte macrophage (CFU-GM) and erythroid (BFU-E) colonies infused per kg patient weight.

(a) **Bone marrow harvesting** formerly was the traditional method of collecting cells for HCT. Marrow is removed from the posterior superior iliac crests with the patient in the prone position under spinal or general anesthesia. In the typical harvest, 1000 mL of marrow is aspirated (10–15 mL/kg patient weight), which requires manually entering the bone marrow space about 100 times. This procedure usually is performed under general anesthesia.

(b) **Blood progenitor cell harvesting** is clearly an easier way to collect stem cells than traditional bone marrow harvests in the operating room. Today, nearly all autologous HCT transplants use blood progenitor cells as the graft source.

   (i)   Early progenitors cells are normally found in low levels in the peripheral blood but stimuli such as marrow recovery after chemotherapy and use of other agents results in a significant release of these cells into the blood. Chemotherapy injures the marrow and alters the normal equilibrium of stem cells between marrow and blood. Hematopoietic growth factors such as granulocyte colony-stimulating factor (G-CSF), alone or after chemotherapy administration, also results in the release of significant numbers of these cells from the marrow. The new agent, plerixafor, works by disrupting the CXCR4 and SDF-1 lineage between the progenitor and the marrow stromal cell that keeps cells tethered in the marrow microenvironment.

   (ii) The blood progenitor cells are collected from the peripheral blood using an apheresis instrument that removes the cells by a centrifugation density gradient and returns the unwanted blood cells and plasma back to the patient. This process usually takes about 2–3 hours and about 12–18 liters of blood are processed in the procedure.

2. **Cryopreservation of cells.** The collected bone marrow or blood progenitor cells are suspended in a balanced salt solution containing the cryoprotectant dimethyl sulfoxide (DMSO) and are cryopreserved in liquid nitrogen. The dimethyl sulfoxide is protective by helping prevent ice crystallization

Table 26.3 Consequences of high-dose chemo-radiation therapy in autologous HCT	
Hematologic consequences	*Other consequences*
Marrow aplasia	Mucositis
Immunosuppression, i.e., opportunistic infection	Alopecia
Thrombocytopenia, i.e., serious hemorrhage	Lung injury
	Nausea and vomiting despite antiemetics
	Liver veno-occlusive disease
	Rashes
	Hyponatremia
	Hemorrhagic cystitis
	Cardiomyopathy
	Renal insufficiency

in the cell during the freezing process. The cells can remain viable at liquid nitrogen temperatures for at least 5 years.

3. **Conditioning (the high-dose chemo-radiation therapy preparative regimen).** In the autologous transplant setting, the preparative regimen, which consists of high-dose chemotherapy and/or total-body irradiation (TBI), is administered first in an attempt to eliminate the malignant disease. In contrast to allogeneic transplantation (see Section III), for autologous transplantation immunosuppression is not required to prevent graft-versus-host disease (GVHD). The dose-limiting toxicity of the chemotherapy drugs chosen primarily affects the marrow. If the dose-limiting toxicity of the chemotherapy drugs affects other organ systems (i.e., vincristine causes damage to the peripheral nervous system), stem cell infusion will not prevent toxicity. Conditioning lasts several days and has both hematologic and other consequences (Table 26.3).

4. **HCT.** Of all of the steps of the transplant process, this is the most anticlimactic (in contrast to solid organ transplants). The transplant involves intravenous infusion of collected bone marrow or blood progenitor cells. The cryopreserved stem cells are thawed and then infused intravenously, similar to a blood transfusion. Through a complex process, cells recognize the marrow microenvironment and "home" from the peripheral circulation to the now-empty marrow space. The cryoprotectant dimethyl sulfoxide is eliminated via the lungs.

5. **Recovery.** The infused cells require time to regenerate the marrow and during this time the patient requires considerable intensive supportive care. The patient is anemic, neutropenic (white blood cells [WBCs] <500/μL), and thrombocytopenic (i.e., pancytopenic). The high-dose chemotherapy additionally has caused breakdown of the normal mucosal barriers in the mouth and gut that increases susceptibility to infectious complications. The mucosal damage to the mouth causes painful ulcerations and limits the ability to eat. Many patients require continuous infusions of opioids. Recovery lasts approximately 2–3 weeks.

(a) **Required supportive care during recovery:**
  (i) Transfusions. Red blood cell (RBC) transfusions are used to keep the hematocrit over 25%, higher in symptomatic patients. Platelet transfusions are used to keep the platelet count above 10,000/μL to minimize bleeding; platelet transfusions may be required at a higher threshold in patients who demonstrate a hemorrhagic diathesis. All blood products are irradiated to prevent engraftment of lymphocytes from the transfused unit that may cause the highly fatal syndrome transfusion-associated GVHD.
  (ii) Cytokine support. Use of G-CSF (filgrastim) hastens marrow recovery, particularly WBC count.
(b) **Possible complications during recovery:**
  (i) **Infections.** When the neutrophil count drops below 500/μL there is a marked increased susceptibility to bacterial and fungal infections. The disturbance of the mucosal barrier due to the conditioning regimen and use of intravascular access devices add to the patient's risk of infection. The longer the neutropenic period, the higher the infectious risk. In most autologous HCT settings, neutrophil recovery occurs within two weeks. The use of prophylactic antibacterial and antifungal agents, recombinant cytokines and peripheral blood progenitor cells dramatically has decreased the incidence of severe infections.
    • The major infections encountered in autologous HCT transplants are Gram-negative and Gram-positive bacterial infections and fungal infections, due particularly to *Candida* sp. and *Aspergillus* sp.
    • Herpes simplex virus (HSV) infections of the perioral area previously were a common cause of morbidity and rarely mortality, but the use of prophylactic acyclovir therapy has dramatically decreased this infectious process.
  (ii) **Veno-occlusive disease of the liver.** This small-vessel liver disease results from chemotherapy-induced liver injury and is related to the intensity of the preparative regimen. It usually presents within the first two to three weeks of the HCT manifest as tender hepatomegaly, jaundice, and fluid retention. It is reversible in most cases; however, fatalities may result from progressive liver damage and extreme fluid imbalances with respiratory failure.
  (iii) **Idiopathic pneumonia syndrome and diffuse alveolar hemorrhage.** These complications may occur within the first 2 weeks after the transplant but may not appear until later, i.e., 1–2 months after HCT and may take many months to resolve. Possible causes include lung toxicity from chemotherapy or irradiation and viral infections.
6. **Engraftment.** Engraftment is the period when production of WBCs, RBCs, and platelets by the marrow resumes. The time to a neutrophil count

recovery, the usual engraftment standard, has been accelerated with the use of recombinant cytokines (e.g., G-CSF) and infusion of blood progenitor cells rather than bone marrow. Median time to a neutrophil count of 500/µL usually is 10–12 days as compared to 18 days or more when bone marrow was used without hematopoietic growth factor support. In uncomplicated HCT procedures, the median time to platelet transfusion and RBC transfusion independence usually is two weeks.

C. Outcomes of autologous stem cell transplantation

Outcomes depend on the underlying disease and the status of the disease at the time of transplant.

1. When comparing autologous and allogeneic HCT for similar diseases, the following appear to be true:
   (a) Treatment-related mortality is less with autologous transplants (typically <3% during the first 100 days post-transplant).
   (b) Relapse rates are higher with autologous transplants (up to 70% of all patients).
2. The major cause of death in autologous HCT is relapse of disease.
3. A long-term complication in autologous HCT, rarely observed in allogeneic HCT, is secondary myelodysplastic syndrome (MDS)/acute myeloid leukemia (AML), now categorized by the World Health Organization (WHO) as therapy-related myeloid neoplasms (t-MN). For a variety of reasons, lymphoma patients appear to be at greatest risk. It remains unclear what treatment is most responsible for the development of treatment-related MDS (t-MDS) or treatment-related acute myeloid leukemia (t-AML), i.e., the initial therapy for the malignancy or the high-dose chemotherapy or chemo-radiation therapy.

D. Advantages and disadvantages of autologous HCT

1. **Advantages:**
   (a) **A readily available source of blood progenitors or bone marrow**, i.e., the patient is the donor.
   (b) **Low treatment-related mortality:**
       (i)   The mortality rate 100 days after the HCT presently is approximately 0.5%.
       (ii) The 100 day mortality rate for allogeneic HCT often is 25% and can be as high as 40% in some high-risk groups.
   (c) **Low toxicity:**
       (iii) Unlike allogeneic HCT, no immunologic barriers must be crossed with an autologous HCT.
       (iv) As there is no GVHD, immunosuppressive medications given after allogeneic HCT, such as cyclosporine and tacrolimus, are unnecessary and hence post-transplant infectious complications are fewer.
       (v)   Graft rejection (failure of the infused cells to engraft) is rare.

2. **Disadvantages:**
    (a) **Tumor contamination:**
        (i) The cryopreserved graft may contain viable tumor cells.
        (ii) When infused into the patient, these tumor cells may contribute to relapse after HCT.
    (b) **Lack of an allogeneic antitumor effect:**
        There is no graft-versus-tumor (GVT) effect, a major feature with allogeneic HCT (see "3. Benefit of donor T cells", below). The tumor cell killing effect depends entirely on the transplant conditioning regimen (high-dose chemotherapy or chemo-radiation therapy).

III. Allogeneic hematopoietic cell transplantation

A. Overview

Allogeneic HCT is the administration of chemotherapy or chemo-radiation therapy to eliminate a malignant or non-malignant disease followed by infusion of normal donor-derived bone marrow or blood progenitor cells. The donor graft is obtained from an HLA-matched or HLA-mismatched family member (usually a sibling) or an unrelated donor (URD). In recent years it was recognized, using a dog animal model, that employing somewhat less intensive cytotoxic agent therapy could induce a sufficient immunosuppression effect to facilitate the engraftment of allogeneic cells. In contrast to a myeloablative HCT, this strategy was termed reduced-intensity conditioning (RIC) or non-myeloablative (NMA) conditioning. The advantage to this approach is that much older patients (usually >60 years) could undergo HCT with relatively greater safety. Also, patients who are otherwise good HCT candidates but ineligible for a myeloablative conditioning HCT due to one or more comorbid illnesses (cardiomyopathy, lung dysfunction, renal insufficiency, etc.) could be candidates for a RIC or NMA conditioning HCT as less organ injury is incurred using a less intensive cytotoxic therapy approach. The engrafted cells still act as effector cells and mediate GVT effects.

B. Indications for allogeneic HCT

1. **Malignancy:**
    (a) The most common use of allogeneic HCT is for hematologic malignancies, such as acute myeloid leukemia, acute lymphoblastic leukemia, myelodysplastic syndrome, non-Hodgkin lymphoma and multiple myeloma.
    (b) The curative potential of allogeneic HCT relies on three concepts:
        (i) Higher doses of chemotherapy may overcome the resistance to standard chemotherapy of some aggressive tumor cells as well as completely ablate or eliminate host bone marrow cells. In this setting the infusion of donor hematopoietic progenitor cells after high-dose chemotherapy or chemo-radiation therapy functions as a "biologic marrow rescue".

(ii) Infusion of normal donor marrow or blood progenitor cells after high-dose chemotherapy re-establishes normal hematopoiesis.

(iii) Perhaps most important, the donor cells eliminate the patient's tumor through immunologic mechanisms, the GVT effect; relapse rates will be lower than in autologous HCT because viable tumor cells that remain despite high-dose chemotherapy can be eradicated by this cellular effect.

(c) The decision as to when to proceed with allogeneic HCT varies by disease and stage.

(i) For some acute myeloid leukemia (AML) patients such as those with unfavorable cytogenetics, allogeneic HCT is the only curative therapy and is therefore recommended for all patients under age 55 years.

(ii) In acute lymphocytic leukemia, many patients (especially children) are cured with conventional chemotherapy. Therefore, transplantation is recommended only for patients who relapse after standard therapy or patients who have features that indicate they are at a high risk for relapse.

(d) The cure rate of allogeneic HCT after relapse is lower than during remission, and not all patients can achieve another remission after relapse. Allogeneic HCT is offered as an option in relapse only rarely.

2. **Bone marrow failure.** Allogeneic HCT remains the treatment of choice for young patients with severe aplastic anemia, particularly those who do not respond to immunosuppressive therapy.

3. **Inherited disorders:**

(a) **Hematopoiesis.** This category consists of a variety of rare congenital disorders. Although uncommon conditions, transplantation in this group demonstrates that any disease involving a hematopoietic stem cell or its progeny can be cured through an allogeneic HCT transplant. These diseases are caused by the developmental absence or abnormality of a specific lineage of cells derived from the lympho-hematopoietic stem cell.

(i) **Immunodeficiency diseases:**
- Severe combined immunodeficiency is a heterogeneous group of lethal disorders of T and B lymphocytes that predispose the patient to life-threatening infections.
- Wiskott–Aldrich syndrome is an X-linked recessive disorder characterized by T-cell immunodeficiency.
- Osteopetrosis is a rare disease that is a result of dysfunctional osteoclasts (specialized macrophages derived from the marrow stem cell).

(ii) **Hemoglobinopathies:**
- This category includes severe disorders of hemoglobin synthesis, such as sickle cell disease and thalassemia.
- In European countries, allogeneic HCT transplant is more frequently used for these diseases than in the United States.

(b) Storage diseases. This disease category includes a number of rare disorders in which an enzyme deficiency leads to an accumulation of toxic endogenous products normally degraded and eliminated by the body macrophages. The buildup of these derivatives leads to a wide range of irreversible neurologic disorders, such as Hurler syndrome, Hunter syndrome, and mucopolysaccharidoses. HCT provides the deficient enzyme in blood cells that can overcome the target organ's enzyme deficiency. The transplant usually must be completed before the patient becomes symptomatic and the damage irreversible.

C. Immunologic aspects of allogeneic HCT

1. **Human leukocyte antigen (HLA) system**

   (a) A donor for the transplant is determined by the matching of HLA proteins, transmembrane proteins that function normally in antigen recognition of foreign agents (e.g., viruses, bacteria). This system is important for immunologic recognition of "non-self", i.e., foreign tissues. They bind to protein fragments and present these fragments (antigens) to T cells, which results in T-cell activation via the T-cell receptor (TCR).

   (b) HLA proteins are encoded by genes of the major histocompatibility complex (MHC) on chromosome 6. A set of four (4) molecules on each chromosome (A, B, C and the D complex DR/DP/DQ) defines a haplotype. Humans inherit a separate haplotype from each parent and each haplotype is co-dominantly expressed on the cell surface, i.e., everyone has a pair of these four molecules. Hence, the "optimal match" situation for an allogeneic HCT is when there is matching at all four pairs of molecules, to which people refer as an "8/8 match". Lesser degrees of matching are associated with worse patient outcomes.

   (c) Each HLA antigen is polymorphic, with hundreds of different alleles for each of the three antigens, making the typing process complex.

   (i) The A, B and C antigens, known as the class I antigens, are usually expressed on all cell types except erythrocytes. The C antigen is located physically between A and B; if A and B are matched, C also most likely would be inherited. Sometimes separate typing for the C antigen is not performed, except in URD HCT in which C mismatching may profoundly affect overall survival and graft-versus-host disease (GVHD) (see below).

   (ii) The class II antigens, or DR/DP/DQ antigens, are usually limited to B cells, monocytes, dendritic cells, and some activated T cells.

   (iii) Antigen disparity can be at the level of minor histocompatibility antigens (miHA), inherited differently. In the setting of an MHC matched but miHA mismatched HCT, GVHD can occur. Some miHAs such as HA-1, HA-2, HB-1, and BCL2A1 are primarily found on hematopoietic cells, whereas some others such as the H-Y antigens, HA-3, HA-8, and UGT2B17 are ubiquitous.

       (iv)   The severity of acute GVHD is directly related to the degree of MHC mismatch.

2. **Finding a suitable donor:**

   (a) The most desirable source of hematopoietic cells is a "full" HLA-matched sibling, i.e., 8/8 matching as described above for the HLA-A, B, C and D complex pairs. As the haplotypes are inherited in co-dominant Mendelian fashion, each full sibling has a 25% chance of matching. Sometimes other close relatives are matches, especially in cases of consanguinity.

   (b) If no immediate family members match, there are registries of normal donors who have agreed to donate blood and marrow to patients who need transplants. These unrelated donors are less likely to match for miHA, which can cause immunologic reactions between donor and recipient.

   (c) Umbilical cord blood (UCB) also is an emerging graft source. For UCB transplantation, often only three of the HLA pairs are evaluated (the HLA-C loci are omitted), leading to only six (6) loci to be matched. Although this type of donor product often is matched only at 4/6 loci, the cells are immunologically naïve and are less likely to be associated with GVHD. Specifically, for a given degree of HLA matching, the incidence of GVHD is reduced compared to a matched unrelated donor (MUD) adult donor yet there is a retained graft-versus-malignancy effect.

3. **Benefits of infusing donor T cells.** The harvesting of hematopoietic progenitors, either from the peripheral blood or from the marrow, mixes mature WBCs with progenitors and some stem cells in the collection bag. Mature T lymphocytes are the principal effectors of cell-mediated immunity; many of the therapeutic benefits and toxicities of allogeneic HCT transplant are derived from immunologic reactions between donor T cells and recipient cells.

   (a) **Engraftment.** Donor T cells appear to facilitate engraftment. These cells, in part, eliminate remaining elements of host immune cells that survive conditioning and might reject the donor graft. Depletion of donor T cells before allogeneic HCT transplant significantly increases the risk of graft failure.

   (b) **Graft versus leukemia effect.** Most allogeneic HCT are performed for malignancies that do not completely respond, or will relapse after exposure, to conventional doses of chemoradiotherapy. Donor T cells are capable of recognizing and eliminating residual malignant cells in the host. Both CD4+ and CD8+ cells contribute to this graft versus leukemia effect in animal models, although the relative importance of specific subsets in clinical transplantation is not yet clear. Depletion of most donor T cells increases the risk of relapse in many situations. If a patient's disease recurs after HCT, sometimes infusion of additional donor leukocytes (known as donor leukocyte infusion, or DLI) can again eradicate the malignancy.

(c) **Immunologic reconstitution.** The thymus involutes with increasing age. Reconstitution of the immune system is slower after allogeneic than after autologous HCT. T cells are the last of the immune cells to recover. T-cell depletion further retards the pace of T-cell reconstitution, making recipients even more prone to reactivation of latent viral infections, including cytomegalovirus (CMV), adenovirus (Bk), varicella-zoster virus (VZV) and others.

4. Disadvantages of infusing donor T cells. GVHD is the greatest disadvantage from the presence of donor T cells.

(a) **Overview of graft-versus-host disease (GVHD)**

Described more than 50 years ago by Billingham, GVHD is a complex and intricate syndrome resulting from a consequence of interactions between the donor and host innate and adaptive immune responses. This interaction of donor T cells with antigen presenting cells (APCs), essentially the "sensors" for acute GVHD, is regulated positively or negatively by numerous cytokines, chemokines and immune cell subsets.

(i)   Three conditions are necessary for the development of GVHD:
  • An immunocompetent graft (i.e., one containing donor T cells).
  • Histocompatibility (minor or major) differences between donor and recipient.
  • A recipient who cannot mount an immune response to the graft.

(ii)   The chemoradiotherapy used to condition HCT recipients and the large number of T cells within the graft combine to make allogeneic HCT the most common setting for acute GVHD. Without additional immunosuppression after administration of the donor graft, more than 90% of allogeneic HCT recipients would develop significant GVHD, even from HLA-identical siblings (in this case due to differences in minor histocompatibility antigens between siblings).

(iii)   Other individuals at risk for GVHD (Table 26.4) are recipients of blood transfusions that contain WBCs (including lymphocytes). Normal individuals who are heterozygous for HLA proteins will not reject lymphocytes transfused from a donor who is homozygous for one of the recipient's haplotypes. If the donor lymphocytes that are not rejected recognize HLA antigens of the host's other haplotype, GVHD may develop. This syndrome is known as transfusion-associated GVHD and is more common in "inbred populations" who share many antigens. GVHD also may develop in patients who received directed blood donation but are not otherwise compromised (e.g., transfusion from an HLA-homozygous mother to a heterozygous child). External irradiation of blood products prevents lymphocytes from proliferating; therefore, all immunocompromised patients must receive irradiated blood products.

Table 26.4 Procedures associated with a high risk of GVHD

Hematopoietic cell transplantation	Patients receiving no GVHD prophylaxis
	Older patient age
	Recipients of HLA-non-identical grafts
	Recipients of grafts obtained from allosensitized donors
Solid organ transplant	Recipients of organs containing lymphoid tissue, i.e., small-bowel transplant
Transfusion of unirradiated blood products	Neonates and fetuses
	Patients with congenital immunodeficiency syndromes
	Patients receiving immunosuppressive chemo-radiation therapy
	Patients receiving directed blood donations from partially HLA-identical, HLA-homozygous donors

GVHD, graft-versus-host disease; HLA, human leukocyte antigen.

(iv) Time of onset. GVHD that occurs before day 100 traditionally has been termed acute GVHD although recently, "late onset" (>100 days) acute GVHD has been described more frequently, especially after RIC and non-myeloablative conditioning regimens. Acute GVHD primarily affects the epithelial cell component of three target organs: skin, gastrointestinal (GI) tract, and liver, often simultaneously. GVHD that occurs after day 100 usually is termed *chronic* GVHD and can affect both mesenchymal as well as epithelial tissues including the skin, GI tract, liver, eyes, lungs, and joints.

(v) Once established, GVHD is difficult to treat, and severe cases are usually fatal. The mainstay of therapy is high-dose steroids.

(b) **Pathophysiology of acute GVHD.** The pathophysiology of acute GVHD can be considered using a framework a model that breaks down this syndrome mechanistically into three sequential phases. While clearly not a step-wise process occurring in discrete stages, this model is conceptually useful.

(i) **Phase one.** The earliest phase of acute GVHD starts before the donor cells are infused. The transplant-conditioning regimen damages and activates host tissues (e.g., intestinal mucosa, liver) that secrete inflammatory cytokines that can up-regulate adhesion molecules and MHC antigens. This sequence enhances recognition of host allogeneic antigens by mature donor T cells contained in the graft.

(ii) **Phase two.** During this phase of acute GVHD, host antigen presenting cells interact with and activate donor T cells that then proliferate and differentiate. When donor and recipient are not MHC identical, donor T cells can recognize host MHC molecules as foreign and the resultant graft-versus-host reaction can be dramatic. In the setting of MHC identical recipient and donor, different peptides bound to the MHC are recognized by the T cell and its T cell receptor (TCR). The T cells secrete interleukin-2 (IL-2) and interferon-γ (type 1 cytokines) as critical mediators of acute GVHD.

(iii) Phase three. This component is the effector phase of acute GVHD. In addition to the activated donor T cells, mononuclear phagocytes, primed by cytokines during phases one and two above, play an important role in this third phase of acute GVHD. Monocytes receive a second, triggering signal to secrete the inflammatory cytokines tumor necrosis factor-α (TNF-α), interleukin-l (IL-1) and IL-6. Toll-like receptors (TLR) recognize pathogen-associated molecular patterns (such as lipopolysaccharide, i.e., endotoxin) released during conditioning and initiate cellular signaling pathways leading to secretion of these proinflammatory cytokines. Lipopolysaccharide (endotoxin) from conditioning regimen-damaged intestinal mucosa stimulates gut-associated lymphocytes and macrophages. TNF-α may directly cause tissue injury by inducing either necrosis or apoptosis (programmed cell death) of target cells. Thus, the induction of inflammatory cytokines may synergize with the cellular damage caused by cytotoxic T cells and natural killer cells, resulting in the amplification of local tissue injury.

(c) **Clinical grading of acute GVHD.** This syndrome, in some ways a complex immune response that has gone awry, is graded 0 through IV (Glücksberg grade) or A through D (IBMTR grade) based on organs involved and extent (stage) of involvement. Patient outcome significantly deteriorates with increasing grade of acute GVHD. Table 26.5

Table 26.5 Clinical grading of acute GVHD

IBMTR Grade	Glücksberg Grade	Skin	GI	Liver
A	I	1	0	0
B	I	2	0	0
B	II	0–2	1	0–1
B	II	0–2	0–1	1
C	II	3	1	0–1
C	II	3	0–1	1
C	II	3	0	0
B	III	0–2	2	0–2
B	III	0–2	0–2	2
C	III	0–3	0–3	2–3
C	III	3	2–3	0–3
D	III	0–3	0–3	4
D	IV	0–3	4	0–4
D	IV	4	0–4	0–4

Adapted with permission from J-Y Cahn et al. Blood 2005;106:1495–500.

illustrates the complex grading system used to score the extent of acute GVHD. The two most commonly used scales, the IBMTR and the Glücksberg, are shown. In each case, a value is given for the degree of involvement for the three major affected organs: skin, GI (gastrointestinal) tract and liver. If a patient has several organs involved, or one organ that is severely involved, the overall score or "grade" is higher, which predicts a worse patient outcome. The IBMTR Grading scale scores acute GVHD from the lowest ("A") to the highest ("D") grade. The Glücksberg Grading employs a numeric system from "I" as the lowest to "IV" for the highest grade.

(d) Prevention of acute GVHD. All allogeneic HCT recipients are treated with immunosuppressive agents before graft infusion as prophylaxis against GVHD. Usually at least two classes of drugs are used together.

    (i) **Tacrolimus (FK-506) or cyclosporine, so-called calcineurin inhibitors.** These compounds are extremely immunosuppressive and block TCR signaling pathways; only one, (not both), is used. These agents also are very toxic drugs, particularly to the kidneys, which additionally may be weakened by antibiotics. Treatment usually lasts at least 6 months after transplant.

    (ii) **Methotrexate (MTX).** A dihydrofolate reductase inhibitor, MTX inhibits expansion of all actively dividing cells. MTX is most effective when several doses are given within the first 2 weeks after HSC transplant, the time of maximal donor T-cell response to host antigens. Thus, MTX slows expansion of donor T-cell clones but also that of donor hematopoietic stem cells and engraftment often is slowed by several days when MTX is used.

    (iii) **Corticosteroids.** These agents, including prednisone and prednisolone, possess potent immunosuppressive properties among many other side effects and can induce apoptosis and lyse lymphocytes. They also inhibit production of inflammatory cytokines that mediate GVHD. Use of this group of drugs usually is reserved for treatment of GVHD that develops despite prophylaxis.

(e) Treatment of acute GVHD. Depending on the graft source and other factors, one-third to two-thirds of patients will develop GVHD despite prophylaxis with immunosuppressive agents. If involvement is confined only to skin, i.e., grade I, usually only topical corticosteroid therapy is applied to the skin, or lower doses of prednisone ($\leq$1 mg/kg/d). If involvement is more extensive in skin or the GI tract, liver, or combinations are involved, higher doses of prednisone 2 mg/kg/day are administered. Often patients respond and the prednisone dose is slowly tapered off. Patients in whom acute GVHD does not respond to prednisone are considered "steroid-refractory", a poor prognostic situation. These patient usually succumb either to progressive organ dysfunction due to GVHD (despite the addition of other potent immunosuppressants), or they develop fatal opportunistic infections.

(f) Chronic GVHD. This syndrome cannot be prevented and can evolve after acute GVHD (progressive), or develop in the absence of acute GVHD (*de novo*). Chronic GVHD is most difficult to treat and a variety of agents are utilized as there is no single preferred therapy. Patients are at markedly increased risk of opportunistic infection despite having adequate neutrophil blood counts fatal infection due to fungal, viral and bacterial organisms are not uncommon. In some patients, a state of "tolerance" develops after years and chronic GVHD ultimately may subside.

D. Phases of allogeneic stem cell transplantation

1. **Conditioning.** Before HCT, the patient receives high-dose chemotherapy or chemo-radiation therapy, the two-fold purpose to eliminate malignant and prevent the host from rejecting the graft.
   (a) Cytoreduction. While chemotherapy and radiation therapy kill tumor cells, this treatment also eliminates the patient's normal or abnormal stem cells. The most common preparative regimens are high-dose cyclophosphamide and total body irradiation (TBI), or high doses of busulfan and cyclophosphamide. These combinations have broad anti-tumor activity.
   (b) Immunosuppression. Conditioning also is immunosuppressive. To allow engraftment of the new HSCs, the patient's endogenous lymphocytes must be suppressed so as not to reject the new stem cells.
2. **Transplant.** The donor graft cells are infused intravenously as with a blood transfusion. The progenitor cells "traffic" or "home" to the appropriate places in the bone marrow where they take up residence and proliferate
3. **Recovery.** This period of intensive supportive care is similar to the recovery period in autologous HCT. High-dose chemotherapy and radiation therapy eliminates normal marrow function as well as causes reversible damage to many organs, including the skin, GI tract, lungs and liver.
   (a) Aggressive supportive care is crucial for long-term success as most toxicities are reversible, i.e., sophisticated support provides the time necessary for host organ regeneration and recovery.
      (i) Transfusions. There is a obligate period of aplasia while awaiting marrow recovery, during which time patients require RBC and platelet transfusions. Prolonged neutropenia predisposes patients to a multitude of bacterial infections and routine granulocyte transfusions are impractical and reserved for special circumstances.
      (ii) Cytokine support. Hematopoietic growth factors (e.g., G-CSF) usually are given to hasten neutrophil recovery after HCT.
   (b) Complications during recovery:
      (i) Infections. As patients are neutropenic or are receiving potent immunosuppressive GVHD prophylaxis agents when they have engrafted and are not neutropenic, they are susceptible to a

variety of infections. Additionally, much earlier in their disease course, patients may have required broad-spectrum antibiotics to prevent or treat infection that subsequently could lead to micro-organism resistance or resulted in internal organ injury when re-challenged with antibiotics. In the course of HCT, bacterial infections may develop during the neutropenic period. Further, a super-infection with bacteria may develop later as patients are receiving immunosuppressants; the slow immune reconstitution and defects in cellular and humoral immunity (hypogammaglobulinemia) also contribute. The lack of a fully functioning immune system often leads to re-activation or active viral infections and unusual or opportunistic infections fungal infections. In addition to these deficiencies, the normal barriers that prevent entry of micro-organisms (e.g., skin, GI tract, respiratory epithelium, etc.) have been damaged. Prompt recognition and institution of various antibacterials and the judicious use of antiviral and antifungal agents greatly lessens the risk of these infections.

- **Bacterial infections.** During the period of neutropenia (blood granulocyte count <500/μL), common bacterial infections include Gram-positive cocci (usually *Staphylococcus epidermidis* from central venous catheter devices and *Staphylococcus aureus*) and Gram-negative rods (*E. coli, Klebsiella* sp. and occasionally *Pseudomonas* sp. from the GI tract and respiratory tract).
- **Viral infections.** Several viruses including CMV, HSV, VZV, adenovirus and respiratory syncytial virus can be fatal after HCT. Serious damage from CMV and HSV can be are prevented via of prophylactic antiviral therapy (e.g., ganciclovir, acyclovir). Other viruses are much more difficult to treat. Viral infections occur more frequently after allogeneic HCT than after autologous HCT.
- **Fungal infections.** Candidiasis and aspergillosis are less common but often fatal infections in patients after HCT. Strategies for prophylaxis of candidiasis with fluconazole therapy have been beneficial but ineffective for aspergillosis; agents with significant activity against this pathogen include voriconazole, micafungin and the latest agent, posaconazole. One of these agents should be utilized when patients are receiving corticosteroids to prevent or treat active GVHD.

(ii) **GI tract.** Both conditioning and GVHD damage the GI tract. Use of multiple antibiotics during HCT also changes bacterial flora (e.g., *Clostridium difficile* entero-colitis). Parenteral nutrition frequently is administered after allogeneic HCT but the data supporting this routine practice are not overly compelling.

(iii) **Liver.** Both hepatic veno-occlusive disease (also known as sinusoidal obstruction syndrome) and GVHD (acute and chronic) cause liver disease. Veno-occlusive disease usually results from liver injury induced by the conditioning regimen most often occurs within the first 2–3 weeks after both allogeneic and autologous HCT. A new agent defibrotide appears to be extremely effective in severe cases of hepatic veno-occlusive disease. Many antibiotic medications such as voriconazole also can be associated with liver injury.

(iv) **Lungs.** Both autologous and allogeneic HCT may result in damage to the lungs. Viral, fungal, and bacterial infections are common but pathogens are identified in only 50% of cases; the remaining cases are probably immunologic or injury from the preparative regimen, e.g., interstitial pneumonia, idiopathic pneumonia syndrome, diffuse alveolar hemorrhage. The lungs are a target of both acute and chronic GVHD and patients are at risk for a progressive, serious lung injury known as bronchiolitis obliterans.

(v) **Immune system.** Reconstitution after HCT is slowed by the use of immunosuppressive agents to prevent GVHD, or by active GVHD itself. Infusions of prophylactic IV immunoglobulin for hypogammaglobulinemia are recommended for the first few months after transplant and prophylactic oral antibiotics such are penicillin may be required for many months and sometimes years in patients with chronic GVHD due to the ever-present risk of serious infection. Patients also are at risk for *Pneumocystis jirovecii* pneumonia due to immunosuppression and cellular immune deficiency and require prophylaxis therapy with trimethoprim-sulfamethoxazole or dapsone.

(vi) **Graft-versus-host disease.** GVHD, caused by immunologic activation of the infused donor T cells against the patient's organs, remains the major complication after allogeneic HCT. This syndrome, however, may be associated with a graft-versus-tumor effect and hence may have a beneficial as well as a detrimental effect.

(vii) **Late effects.** Even survivors of HCT have a reduced life expectancy compared to age-matched controls in the general population. Malignancy can recur and patients are at increased risk for second malignancy. Other late consequences include iron overload (due to numerous RBC transfusions), endocrine insufficiency (especially thyroid disorders), osteoporosis and cataracts. In many ways, HCT can be viewed as an acceleration of the aging process.

E. Outcomes of allogeneic stem cell transplantation

Patient outcome is complex and depends upon patient-, disease- and treatment-related factors including the underlying disease and stage at time of transplant, previous therapy given and the type of transplant (HLA-identical family member donor versus HLA-nonidentical family member donor versus HLA-identical unrelated donor). A few general observations:

1. The later in the disease course the HCT occurs, the lower the survival rate.
2. Unrelated transplants generally do not fare as well as sibling-matched transplants because of increased incidence of GVHD and infections.
3. Relapses still may occur, even years later, although the relapse rates are lower with allogeneic than with autologous HCT.
4. The transplant-related mortality rate at day 100 is approximately 20–30%, depending on how closely the donor and recipient are matched. The most frequent causes of death include relapse, GVHD and infection.

IV. Summary

HCT is a curative therapy for a number of hematologic disorders, both malignant and nonmalignant. Autologous HCT transplants have fewer immunologic complications but have higher rates of relapse after transplant. Allogeneic HCT have lower rates of relapse but have more immunologic complications, including GVHD, which can be fatal. Advances in HLA typing, supportive care, and newer immunosuppressive agents significantly have improved long-term survival rates after HCT over the past 10 years.

Further reading

Bensinger W, DiPersio JF, McCarty JM. Improving stem cell mobilization strategies: future directions. Bone Marrow Transplant 2009;43:181–95.

Craddock CF. Full-intensity and reduced-intensity allogeneic stem cell transplantation in AML. Bone Marrow Transplant 2008;41:415–23.

Ferrara JL, Levine JE, Reddy P, Holler E. Graft-vs-host-disease. Lancet 2009;373:1550–61.

Hiemenz JW. Management of infections complicating allogeneic hematopoietic stem cell transplantation. Semin Hematol 2009;46:289–312.

Pihusch M. Bleeding complications after hematopoietic stem cell transplantation [review]. Semin Hematol 2004;41(suppl 1):93–100.

Rizzo JD, Wingard JR, Tichelli A, et al. Recommended screening and preventive practices for long-term survivors after hematopoietic cell transplantation: joint recommendations of the European Group for Blood and Marrow Transplantation, the Center for International Blood and Marrow Transplant Research, and the American Society of Blood and Marrow Transplantation. Biol Blood Marrow Transplant 2006;12:138–51.

Schoemans H, Theunissen K, Maertens J, et al. Adult umbilical cord blood transplantation: a comprehensive review. Bone Marrow Transplant 2006;38:83–93.

Tichelli A, Rovó A, Gratwohl A. Late pulmonary, cardiovascular, and renal complications after hematopoietic stem cell transplantation and recommended screening practices. Hematology Am Soc Hematol Educ Program 2008:125–33.

Tomblyn M, Lazarus HM. Donor lymphocyte infusions. The long and winding road. Bone Marrow Transplant 2008;42:569–79. Burns LJ. Late effects after autologous hematopoietic cell transplantation. Biol Blood Marrow Transplant 2008;15(1 Suppl):21–4.

27 Atlas of Hematology Slides

Alvin H. Schmaier

Case Western Reserve University, University Hospitals Case Medical Center, Cleveland, OH, USA

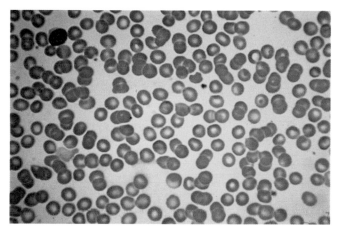

1. Medium-power light microscopic view of a normal peripheral blood smear showing normochromic, normocytic red blood cells, a small lymphocyte, and adequate numbers of platelets. The area of central pallor on the red blood cells comprises one third the diameter of the cell. The diameter of the nucleus of the small lymphocytes is approximately equal to the diameter of the red blood cell. This slide and all the other slides in this Atlas are stained with Wright–Giemsa stain, the traditional stain for examination of the peripheral blood smear. *This slide is from the American Society of Hematology Slide Bank CD prepared by the Center for Educational Resources, University of Washington, 1998.*

Concise Guide to Hematology, First Edition. Edited by Alvin H. Schmaier, Hillard M. Lazarus.
© 2012 Blackwell Publishing Ltd. Published 2012 by Blackwell Publishing Ltd.

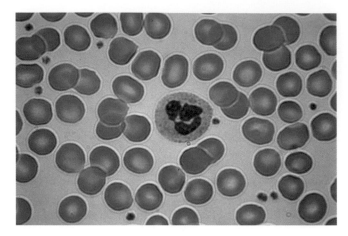

2. High-power view of a normal polymorphonuclear leukocyte (PMN, neutrophil). The nucleus consists of three lobes and the cytoplasm has mild granularity that is characteristic of a typical neutrophil. *This slide is from the American Society of Hematology Slide Bank CD prepared by the Center for Educational Resources, University of Washington, 1998.*

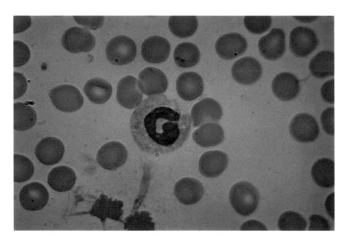

3. High-power view of the band form of the neutrophil is shown. The nucleus is non-segmented in contrast to the mature form. The cytoplasm has mild granularity as seen in the mature granulocyte. *This slide is from the American Society of Hematology Slide Bank CD prepared by the Center for Educational Resources, University of Washington, 1998.*

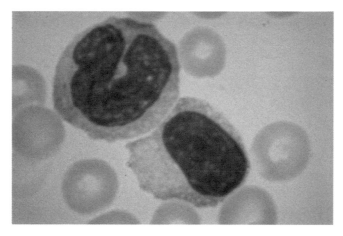

4. High-powered view of a normal monocyte with a large, lobulated nucleus. It is next to a large lymphocyte with an abundant, agranular cytoplasm. *This slide is from the American Society of Hematology Slide Bank CD prepared by the Center for Educational Resources, University of Washington, 1998.*

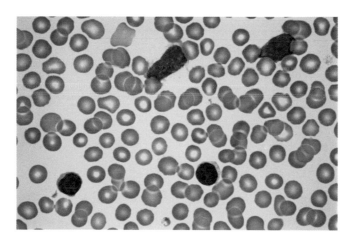

5. Medium-powered view of two normal small lymphocytes with round nucleus and scant cytoplasm and two large, atypical, reactive lymphocytes. Often times with reactive lymphocytes, red blood cells make indentations on the lymphocytes' cytoplasm. *This figure is the courtesy of Dr. William Finn, Department of Pathology, University of Michigan.*

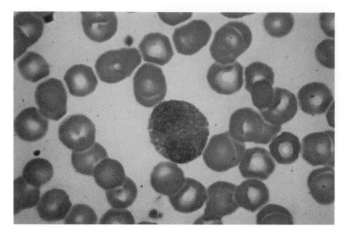

6. High-powered view of a normal two-lobed eosinophil. The cytoplasm contains prominent azurophilic granules. *This slide is from the American Society of Hematology Slide Bank CD prepared by the Center for Educational Resources, University of Washington, 1998.*

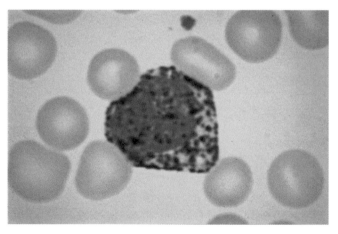

7. High-powered view of a normal basophil with prominent basophilic cytoplasmic granules that obscure the nucleus. *This slide is from the American Society of Hematology Slide Bank CD prepared by the Center for Educational Resources, University of Washington, 1998.*

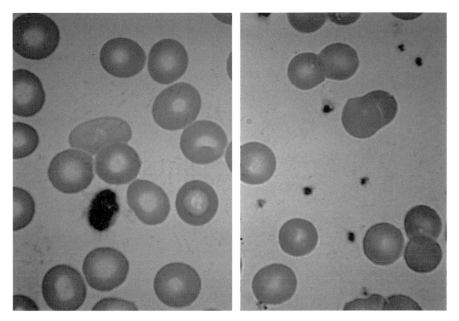

8. A high-powered view of a large platelet on the left and normal-sized platelets on the right. Large platelets contain basophilic, granular cytoplasm. *This slide is from the American Society of Hematology Slide Bank CD prepared by the Center for Educational Resources, University of Washington, 1998.*

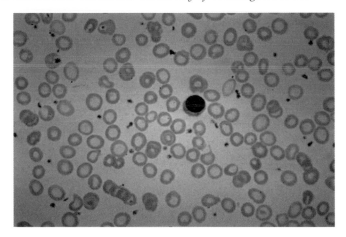

9. Medium-powered view of a hypochromic, microcytic red blood cells. The area of central pallor is greater than one third the diameter of the cell. This fact is the definition of hypochromia. The diameter of the erythrocytes is smaller than the diameter of the nucleus of the small lymphocyte pictured in this figure, reflecting low red cell volume (microcytosis). The platelet count on this smear is normal or increased. This smear is characteristic of iron deficiency anemia. *This slide is from the American Society of Hematology Slide Bank CD prepared by the Center for Educational Resources, University of Washington, 1998.*

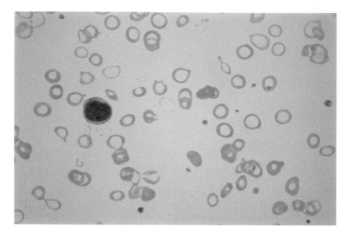

10. Medium-powered view of markedly hypochromic and microcytic red blood cells. As the patient becomes more anemic, the peripheral blood smear will show increased variation in size (anisocytosis) and shape (pokilocytosis). The pronounced area of central pallor is also noted. *This slide is from the American Society of Hematology Slide Bank CD prepared by the Center for Educational Resources, University of Washington, 1998.*

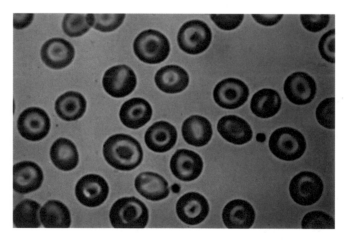

11. High-powered view of erythrocytes with target cells that are cells with a central appearance of membrane. Target cells arise under conditions of reduced intracellular hemoglobin (e.g. thalassemias or hemoglobin C trait and disease) or in conditions where there is excess red blood cell membrane in relation to the contents of the cells (e.g. liver disease). *This slide is from the American Society of Hematology Slide Bank CD prepared by the Center for Educational Resources, University of Washington, 1998.*

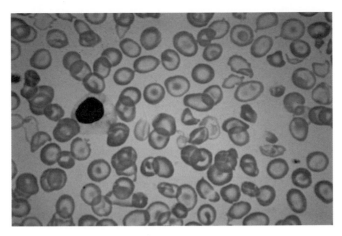

12. Medium-powered view of targeted hypochromic, microcytic red blood cells that are scattered throughout the smear. Most of the red blood cells have a cell diameter smaller than the nucleus of the lymphocyte. This smear is characteristic of what one would see in some of the thalassemias. *This slide is from the American Society of Hematology Slide Bank CD prepared by the Center for Educational Resources, University of Washington, 1998.*

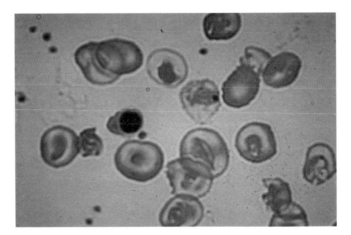

13. High-powered view of severely hypochromic, targeted red blood cells with the presence of a nucleated red blood cell. This smear is characteristic of homozygous beta thalassemia or Cooley's anemia. *This figure is the courtesy of Dr. William Finn, Department of Pathology, University of Michigan.*

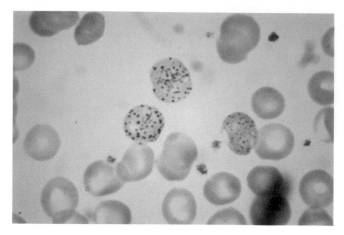

14. High-powered view of red blood cells showing prominent dark stained deposits with a stippled appearance in their cytoplasm. This feature is called basophilic stippling. It represents pathologic aggregates of ribosomes seen in disorders of hemoglobin synthesis such as thalassemia, hemoglobinopathy, lead poisoning, and myelodysplastic syndromes. *This slide is from the American Society of Hematology Slide Bank CD prepared by the Center for Educational Resources, University of Washington, 1998.*

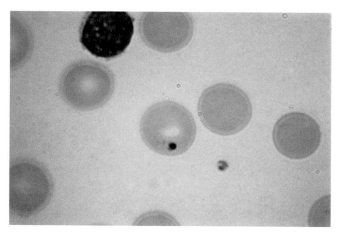

15. The dark dot of material seen in the lower portion of the central red blood cell is a Howell–Jolly body. It is a small remnant of the red blood cell nucleus. It is characteristically seen in post-splenectomy states or when a patient may have developed functional asplenia. *This slide is from the American Society of Hematology Slide Bank CD prepared by the Center for Educational Resources, University of Washington, 1998.*

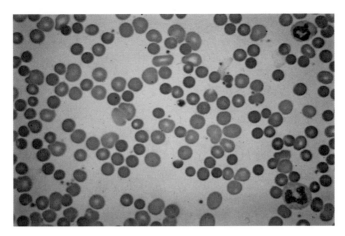

16. Low-power view of red blood cells with a loss of the area of central pallor. These cells are called spherocytes. They can arise from defects in the proteins that constitute red blood cell membranes or when the red blood cells are coated with immunoglobulin or complement and remodeled after traversing the spleen. *This slide is from the American Society of Hematology Slide Bank CD prepared by the Center for Educational Resources, University of Washington, 1998.*

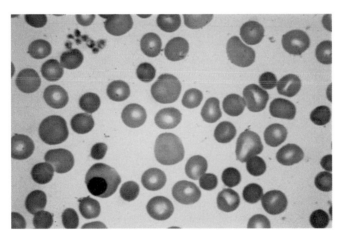

17. Medium-powered view of spherocytes of varying sizes. Also a nucleated red blood cell is present. This smear is characteristic of that seen in a warm (IgG) antibody-mediated hemolytic anemia. *This slide is from the American Society of Hematology Slide Bank CD prepared by the Center for Educational Resources, University of Washington, 1998.*

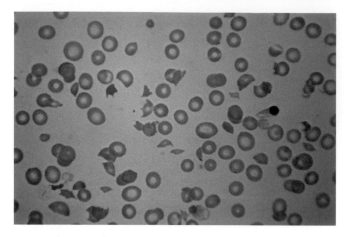

18. Low-powered view of a peripheral blood smear showing variation in the size (anisocytosis) and shape (pokilocytosis) of red blood cells. Some of the red blood cells appear broken apart and fragmented (schistocytes). The crescent-shaped, fragmented cells are called helmet cells. This smear is characteristic of intravascular destruction of red blood cells as is seen in a micro-angiopathic hemolytic anemia from any etiology. *This slide is from the American Society of Hematology Slide Bank CD prepared by the Center for Educational Resources, University of Washington, 1998.*

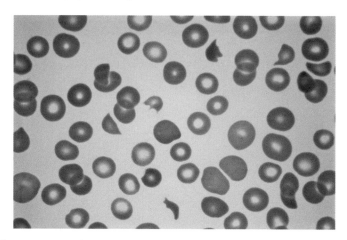

19. Medium-powered view of fragmented red blood cells with helmet cells and schistocytes. Some of the red blood cells have a different shade of color (polychromasia). Polychromasia indicates the presence of younger red blood cells that have remnant ribosomes present in their cytoplasm. Its presence indicates a bone marrow producing and releasing young red blood cells to compensate for peripheral destruction or loss as seen in severe hemolytic anemias (i.e. anemias with shortened red blood cell survival) or brisk hemorrhage. *This figure is the courtesy of Dr. William Finn, Department of Pathology, University of Michigan.*

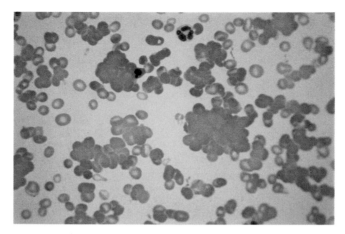

20. Low-powered view of clumps of red blood cells as seen with IgM (cold antibody) agglutinin disease. Cells agglutinate or form clumps on the peripheral blood smear as result of exposure to cooler peripheral temperatures. The agglutinated red blood cells can appear as a large smudge on the peripheral blood smear. *This slide is from the American Society of Hematology Slide Bank CD prepared by the Center for Educational Resources, University of Washington, 1998.*

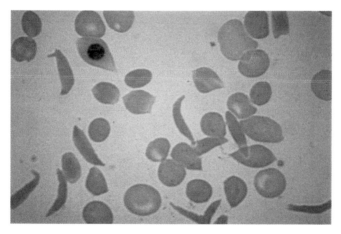

21. High-powered view of crescent shaped sickle cells that are characteristic of sickle cell disease. A nucleated red blood cell also is present in the peripheral blood smear. *This slide is from the American Society of Hematology Slide Bank CD prepared by the Center for Educational Resources, University of Washington, 1998.*

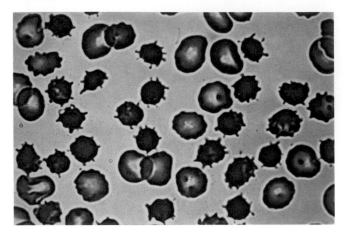

22. Medium-powered view of spiculated spherocytes (acanthocytes) seen in spur cell anemia associated with liver disease or in abetalipoproteinemia. Acanthocytes indicate abnormal lipid ratios in the red blood cell membrane and are formed as a result of "conditioning" a less fluid red cell membrane as it transverses a functioning spleen. *This slide is from the American Society of Hematology Slide Bank CD prepared by the Center for Educational Resources, University of Washington, 1998.*

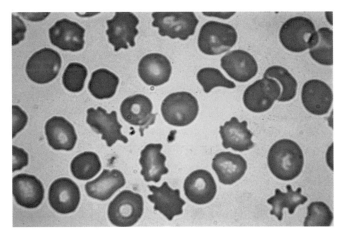

23. High-powered view of misshaped red blood cells (pokilocytosis). Cells with these bizarre shapes are seen in various metabolic states such as hypothyroidism, hypoparathyroidism, liver disease and membrane protein abnormalities. *This slide is from the American Society of Hematology Slide Bank CD prepared by the Center for Educational Resources, University of Washington, 1998.*

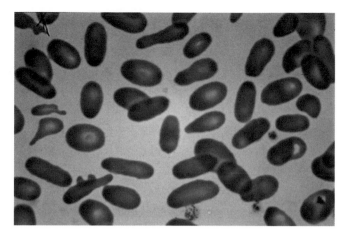

24. High-powered view of ovalocytosis that results from a defect in the membrane proteins of the cell as seen in hereditary disorders such as hereditary ovalocytosis. *This slide is from the American Society of Hematology Slide Bank CD prepared by the Center for Educational Resources, University of Washington, 1998.*

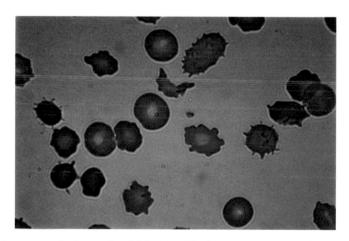

25. High-powered view of red blood cells from a patient with renal failure. The central red blood cell with crenated edges is called a burr cell. The smear also shows other red blood cells that are spiculated acanthocytes and a spiculated fragmented cell. *This slide is from the American Society of Hematology Slide Bank CD prepared by the Center for Educational Resources, University of Washington, 1998.*

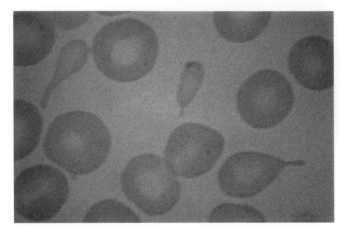

26. High-powered view of a misshapen red blood cell that looks like a tear drop. Tear drop cells are seen in patients with myeloproliferative disorders or other causes of marrow fibrosis or extramedullary hematopoiesis. *This slide is from the American Society of Hematology Slide Bank CD prepared by the Center for Educational Resources, University of Washington, 1998.*

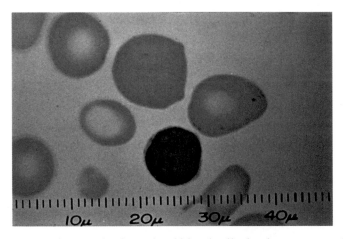

27. High-powered view of enlarged red blood cells that have a mean diameter greater than the nucleus of the small lymphocyte. These red blood cells are macroovalocytes that can be seen in B$_{12}$ or folate deficiency. *This slide is from the American Society of Hematology Slide Bank CD prepared by the Center for Educational Resources, University of Washington, 1998.*

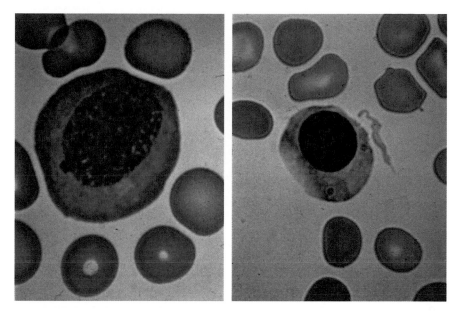

28. High-powered view of megaloblastic nucleated red blood cells as seen in B$_{12}$ or folate deficiency. These cells are not normally seen in the peripheral blood. The larger cell is an early polychromatophilic normoblast; the smaller cell is an orthochromatophilic normoblast. In both cells, the nuclear chromatin pattern is more open than the tightly packed chromatin in equivalent staged normoblasts in normal individuals. *This slide is from the American Society of Hematology Slide Bank CD prepared by the Center for Educational Resources, University of Washington, 1998.*

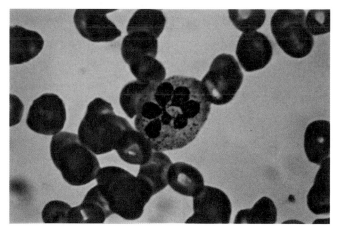

29. Medium-powered view of a megaloblastic, hypersegmented polymorphonuclear leukocyte. This cell with ≥5 nuclear lobes is characteristic of B$_{12}$ or folate deficiency. *This slide is from the American Society of Hematology Slide Bank CD prepared by the Center for Educational Resources, University of Washington, 1998.*

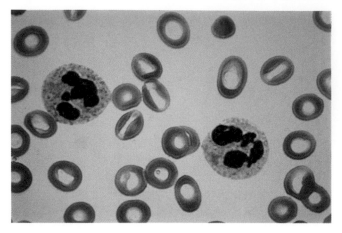

30. Medium-powered view of two polymorphonuclear leukocytes with bluish bodies in their cytoplasm. These bluish inclusion bodies are called Döhle bodies and are aggregates of rough endoplasmic reticulum in individuals who have had a recent microbial infection or other acute inflammatory condition. *This slide is from the American Society of Hematology Slide Bank CD prepared by the Center for Educational Resources, University of Washington, 1998.*

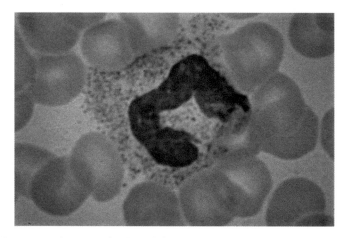

31. High-powered view of a band form of a polymorphonuclear leukocyte with prominent granules in its cytoplasm. These granules are called toxic granulation and are seen during infections in individuals. *This slide is from the American Society of Hematology Slide Bank CD prepared by the Center for Educational Resources, University of Washington, 1998.*

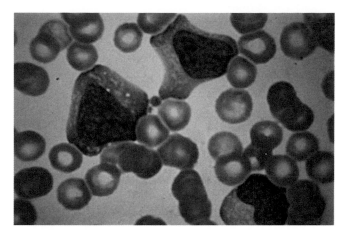

32. High-powered view of two large lymphocytes seen in an individual with a recent viral infection or infectious mononucleosis. In large lymphocytes, the cytoplasm of the cell is often indented by adjacent red blood cells. The single leukocyte on the edge of the figure is a monocyte. *This slide is from the American Society of Hematology Slide Bank CD prepared by the Center for Educational Resources, University of Washington, 1998.*

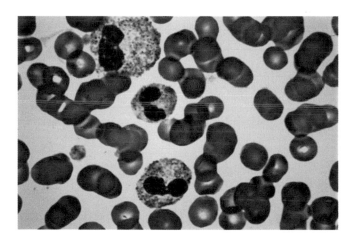

33. Medium-powered view of three two-lobed polymorphonuclear leuko-cytes. These cells have the Pelger–Hüet anomaly. This entity can be seen as a benign congenital abnormality (the true Pelger–Hüet anomaly) or can arise secondarily in both reactive conditions (e.g. mycoplasma infection, drug effects) or neoplastic conditions (e.g. myelodysplastic or myeloproliferative syndromes or acute leukemia). Such acquired Pelger–Hüet-like changes are called "Pseudo-Pelger–Hüet". *This figure is the courtesy of Dr. William Finn, Department of Pathology, University of Michigan.*

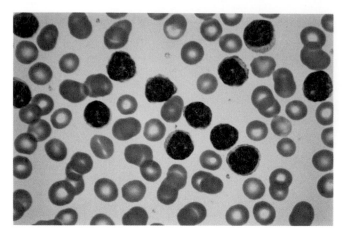

34. Medium-powered view of multiple small lymphocytes. The presence of cells like this in the peripheral blood is characteristic of chronic lymphocytic leukemia. *This figure is the courtesy of Dr. William Finn, Department of Pathology, University of Michigan.*

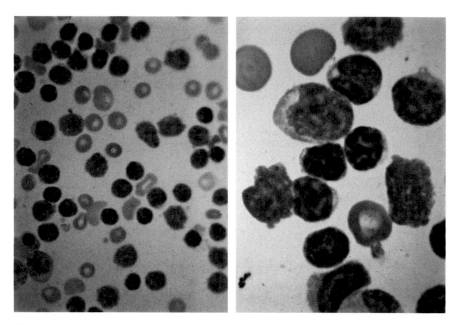

35. On one side, a low-powered view of small and large lymphocytes seen in chronic lymphocytic leukemia. On the other side is a high-powered view of the same cells. In certain instances, an outline of a degenerated cell is seen on the smear. These degenerated cells are called smudge cells and are characteristic of but not specific for chronic lymphocytic leukemia. *This slide is from the American Society of Hematology Slide Bank CD prepared by the Center for Educational Resources, University of Washington, 1998.*

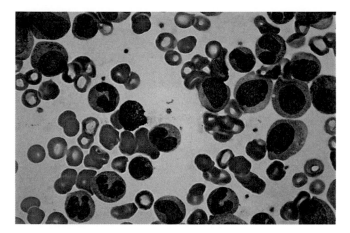

36. Medium-powered view showing an array of granulocytic precursors in the peripheral blood. The smear shows polymorphonuclear leukocytes, bands, metamyelocytes, myelocytes, and a promyelocyte. It also shows an increase in basophils. This smear is characteristic of chronic myelogenous leukemia. *This figure is the courtesy of Dr. William Finn, Department of Pathology, University of Michigan.*

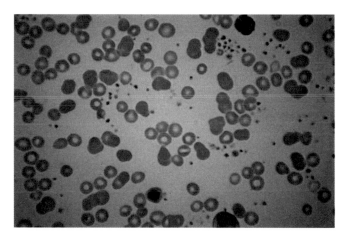

37. Low-powered view of peripheral blood showing an increase in platelets in clumps, a nucleated red blood cell, and myeloblast. This smear is from a patient with essential thrombocythemia. *This slide is from the American Society of Hematology Slide Bank CD prepared by the Center for Educational Resources, University of Washington, 1998.*

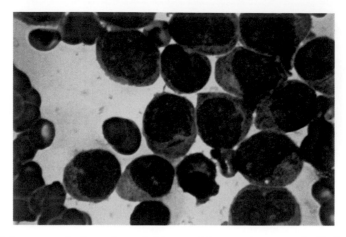

38. A high-powered view of myeloblasts with prominent nucleoli. One of the myeloblasts contains an Auer rod (a stick-like structure in the cytoplasm), others have granular cytoplasm. This smear is characteristic of acute myelogenous leukemia (M1 morphology). *This figure is the courtesy of Dr. William Finn, Department of Pathology, University of Michigan.*

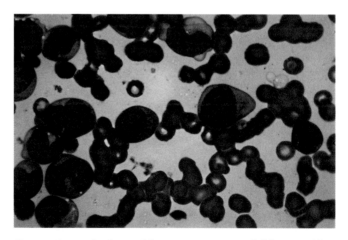

39. A medium-powered view of homogenous myeloblasts with prominent nucleoli. Some of the nuclei are folded. This smear is characteristic of acute monocytic leukemia (M4/M5 morphology). *This figure is the courtesy of Dr. William Finn, Department of Pathology, University of Michigan.*

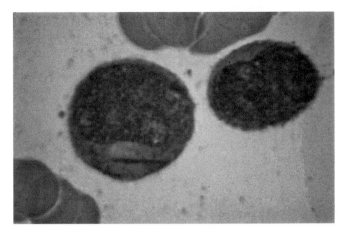

40. A high-powered view of bone marrow from a patient with acute myeloid leukemia showing two large primitive myeloblasts with very prominent granules and the presence of an Auer rod. Auer rods are only seen in malignant proliferations of myeloid cells. *This slide is from the American Society of Hematology Slide Bank CD prepared by the Center for Educational Resources, University of Washington, 1998.*

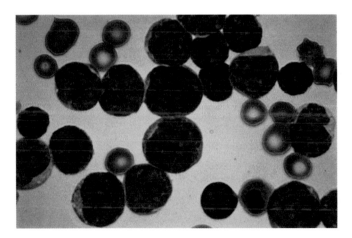

41. A high-powered view of primitive cells in the peripheral blood. Many of these cells have nucleoli. The large nuclear to cytoplasmic ratio of the blasts is characteristic of acute lymphocytic leukemia. *This slide is from the American Society of Hematology Slide Bank CD prepared by the Center for Educational Resources, University of Washington, 1998.*

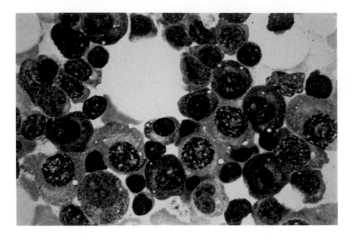

42. A bone marrow specimen showing a syncytium of plasma cells with an eccentric nucleus, clumped nuclear chromatin in the nucleus, prominent nucleoli and perinuclear Golgi apparatus. This smear is characteristic of multiple myeloma. *This figure is the courtesy of Dr. William Finn, Department of Pathology, University of Michigan.*

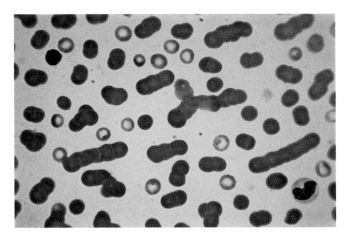

43. A low-power peripheral blood smear showing a stacking of red blood cells. This entity called rouleaux is characteristic of hypergammaglobulinemic states such as multiple myeloma. *This slide is from the American Society of Hematology Slide Bank CD prepared by the Center for Educational Resources, University of Washington, 1998.*

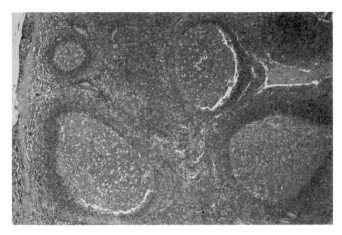

44. A low-powered view of well-formed germinal centers of a hyperplastic lymph node cross section. The follicular architecture is intact. *This figure is the courtesy of Dr. William Finn, Department of Pathology, University of Michigan.*

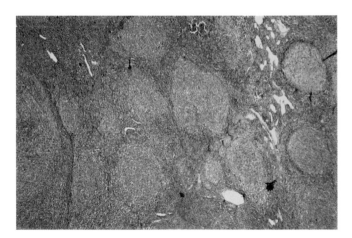

45. A low-powered view of a follicular lymphoma showing increased number of follicles with crowding of the germinal centers. *This figure is the courtesy of Dr. William Finn, Department of Pathology, University of Michigan.*

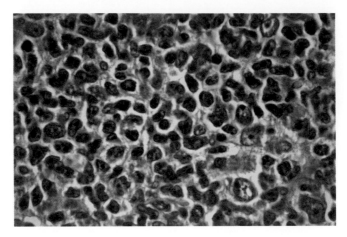

46. A high-powered view of a neoplastic follicle in follicular lymphoma, showing a monotonous population of "small cleaved" lymphocytes. *This figure is the courtesy of Dr. William Finn, Department of Pathology, University of Michigan.*

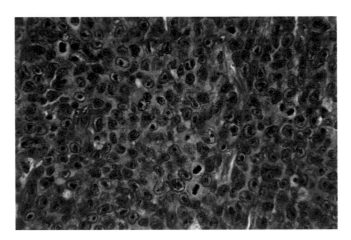

47. A medium-powered view of a diffuse, large B-cell lymphoma. *This figure is the courtesy of Dr. William Finn, Department of Pathology, University of Michigan.*

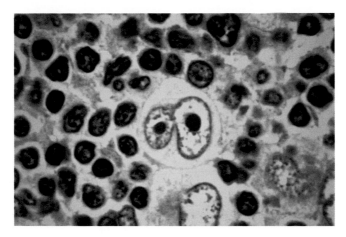

48. A high-powered view of a Reed–Sternberg cell from a lymph node involved with Hodgkin's disease. Note the characteristic bilobed nucleus with prominent nucleoli. *This figure is the courtesy of Dr. Bertrum Schnitzer, Department of Pathology, University of Michigan.*

Index

Page numbers in bold refer to tables. Page numbers in italic refer to figures.

Concise Guide to Hematology, First Edition. Edited by Alvin H. Schmaier, Hillard M. Lazarus.
© 2012 Blackwell Publishing Ltd. Published 2012 by Blackwell Publishing Ltd.